Ischemic Heart Disease in the Context of Different Comorbidities

Ischemic Heart Disease in the Context of Different Comorbidities

Editors

Irina-Iuliana Costache
Bogdan-Mircea Mihai
Minerva Codruta Badescu

MDPI • Basel • Beijing • Wuhan • Barcelona • Belgrade • Manchester • Tokyo • Cluj • Tianjin

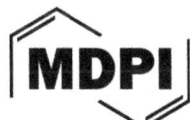

Editors

Irina-Iuliana Costache
Department of Internal
Medicine and Cardiology
"Grigore T. Popa" University
of Medicine and Pharmacy
Iasi
Romania

Bogdan-Mircea Mihai
Head of Diabetes, Nutrition
and Metabolic Diseases Unit
"Grigore T. Popa" University
of Medicine and Pharmacy
Iasi
Romania

Minerva Codruta Badescu
Department of Internal
Medicine
"Grigore T. Popa" University
of Medicine and Pharmacy
Iasi
Romania

Editorial Office
MDPI
St. Alban-Anlage 66
4052 Basel, Switzerland

This is a reprint of articles from the Special Issue published online in the open access journal *Life* (ISSN 2075-1729) (available at: www.mdpi.com/journal/life/special_issues/ischemic_heart_disease_life).

For citation purposes, cite each article independently as indicated on the article page online and as indicated below:

LastName, A.A.; LastName, B.B.; LastName, C.C. Article Title. *Journal Name* **Year**, *Volume Number*, Page Range.

ISBN 978-3-0365-5810-3 (Hbk)
ISBN 978-3-0365-5809-7 (PDF)

© 2022 by the authors. Articles in this book are Open Access and distributed under the Creative Commons Attribution (CC BY) license, which allows users to download, copy and build upon published articles, as long as the author and publisher are properly credited, which ensures maximum dissemination and a wider impact of our publications.

The book as a whole is distributed by MDPI under the terms and conditions of the Creative Commons license CC BY-NC-ND.

Contents

About the Editors vii

Preface to "Ischemic Heart Disease in the Context of Different Comorbidities" ix

Irina-Iuliana Costache, Bogdan-Mircea Mihai and Minerva Codruta Badescu
Ischemic Heart Disease in the Context of Different Comorbidities
Reprinted from: *Life* **2022**, *12*, 1558, doi:10.3390/life12101558 1

Adina Carmen Ilie, Sabinne Marie Taranu, Ramona Stefaniu, Ioana Alexandra Sandu, Anca Iuliana Pislaru and Calina Anda Sandu et al.
Chronic Coronary Syndrome in Frail Old Population
Reprinted from: *Life* **2022**, *12*, 1133, doi:10.3390/life12081133 5

Sabina Andreea Leancă, Daniela Crișu, Antoniu Octavian Petriș, Irina Afrăsânie, Antonia Genes and Alexandru Dan Costache et al.
Left Ventricular Remodeling after Myocardial Infarction: From Physiopathology to Treatment
Reprinted from: *Life* **2022**, *12*, 1111, doi:10.3390/life12081111 19

Minerva Codruta Badescu, Oana Viola Badulescu, Dragos Viorel Scripcariu, Lăcrămioara Ionela Butnariu, Iris Bararu-Bojan and Diana Popescu et al.
Myocardial Ischemia Related to Common Cancer Therapy—Prevention Insights
Reprinted from: *Life* **2022**, *12*, 1034, doi:10.3390/life12071034 43

Victorita Sorodoc, Oana Sirbu, Catalina Lionte, Raluca Ecaterina Haliga, Alexandra Stoica and Alexandr Ceasovschih et al.
The Value of Troponin as a Biomarker of Chemotherapy-Induced Cardiotoxicity
Reprinted from: *Life* **2022**, *12*, 1183, doi:10.3390/life12081183 65

Georgiana-Diana Cazac, Cristina-Mihaela Lăcătușu, Cătălina Mihai, Elena-Daniela Grigorescu, Alina Onofriescu and Bogdan-Mircea Mihai
New Insights into Non-Alcoholic Fatty Liver Disease and Coronary Artery Disease: The Liver-Heart Axis
Reprinted from: *Life* **2022**, *12*, 1189, doi:10.3390/life12081189 83

Irina Gîrleanu, Anca Trifan, Laura Huiban, Cristina Muzîca, Oana Cristina Petrea and Ana Maria Sîngeap et al.
Ischemic Heart Disease and Liver Cirrhosis: Adding Insult to Injury
Reprinted from: *Life* **2022**, *12*, 1036, doi:10.3390/life12071036 109

Alina Ecaterina Jucan, Otilia Gavrilescu, Mihaela Dranga, Iolanda Valentina Popa, Bogdan Mircea Mihai and Cristina Cijevschi Prelipcean et al.
Ischemic Heart Disease in Patients with Inflammatory Bowel Disease: Risk Factors, Mechanisms and Prevention
Reprinted from: *Life* **2022**, *12*, 1113, doi:10.3390/life12081113 123

Amalia-Stefana Timpau, Radu-Stefan Miftode, Daniela Leca, Razvan Timpau, Ionela-Larisa Miftode and Antoniu Octavian Petris et al.
A Real Pandora's Box in Pandemic Times: A Narrative Review on the Acute Cardiac Injury Due to COVID-19
Reprinted from: *Life* **2022**, *12*, 1085, doi:10.3390/life12071085 137

Ștefania Teodora Duca, Adriana Chetran, Radu Ștefan Miftode, Ovidiu Mitu, Alexandru Dan Costache and Ana Nicolae et al.
Myocardial Ischemia in Patients with COVID-19 Infection: Between Pathophysiological Mechanisms and Electrocardiographic Findings
Reprinted from: *Life* **2022**, *12*, 1015, doi:10.3390/life12071015 . . . . **161**

Raluca Ecaterina Haliga, Bianca Codrina Morărașu, Victorița Șorodoc, Cătălina Lionte, Oana Sîrbu and Alexandra Stoica et al.
Rare Causes of Acute Coronary Syndrome: Carbon Monoxide Poisoning
Reprinted from: *Life* **2022**, *12*, 1158, doi:10.3390/life12081158 . . . . **181**

Lăcrămioara Ionela Butnariu, Laura Florea, Minerva Codruta Badescu, Elena Țarcă, Irina-Iuliana Costache and Eusebiu Vlad Gorduza
Etiologic Puzzle of Coronary Artery Disease: How Important Is Genetic Component?
Reprinted from: *Life* **2022**, *12*, 865, doi:10.3390/life12060865 . . . . **193**

About the Editors

Irina-Iuliana Costache

Irina-Iuliana Costache is Professor in Cardiology and Internal Medicine at the Faculty of Medicine, "Grigore T. Popa" University of Medicine and Pharmacy, Iasi, Romania and a senior physician in internal medicine and cardiology at "Sf. Spiridon" County Emergency Clinical Hospital, Cardiology Clinic, Iasi, Romania. She is a respected and awarded member of the National and European Society of Cardiology. Professor Costache's academic activity is extensive and remarkable through a large number of published books and journal articles with a high scientific impact. Her main focus is cardiovascular disease, especially ischemic heart disease, arterial hypertension, valvular diseases, pulmonary embolism and heart failure.

She has a great amount of experience in echocardiography and the management of cardiac emergencies. Through direct involvement in numerous clinical trials, she made a substantial contribution to understanding the mechanisms of cardiovascular diseases and the effects of modern pharmacological therapies.

Bogdan-Mircea Mihai

Bogdan-Mircea Mihai is Professor in Diabetes, Nutrition and Metabolic Diseases, Head of Diabetes, Nutrition and Metabolic Diseases Unit at the Faculty of Medicine, "Grigore T. Popa" University of Medicine and Pharmacy, Iasi, Romania. He is also a senior physician in internal medicine and senior physician in diabetes, nutrition and metabolic diseases at "Sf. Spiridon" County Emergency Clinical Hospital, Iasi, Romania. Professor Mihai has a special contribution, awarded at the national level, to the study of diabetes, made concrete through numerous books and publications in journals with high impact in the international scientific community. He has extensive experience in the management of diabetes, including its cardiovascular and renal complications, and metabolic diseases at the intersection of obesity, dyslipidemias, metabolic syndrome, and nonalcoholic fatty liver disease.

Minerva Codruta Badescu

Minerva Codruta Badescu is MD, PhD, lecturer at "Grigore T. Popa" University of Medicine and Pharmacy, Iasi, Romania and senior physician in internal medicine at "Sf. Spiridon" County Emergency Clinical Hospital, IIIrd Internal Medicine Clinic, Iasi, Romania. She is a valuable member of the academic community, being involved in many universities and postgraduate educational programs and research projects. She is the author of numerous book chapters and articles in prestigious international journals, the main field of interest being cardiovascular diseases with arterial and venous thrombosis as their substrate. She also focuses on the management of antithrombotic therapy in difficult and complex clinical scenarios, such as thrombophilic states or congenital bleeding disorders. Dr Badescu was awarded three times for her peer-review activity.

Preface to "Ischemic Heart Disease in the Context of Different Comorbidities"

Cardiovascular diseases are the most important health problem of modern times and have a pandemic spread. There are many structural and functional cardiac abnormalities and their clinical expression is very wide, from the complete absence of symptoms to chest pain and dyspnea, syncope, hemodynamic instability and death. Among cardiovascular diseases, ischemic heart disease ranks as the most prevalent and causes almost one-third of deaths worldwide.

The field of cardiology is very dynamic, constantly evolving and improving. Our knowledge about myocardial ischemia is deepening every day, as major progress is made both in understanding its pathophysiological substrate and in improving diagnostic algorithms and therapeutic protocols.

Myocardial ischemia is the fundamental substrate of acute and chronic coronary syndromes. Beyond this significant role, its importance also resides in the coexistence with many pathological conditions, in which myocardial ischemia appears either as an associated factor or a consequence.

Firstly, the diagnosis of myocardial ischemia in the context of non-cardiac comorbidities can be a challenge for the clinician, who has the difficult task of choosing from many options the appropriate paraclinical investigations-ECG, biomarkers, stress tests, invasive and non-invasive imaging procedures-to establish a correct diagnosis.

Secondly, the high incidence and severe prognosis of myocardial ischemia highlight the need for continuous research in the field, to optimize the diagnosis and treatment and to improve the prognosis and survival of the patients.

Thirdly, atherosclerotic disease as a whole and myocardial ischemia, in particular, is frequently associated with a complex metabolic background. Innovative therapies bring important benefits, providing protection against atherosclerotic disease and significantly reducing major adverse cardiovascular events in dedicated clinical trials.

To summarize, these were the main reasons why we chose this broad topic. We aimed to form a team of specialists whose advanced experience allows us to understand the complex mechanisms of the bidirectional relationship between myocardial ischemia and various pathologies. Only by working as a strong team can we identify the best diagnostic and therapeutic solutions for our patients. We believe that our goal was fully achieved, and we express our deepest gratitude to our colleagues, who shared their knowledge and experience.

Irina-Iuliana Costache, Bogdan-Mircea Mihai, and Minerva Codruta Badescu
Editors

Editorial
Ischemic Heart Disease in the Context of Different Comorbidities

Irina-Iuliana Costache [1,2,*], Bogdan-Mircea Mihai [3,4] and Minerva Codruta Badescu [1,5]

1. Department of Internal Medicine, "Grigore T. Popa" University of Medicine and Pharmacy, 16 University Street, 700115 Iasi, Romania
2. Cardiology Clinic, "St. Spiridon" County Emergency Clinical Hospital, 1 Independence Boulevard, 700111 Iasi, Romania
3. Unit of Diabetes, Nutrition and Metabolic Diseases, "Grigore T. Popa" University of Medicine and Pharmacy, 16 University Street, 700115 Iasi, Romania
4. Clinical Center of Diabetes, Nutrition and Metabolic Diseases, "St. Spiridon" County Emergency Clinical Hospital, 1 Independence Boulevard, 700111 Iasi, Romania
5. III Internal Medicine Clinic, "St. Spiridon" County Emergency Clinical Hospital, 1 Independence Boulevard, 700111 Iasi, Romania
* Correspondence: irina.costache@umfiasi.ro

Ischemic heart disease (IHD) is a leading cause of morbidity and mortality worldwide. Since coronary atherosclerosis is its main substrate, IHD generally affects the geriatric population [1]. As aging is associated with an increased number of comorbidities, IHD further negatively influences these patients' quality of life and longevity.

Ilie et al. debated the strong relationship between frailty and chronic coronary syndromes [2]. They discussed the mechanisms of the bidirectional interaction between frailty—a complex geriatric syndrome with many phenotypes—and increased risk of ischemic coronary events. They also highlighted the key roles of sarcopenia, systemic inflammation, endothelial dysfunction, and impaired lipid and glucose metabolisms. The authors also provided useful guidance for risk assessment, diagnosis, and treatment of old and frail patients with stable IHD.

Epidemiological studies have shown a decrease in the age at which risk factors for atherosclerosis begin to accumulate. In this context, the age at which the incidence and prevalence of IHD begin to increase has shifted to younger ages, causing the impact of the disease on public health to become even greater [3]. Approximately 1.72% of the world's population is currently affected by IHD, and the prevalence is still rising. As the global distribution map of IHD demonstrates, Eastern European countries contribute by far the highest prevalence [4].

Although myocardial infarction is only the tip of the iceberg, its consequences have a significant negative impact on morbidity and mortality in patients with IHD. Leancă et al. [5] provided an excellent review on adverse cardiac remodeling in survivors of acute myocardial infarction. The authors performed an in-depth analysis of the pathophysiological mechanisms involved in this process, and systematized the complex methods of evaluation by biomarkers and both conventional and high-performance imaging. The main goals of treatment were to avoid the progression of IHD to heart failure and to reduce mortality. The article provides strong evidence to guide individualized treatment aimed at counteracting adverse ventricular remodeling and promoting reverse ventricular remodeling.

Cancer is highly prevalent in the elderly, and cardiac toxicity of antineoplastic agents is currently a topic of major interest. Badescu et al. have shown that some commonly used oncological treatments have adverse effects on coronary arteries, as they induce endothelial dysfunction, coronary artery spasm, thrombosis, and fibrosis [6]. These harmful structural and functional changes lead to cardiovascular events that require reduction or temporary or permanent stop of antineoplastic therapy, and all of these events have a negative impact on cancer outcomes. The authors provided a comprehensive, systematized, structured, and up-to-date analysis of the available literature regarding the optimal measures to mitigate the toxic effects of major antineoplastic therapies on coronary arteries. Sorodoc et al. focused on chemotherapy-induced cardiotoxicity and discussed the value of troponin as a biomarker of myocardial injury in oncologic patients [7]. The authors highlighted that troponin is a sensitive indicator of myocardial injury, as well as a marker for increased risk of developing left ventricular systolic dysfunction and progression to heart failure. The assessment of troponin levels enables early detection of cardiac injury and identification of patients that could benefit from the implementation of prevention measures. Moreover, the authors warn that troponin has no diagnostic value for cardiotoxicity and should not be used to modulate chemotherapy in cancer patients.

The cross-talk between the heart and the liver is the main focus of the articles of Cazac et al. and Gîrleanu et al. Non-alcoholic fatty liver disease reflects a disrupted lipid and carbohydrate metabolism, and it is perceived today as the hepatic manifestation of the metabolic syndrome [8]. The authors emphasize that in the presence of a common pathogenic substrate, this liver disease should be considered a marker of an increased risk for atherosclerotic cardiovascular disease. It is highlighted that patients with non-alcoholic fatty liver disease have an increased prevalence of subclinical atherosclerosis, a higher risk for the development of acute coronary syndromes (ACS), a need for more revascularization procedures, and an increased risk of fatal and non-fatal cardiovascular outcomes.

Vascular inflammation, endothelial dysfunction, and procoagulant status are present in both liver cirrhosis and coronary artery disease [9]. Along with the main pathogenic mechanisms, the authors discuss the specifics of the diagnosis and treatment of IHD in cirrhotic patients, taking into account the fragile balance between thrombosis and bleeding, as well as the limited amount of evidence from clinical studies, especially in patients with advanced liver disease.

The link between inflammatory bowel disease and IHD is systemic inflammation. The article by Jucan et al. provides robust data regarding the elevated risk of IHD in inflammatory bowel disease patients, based on an in-depth analysis of the relevant literature [10]. The crucial role of chronic inflammation is extensively debated. The authors showed that the disruption of the intestinal mucosal barrier allows microbial translocation and other endotoxins to reach the blood. These events are followed by multi-pathway activation of systemic inflammation that leads to endothelial dysfunction, changes in the vascular smooth muscle, reduction in vessels elasticity, medial calcification, and atherosclerotic plaque formation and progression.

Cardiovascular complications of the SARS-CoV-2 infection have troubled the medical community for more than two years now, and not all questions have yet been answered. An impressive amount of data was systematized in the article by Timpau et al., covering all known mechanisms by which the infection with COVID-19 causes cardiac injury, expressed as ACS, heart failure, myocarditis, and stress cardiomyopathy [11]. The diagnostic role and prognostic value of inflammation and myocardial damage biomarkers are commented on from the perspective of an in-depth and comprehensive study of the dedicated literature, offering a robust conclusion that guides the practitioners. Duca et al. focused their research on myocardial ischemia in patients with the COVID-19 infection, and highlighted not only its complex pathophysiology, but also the diversity of its electrocardiographic expression [12]. The authors showed that myocardial ischemia is the result of endothelial damage mediated by the virus, cytokine storm caused by hyperactivation of the immune system, and oxygen supply–demand imbalance due to extensive pulmonary lesions. Moreover, they emphasized that the electrocardiographic aspects of myocardial ischemia were generally severe, and occurred even in younger and healthier patients.

A very particular aspect regarding IHD is presented by Haliga et al., namely the ACS precipitated by carbon monoxide (CO) poisoning [13]. This original research article demonstrated that the development of myocardial injury in these patients is the combined result of hypoxia, direct CO-mediated cell damage, coronary spasm, and intracoronary thrombosis. The authors showed that ACSs occur irrespective of the poisoning severity, some in the absence of significant cardiovascular risk factors and in both normal coronary arteries and non-critical atherosclerotic plaques. Among the many interesting results of the study, we want to draw attention to the young age of STEMI patients, with a mean of 27.7 years, and the absence of comorbidities.

As medicine advances and knowledge deepens, one non-modifiable cardiovascular risk factor, namely the genetic substrate, is studied with increased interest. It seems that it will become a major landmark in the implementation of preventive measures in the future. Butnariu et al. provided a state-of-the-art analysis of the data available in the literature on the role of genetic factors in the etiology of IHD [14]. The authors discussed the phenotypic variability and the genetic heterogeneity of the disease, suggesting that genetic and genomic studies may provide the highly sought-after and awaited answers about what makes us unique in the face of the disease. The multiple facets of monogenic and polygenic coronary artery disease are emphasized, with the hope that the identification of individuals at high risk for IHD will be facilitated. The door toward the medicine of the future is now open, and gene therapy strategies no longer seem to be an unattainable desideratum.

We may conclude that this Special Issue excels through multidisciplinarity, integrating into a unified whole the experience of various specialists whose common interest is IHD. We consider that the goal has been fully achieved, and we have succeeded in drawing attention to the multiple diagnostic and therapeutic challenges determined by the association of IHD with a series of comorbidities, as well as providing useful guidance for practice.

Conflicts of Interest: The authors declare no conflict of interest.

References

1. Rodgers, J.L.; Jones, J.; Bolleddu, S.I.; Vanthenapalli, S.; Rodgers, L.E.; Shah, K.; Karia, K.; Panguluri, S.K. Cardiovascular Risks Associated with Gender and Aging. *J. Cardiovasc. Dev. Dis.* **2019**, *6*, 19. [CrossRef] [PubMed]
2. Ilie, A.C.; Taranu, S.M.; Stefaniu, R.; Sandu, I.A.; Pislaru, A.I.; Sandu, C.A.; Turcu, A.M.; Alexa, I.D. Chronic Coronary Syndrome in Frail Old Population. *Life* **2022**, *12*, 1133. [CrossRef] [PubMed]
3. Vikulova, D.N.; Grubisic, M.; Zhao, Y.; Lynch, K.; Humphries, K.H.; Pimstone, S.N.; Brunham, L.R. Premature Atherosclerotic Cardiovascular Disease: Trends in Incidence, Risk Factors, and Sex-Related Differences, 2000 to 2016. *J. Am. Heart Assoc.* **2019**, *8*, e012178. [CrossRef] [PubMed]
4. Khan, M.A.; Hashim, M.J.; Mustafa, H.; Baniyas, M.Y.; Al Suwaidi, S.; AlKatheeri, R.; Alblooshi, F.M.K.; Almatrooshi, M.; Alzaabi, M.E.H.; Al Darmaki, R.S.; et al. Global Epidemiology of Ischemic Heart Disease: Results from the Global Burden of Disease Study. *Cureus* **2020**, *12*, e9349. [CrossRef] [PubMed]
5. Leancă, S.A.; Crisu, D.; Petris, A.O.; Afrasanie, I.; Genes, A.; Costache, A.D.; Tesloianu, D.N.; Costache, I.I. Left Ventricular Remodeling after Myocardial Infarction: From Physiopathology to Treatment. *Life* **2022**, *12*, 1111. [CrossRef] [PubMed]
6. Badescu, M.C.; Badulescu, O.V.; Scripcariu, D.V.; Butnariu, L.I.; Bararu-Bojan, I.; Popescu, D.; Ciocoiu, M.; Gorduza, E.V.; Costache, I.I.; Rezus, E.; et al. Myocardial Ischemia Related to Common Cancer Therapy-Prevention Insights. *Life* **2022**, *12*, 1034. [CrossRef] [PubMed]
7. Sorodoc, V.; Sirbu, O.; Lionte, C.; Haliga, R.E.; Stoica, A.; Ceasovschih, A.; Petris, O.R.; Constantin, M.; Costache, I.I.; Petris, A.O.; et al. The Value of Troponin as a Biomarker of Chemotherapy-Induced Cardiotoxicity. *Life* **2022**, *12*, 1183. [CrossRef] [PubMed]
8. Cazac, G.D.; Lacatusu, C.M.; Mihai, C.; Grigorescu, E.D.; Onofriescu, A.; Mihai, B.M. New Insights into Non-Alcoholic Fatty Liver Disease and Coronary Artery Disease: The Liver-Heart Axis. *Life* **2022**, *12*, 1189. [CrossRef] [PubMed]
9. Gîrleanu, I.; Irifan, A.; Huiban, L.; Muzica, C.; Petrea, O.C.; Singeap, A.M.; Cojocariu, C.; Chiriac, S.; Cuciureanu, T.; Costache, I.I.; et al. Ischemic Heart Disease and Liver Cirrhosis: Adding Insult to Injury. *Life* **2022**, *12*. [CrossRef] [PubMed]
10. Jucan, A.E.; Gavrilescu, O.; Dranga, M.; Popa, I.V.; Mihai, B.M.; Prelipcean, C.C.; Mihai, C. Ischemic Heart Disease in Patients with Inflammatory Bowel Disease: Risk Factors, Mechanisms and Prevention. *Life* **2022**, *12*, 1036. [CrossRef] [PubMed]
11. Timpau, A.S.; Miftode, R.S.; Leca, D.; Timpau, R.; Miftode, I.L.; Petris, A.O.; Costache, I.I.; Mitu, O.; Nicolae, A.; Oancea, A.; et al. A Real Pandora's Box in Pandemic Times: A Narrative Review on the Acute Cardiac Injury Due to COVID-19. *Life* **2022**, *12*, 1085. [CrossRef] [PubMed]
12. Duca, S.T.; Chetran, A.; Miftode, R.S.; Mitu, O.; Costache, A.D.; Nicolae, A.; Iliescu-Halitchi, D.; Halitchi-Iliescu, C.O.; Mitu, F.; Costache, I.I. Myocardial Ischemia in Patients with COVID-19 Infection: Between Pathophysiological Mechanisms and Electrocardiographic Findings. *Life* **2022**, *12*, 1015. [CrossRef] [PubMed]
13. Haliga, R.E.; Morarasu, B.C.; Sorodoc, V.; Lionte, C.; Sirbu, O.; Stoica, A.; Ceasovschih, A.; Constantin, M.; Sorodoc, L. Rare Causes of Acute Coronary Syndrome: Carbon Monoxide Poisoning. *Life* **2022**, *12*, 1158. [CrossRef] [PubMed]
14. Butnariu, L.I.; Florea, L.; Badescu, M.C.; Tarca, E.; Costache, I.I.; Gorduza, E.V. Etiologic Puzzle of Coronary Artery Disease: How Important Is Genetic Component? *Life* **2022**, *12*, 865. [CrossRef] [PubMed]

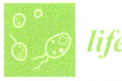 *life*

Review
Chronic Coronary Syndrome in Frail Old Population

Adina Carmen Ilie, Sabinne Marie Taranu *, Ramona Stefaniu, Ioana Alexandra Sandu, Anca Iuliana Pislaru, Calina Anda Sandu, Ana-Maria Turcu and Ioana Dana Alexa

Department of Medical Specialties II, Grigore T. Popa University of Medicine and Pharmacy Iasi, 700115 Iași, Romania; adina.ilie@umfiasi.ro (A.C.I.); ramona.stefaniu@umfiasi.ro (R.S.); ioana0sandu@gmail.com (I.A.S.); pislaru.anca2@gmail.com (A.I.P.); sandu.calina@gmail.com (C.A.S.); ana_turcu2000@yahoo.com (A.-M.T.); ioana.b.alexa@gmail.com (I.D.A.)
* Correspondence: sabinnemarie.taranu@yahoo.com

Abstract: The demographic trend of aging is associated with an increased prevalence of comorbidities among the elderly. Physical, immunological, emotional and cognitive impairment, in the context of the advanced biological age segment, leads to the maintenance and precipitation of cardiovascular diseases. Thus, more and more data are focused on understanding the pathophysiological mechanisms underlying each fragility phenotype and how they potentiate each other. The implications of inflammation, sarcopenia, vitamin D deficiency and albumin, as dimensions inherent in fragility, in the development and setting of chronic coronary syndromes (CCSs) have proven their patent significance but are still open to research. At the same time, the literature speculates on the interdependent relationship between frailty and CCSs, revealing the role of the first one in the development of the second. In this sense, depression, disabilities, polypharmacy and even cognitive disorders in the elderly with ischemic cardiovascular disease mean a gradual and complex progression of frailty. The battery of tests necessary for the evaluation of the elderly with CCSs requires a permanent update, according to the latest guidelines, but also an individualized approach related to the degree of frailty and the conditions imposed by it. By summation, the knowledge of frailty screening methods, through the use of sensitive and individualized tools, is the foundation of secondary prevention and prognosis in the elderly with CCSs. Moreover, a comprehensive geriatric assessment remains the gold standard of the medical approach of these patients. The management of the frail elderly, with CCSs, brings new challenges, also from the perspective of the treatment particularities. Sometimes the risk–benefit balance is difficult to achieve. Therefore, the holistic, individualized and updated approach of these patients remains a desired objective, by understanding and permanently acquiring knowledge on the complexity of the frailty syndrome.

Keywords: frailty; chronic coronary syndrome; elderly

Citation: Ilie, A.C.; Taranu, S.M.; Stefaniu, R.; Sandu, I.A.; Pislaru, A.I.; Sandu, C.A.; Turcu, A.-M.; Alexa, I.D. Chronic Coronary Syndrome in Frail Old Population. *Life* **2022**, *12*, 1133. https://doi.org/10.3390/life12081133

Academic Editor: Alexey V. Polonikov

Received: 23 June 2022
Accepted: 25 July 2022
Published: 27 July 2022

Publisher's Note: MDPI stays neutral with regard to jurisdictional claims in published maps and institutional affiliations.

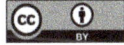

Copyright: © 2022 by the authors. Licensee MDPI, Basel, Switzerland. This article is an open access article distributed under the terms and conditions of the Creative Commons Attribution (CC BY) license (https://creativecommons.org/licenses/by/4.0/).

1. Introduction
1.1. The Demographic Trend of Aging

The old population continues to increase worldwide, being highly influenced by important regressions in the main causes of mortality. The demographic changes are reflected in society, raising the needs and costs of health care yearly. Worldwide, the proportion of people over the age of 65 is expected to exceed 25% by 2030, and in Europe, the number of older people will increase to 152.6 million in 2060 from 87.5 million in 2010 [1]. At the same time, the growing trend of demographic aging is associated with a high prevalence of coronary artery disease (CAD) in both men and women. The mortality risk and morbidity attributed to chronic coronary syndromes are increased due to aging (especially after 75 years) and due to a high incidence of comorbidities (e.g., hypertension, diabetes, chronic kidney disease, etc.).

With global aging, frailty has become a common condition in the old population. Frailty is highly related to the incidence and unfavorable prognosis of atherosclerotic coronary heart disease [2].

The literature reports two-way associations between cardiovascular disease and frailty. Although peripheral arterial disease and heart failure have been more frequently linked to frailty, current studies focus on broader directions, considering the impact and relationship between chronic coronary syndromes and frailty [3].

1.2. Chronic Coronary Syndromes. Definition, Prevalence and Features in Senior Patients

Of all types of cardiovascular diseases, coronary syndrome showed the highest mortality rate, resulting in approximately 659,000 deaths and 805,000 coronary events yearly in the United States [4].

The pathological foundation of coronary heart disease is based on the permanent accumulation of atherosclerotic plaque in the epicardial arteries. It can manifest as obstructive or non-obstructive. Lifestyle regulations, medication and invasive procedures having therapeutic and diagnostic roles can influence the evolution of this process, by stabilizing or regressing the disease. CAD is known by its long periods of stability, but we have to consider the possibility of an acute atherothrombotic event due to plaque rupture or erosion. This event will increase the risk of turning into unstable angina, at any time. Even in apparently silent clinical periods, the disease is usually progressive, and therefore severe. The fact that this pathology implies a dynamic manifestation, we can integrate it in two different clinical presentations known as acute coronary syndromes (ACSs) and chronic coronary syndromes (CCSs) [5,6].

To briefly define chronic coronary syndromes is a challenge, as they are identified by the different evolutionary stages of coronary heart disease, excluding the states in which an acute coronary artery thrombosis dominates the clinical presentation (i.e., ACS) [5,7].

Studies show an increased risk in the old population to develop CCSs. Despite this fact, it seems like this group mostly remains insufficiently diagnosed and treated. The atypical character of the symptoms in a senior patient is recognized, thus delaying the timing of the definite diagnosis [5].

1.3. Frailty. Definition, Prevalence and Features in Senior Patients

Frailty is a geriatric syndrome, encompassing different and complex phenotypes, from the physical to the immunological and cognitive components. Frailty is identified by the state of gradual and absolute decline, regardless of the aspects in which it occurs. Geriatric syndromes such as functional dependence, cognitive impairment and malnutrition are in most cases caused by physical frailty which implies decreased muscle strength, a loss of endurance, decreased physiological function and a decreased ability to adapt to stress. Studies have shown clear interactions between frailty status and the complications of coronary heart disease [2,8,9]. Therefore, the evaluation of frailty in seniors has become an indirect way of assessing the true adverse events associated with chronic coronary syndromes.

Fried et al. proposed five dimensions of frailty, which continue to be the diagnostic criteria for this syndrome: decreased muscle strength, decreased walking speed, fatigue, decreased physical activity and involuntary weight loss [2]. Despite its wide use, the Fried phenotype only assesses the physical component of frailty [10]. Other methods of evaluation assess other components, but the golden standard in diagnosing or assessing frailty is the geriatric evaluation.

There are also revealing data confirming a relationship of interdependence and mutual empowerment between CCSs and frailty. Plurivascular disease (40%), tortuosity and calcifications (80–90%) have been seen in patients 80 years of age with a high prevalence of obstructive coronary heart disease (60%) in autopsy studies [6].

However, there is a predominant tendency in current studies to speculate on a one-way relationship between CCSs and frailty, so it seems that cardiovascular damage predisposes to frailty rather than vice versa [8,11].

2. Pathogeny, Mechanisms and Associated Factors

2.1. Pathophysiology of CCSs and Frailty in Senior Patients

The mechanisms surrounding frailty and cardiac aging require special attention due to their role in senior patients' morbidity, mortality, quality of life and their need for medical assistance and increased medical costs [12].

Frailty often coexists with heart disease due to coexisting pathophysiological changes, aging and numerous comorbidities, all leading to rapid functional decline and sarcopenia. Higher rates of disability, institutionalization and mortality were recorded in senior patients with both frailty and CCSs [12].

In the pathogenesis of CCSs, varied mechanisms were described in which protein degradation, denervation, atrophy and altered fatty acid oxidation played an important role. Moreover, peroxisome proliferation and decreased protein synthesis, commonly in seniors, activate the gamma coactivator-1 alpha receptor (PGC-1α), whose expression is mitochondrial dysfunction. Thus, sarcopenia represented by homeostenosis of muscle metabolism increases predisposition to chronic coronary syndromes. The altered protein, lipid and glucose metabolism (i.e., insulin resistance) and also endothelial dysfunction, a substrate of cardiovascular disease, are precipitated by an ongoing inflammatory process (increased expression of biomarkers), usually encountered in old age [12].

Nicotinamide adenine dinucleotide phosphate (NADPH) oxidase increases the production of reactive oxygen species (ROS) and stimulates the ubiquitin-proteasome system in skeletal muscle, leading to the development of sarcopenia and increasing the occurrence of chronic coronary syndromes [12–15].

Elevated levels of C-reactive protein, Interleukin 6 (IL-6) and tumor necrosis factor alpha (TNF-α) are also linked to the loss of skeletal muscle mass. At the same time, TNF-α/nuclear factor-κB (NF-kB) catalyzes the synthesis of ROS in mitochondria, leading to the degradation of muscle proteins, sarcopenia and increasing the risk for ischemic events [12,16,17].

The loss of muscle mass and function also contributes to ischemic heart damage. Therefore, knowledge of the pathogenesis of sarcopenia at the cellular mechanism level is important. With aging, the pathways leading to sarcopenia, involving myostatin, phosphatidylinositol 3-kinase and lysosomal catabolism, are affected. Consequently, autophagy as a mechanism of cell preservation is inactivated and damaged. Its constituents remain undegraded, resulting in the alteration of the quality and quantity of muscle mass, leading, in time, to cardiovascular conditions [12,18–20].

The abnormal activation of inflammasome NLRP3, a multiprotein signaling complex found in the cytoplasm of the cell, has also been linked to cardiac inflammation, systolic dysfunction and ventricular remodeling that precipitate the onset of ischemic cardiovascular events [12,21–24].

Vascular aging is defined by mechanisms involving oxidative stress, mitochondrial dysfunction, genomic instability and epigenetic alterations. Moreover, lipid metabolism, extracellular matrix, coagulation/hemostasis impairment and inflammation are considered to have an important role in vascular aging. Lots of the predisposing factors for atherosclerosis, such as the damage to deoxyribonucleic acid from endogenous or exogenous sources, can lead to improper endothelial function, mediated by reduced nitric oxide synthase (eNOS) activity. They promote impaired vasodilator phenomena, the frailty of blood vessels and the growth of the intimal wall, ultimately leading to an increased risk for coronary heart disease. Theories of aging illustrate the mediator role of special proteins known as sirtuins (e.g., SIRT1) in endothelial function, whose impairment leads to increased reactive oxygen species (ROS). The ROS determine the development of vascular senescence and atherosclerosis [6,25].

In addition, research revealed that dehydroepiandrosterone, fibroblast growth factors (e.g., FGF-23), growth-differentiating factor-15 and plasma-associated lipokaline linked to neutrophil gelatinase have been involved in the progression of cardiovascular disease in the senior patient [6].

2.2. Implications of Inflammation in the Pathogenesis of CCSs and Frailty

Inflammation, represented by an impaired immune status and changes in function of immune cell subpopulations, is revealed to be closely related to frailty [26].

A meta-analysis of 32 cross-sectional studies in a group of 23,910 old people showed higher levels of inflammation, indicated by elevated serum levels of CRP and IL-6, in those with frailty and pre-frailty compared to those without frailty. At the same time, a positive link between high serum levels of IL-6, CRP and a loss of muscle mass was highlighted, with a reduction in the grip force, and correlations between inflammation and atherosclerosis were reported simultaneously [2,27].

In CCS patients as well as in frail ones, chronic low-grade inflammation, namely a lifetime exposure to the antigen, angiotensin activation, high body mass index, glucose intolerance and redox instability, are predominantly reported. Aside from conventional inflammatory markers, in CCSs and frailty syndrome, thrombotic markers such as factor VIII and D-Dimers are also elevated [28].

Inflammation is a key factor in both CCSs and frailty. In the first one, we already established the role of the inflammatory syndrome in lipoprotein oxidation and plaque activation. In the second, inflammation is shown to activate a catabolic neurohormonal process that implies the redistribution of amino acids from skeletal muscle to other organ systems. This is a cause of sarcopenia, represented by a decrease in muscle mass, with the inherent modification in muscle metabolism and impairment to adapt to stress factors [28,29].

Intermediate monocytes contribute to the proinflammatory status by releasing cytokines (e.g., TNF-α, IL-1β and IL-6) and reactive oxygen species. Alongside elevated lipoprotein levels, they constitute a possible marker for atherosclerosis and increased CVD risk [26].

IL-6 was found to directly activate muscle catabolism by stimulating the ubiquitin-proteome pathway, annihilating the cytoplasm and nucleoprotein in fibrocytes. In this context, the increase in IL-6 is considered an important predictor of decreased motor capacity, especially in older women. Indirectly, the concentrations of growth hormone (GH) and insulin-like growth factor-1 (IGF-1) have lowered, with decreased protein production and sarcopenia [2].

2.3. The Role of Albumin and Vitamin D in the Pathogenesis of CCSs and Frailty

A cohort study by Johansen et al. revealed that for each 1 g/dL increment in serum albumin levels, the frailty grades in senior hemodialysis patients, lowered by 0.4 points, thus suggesting that old patients with increased serum protein concentrations had a decreased rate of frailty [2,30]. These data are sustained by other studies on old, frail and non-frail patients with different comorbidities. Moreover, Dai et al. showed that blood serum albumin concentrations in senior patients with frailty and CCSs were significantly lower than that in pre-frailty and non-frailty patients. Serum albumin, a marker of nutritional status, may be an indicator of frailty in senior patients with chronic coronary syndrome [2].

A 25 (OH) D deficit is a negative prognostic factor in old patients with chronic coronary syndrome. The level of 25 (OH) D can be utilized as a marker to evaluate the gravity of CAD. Recent data have shown its role in predicting frailty [31]. Although results are not very specific, they indicate a link between the genetic mechanism of action of the vitamin D receptor (VDR) and that of cell differentiation and protein production. Thus, when vitamin D is low, adhesion to its receptor decreases simultaneously with muscle mass and strength [2].

The pathophysiological components between aging, frailty and CCSs in old patients are synthetized in Figure 1. There are three major factors contributing to both frailty and CCSs in old persons: normal aging, accelerated aging and inflammation. Each one can be an independent factor for frailty and/or CCSs, but they can also be found together as coexisting factors. Normal aging contributes to both frailty and CCSs and the cited mechanisms are: insulin resistance, increased production and accumulation of oxygen reactive species, normal changes in body composition which appear with aging (sarcopenia, central adiposity), homeostatic dysregulation, energy imbalance, neurodegeneration and hormonal dysregulation and inflammageing. Accelerated aging (which includes premature or aging at a rapid pace induced by diseases, genetic disorders or external factors) contributes to frailty and/or CCSs and the involved mechanisms are: increased oxidative stress, telomere shortening, immunosenescence, reduced autophagy and cellular senescence. Inflammation contributes to frailty and/or CCSs and the involved biomarkers are: C-reactive protein, Interleukin 6, tumor necrosis factor alpha (TNF-α) and nuclear factor-κB (NF-kB). All three factors contribute in varied degrees to both frailty and CCSs. Moreover, frailty is well-documented as being an important independent risk factor for CCSs in old patients and CCSs have a negative impact on frailty in old persons. The association of frailty and CCSs has a negative impact on the evolution of geriatric syndromes (especially cognitive impairment, immobility, delirium and iatrogenesis) and the development of CCS complications (acute coronary syndrome, heart failure and arrythmias). All these aspects imply polypharmacy, increased morbidity and death.

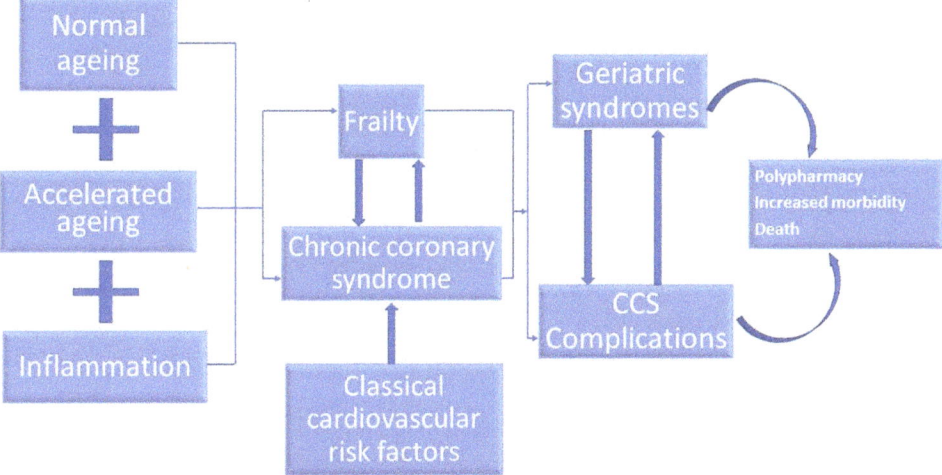

Figure 1. The pathophysiological components between aging, frailty and CCS in old patients. CCS—chronic coronary syndrome.

3. Clinical Presentation and Evaluation of the Frail Senior Patient with CCSs

Diagnosing chronic coronary syndromes in the old aged can be challenging. Senior patients generally have atypical symptoms (e.g., fatigue, dyspnea, nausea, vomiting or postprandial epigastric pain) rather than conventional angina. The presence of hearing or cognitive disorders complicates the anamnesis, and the associated comorbidities delay the diagnosis [6].

Regarding chronic coronary syndromes, the clinical scenarios reported by the latest guidelines are: (i) patients with suspected coronary heart disease and "stable" angina symptoms and/or dyspnea, (ii) patients with a new decompensation of heart failure or left ventricular dysfunction and suspected coronary heart disease, (iii) asymptomatic and symptomatic patients with symptoms stabilized at <1 year after ACS or patients with recent revascularization, (iv) asymptomatic and symptomatic patients > 1 year after initial diagnosis or revascularization, (v) patients with angina pectoris and suspected vasospastic or microvascular angina and (vi) asymptomatic subjects in whom coronary heart disease is detected on screening [5].

All of these are categorized as chronic coronary syndromes but entail various and time-modifiable risks for possible cardiovascular complications. For example, the installation of an ACS can sharply imbalance each of these clinical situations. Risks, in turn, could be precipitated by the improper management of cardiovascular risk factors, inadequate lifestyle adjustments, medical treatment or failure of revascularization. Alternatively, appropriate secondary prevention methods can counterbalance the adverse events of chronic coronary syndromes [5].

Frailty, disability or other processes of the disease that exacerbate fatigue (i.e., pulmonary, skeletal and peripheral artery disease) can veil the perception of the typical symptoms of chronic coronary syndrome by assuming increased oxygen demand for the associated pathologies. Although electrocardiographic anomalies could predict possible negative complications, previous pathologies/abnormalities could limit the usefulness of ECG screening. Transthoracic echocardiography, however, has proven useful in screening for global and segmental ventricular function and structural pathology in old patients [5,6].

There are scarce data about diagnostic and prognostic values of imaging modalities in CCS evaluation in frail old patents compared to the standard population. The few data are for the old and very old population compared to the adult population.

Age influences the validity and reliability of diagnostic tests in CCS patients. In the context of advanced age, exercise stress tests are submaximal undertaken by frail seniors, their diagnostic and prognostic value being less than for young adults. In a study of Newman and Phillips, the sensitivity and specificity of the ECG exercise test in patients aged ≥ 65 years were 85% and 56%, respectively, and data from a metanalysis, including patients regardless of age, reported that the sensitivity and specificity of ECG exercise testing for the diagnosis of stable CAD were 58% and 62%, respectively [32,33]. Independently of age, bicycle echocardiography is more useful clinically than other tests in the diagnosis of CCSs [32]. Generally, stress testing is better at confirming than infirming CCSs [34]. Exercise echocardiography in old patients reveals resting wall motion abnormalities in 36% of the seniors and new or worsening wall motion abnormalities in 41% of patients. Moreover, in the multivariate analysis, exercise echocardiography variables, such as end systolic volume and ejection fraction, added significantly to clinical factors in predicting mortality [35]. Dobutamine stress echocardiography in old patients generally is well-tolerated, but there is a higher risk for side effects. Asymptomatic hypotension occurred more frequently in the elderly (7% in those <55 vs. 13% in the 55–74 age group vs. 25% in those ≥ 75). Moreover, any ventricular arrhythmia was more common in the elderly patient population (26% vs. 30% vs. 41%) [36].

Although angiography is frequently used in CCS diagnosis in seniors, many times it is temporized due to frailty and some associated conditions, such as anemic syndromes and chronic kidney disease, the latter coming with high risk of contrast substance nephropathy [37]. Major vascular complications may occur in 3.6% of older patients undergoing diagnostic coronary angiography [6]. When considering cardiac catheterization, the probability of hemorrhagic, embolic and neurological events and acute renal damage induced by the contrast substance should be considered, all of which are increased in geriatric patients. In addition, the old aged with rheumatological or orthopaedical comorbidities may have issues maintaining clinostats and anesthesia. Thus, an individualized approach, comparing the possible advantages and disadvantages of invasive assessment, is required before advising cardiac catheterization to seniors [5,6].

Exploring the presence and rate of ischemia in old patients needs a careful analysis of the usefulness of the diagnosis, as well as the patient's preferences and objectives of treatment. It is fundamental to establish if the patient in question is eligible for future treatments. A non-invasive diagnostic stress assessment is very important when the subject's likelihood of developing chronic coronary syndrome is intermediate. Pharmacological stress echocardiography and single-photon emission computed tomography (SPECT), including myocardial perfusion imaging (MPI), have been shown to be effective in stratifying risk in these patients. In those non-eligible for testing, vasoactive agents such as adenosine or dobutamine are needed to cause differential coronary flow or ischemia. This medication associates a high level of iatrogeny, favoring adverse effects such as tachyarrhythmias, hypotension and severe myocardial ischemia. However, depending on the degree of frailty, these agents can be used safely in the old aged [5,6].

The role of magnetic resonance imaging in the evaluation of cardiac ischemia in geriatric patients is still being studied. Stress cardiac magnetic resonance strongly predicted cardiovascular events in people older than 70 years in a cohort of 110 patients. In a cohort of 110 patients who undergo stress CMR, 40.9% of the patients tested positive for ischemia. The median follow-up was 26 months, and in this period, there were 35 cardiovascular events. Therefore, a positive stress CMR with a moderate or severe hypoperfusion defect predicted the appearance of cardiovascular events in the follow-up in patients older than 70 years [38].

Coronary CT angiography is a non-invasive imaging method that can objectify the atherosclerotic rate with no need for pharmacological effort or stress testing. Still, senior people may fail to go through with the test due to their inability to hold their breath. Moreover, they are more likely to acquire atrial fibrillation and renal injury compared to young patients [5,6]. Computed tomography coronary angiography performed in an old population was able to exclude obstructive atheroma in 59% of patients. The positive predictive value of CTCA showing obstructive atheroma was between 74 and 89% when compared with invasive angiography [39].

Regarding the diagnosis of frailty, two main models have been proposed in recent decades. The first is the phenotype model proposed by Fried et al., describing frailty in terms of five physical dimensions: (1) unintentional weight loss of at least 4.5 kg in the last year or ≥5% of body weight in the previous year; (2) self-reported exhaustion identified by two questions from the CES-D depression scale; (3) a reduction in the grip force, adapted according to gender and body mass index (BMI); (4) decreased mobility adjusted to gender and height; and (5) low energy consumption related to physical activity based on the subject's self-report on the Minnesota Leisure Time Physical Activity Questionnaire (MTLAQ-short version). The lack of any of these items defines patients as "robust". "Pre-frail" subjects have low scores of one or two, and "frail" patients meet three or more of these criteria [1].

A Canadian study of the frailty index of health and aging (CFI), proposed by Rockwood et al., is based on a cumulative deficit model, comprising 70 items that include clinical signs, symptoms, diseases and comorbidities, in order to construct an individual FI score, compared to the standard one. Various instruments based on these two main models have been used in cardiac rehabilitation [40].

The gold standard for assessing frailty in an old patient remains the Comprehensive Geriatric Assessment (CGA). The CGA consists of a holistic evaluation in different areas of health in seniors, exploring 10 dimensions (cognition, motivation, disability, communication, mobility, balance, bowel/bladder function, nutrition, social ability and comorbidity). The Frailty Index based on a Comprehensive Geriatric Assessment (FI-CGA) is based on the CGA, evaluates the 10 dimensions and classifies patients into three classes of frailty: mild (0–7), moderate (7–13) and severe (>13) [1,41,42].

The different methods in evaluating frailty and its components are described in Table 1 [8].

Table 1. Diagnostic methods of frailty and frailty subtype.

Diagnostic Methods of Frailty	Frailty Subtype				
	Physical	Cognitive	Clinical	Psychological	Social
Fried criteria	x	-	x	-	-
FI-CGA	x	x	x	x	x
CFS	x	-	x	-	-
CSHA-FI	x	x	x	x	-
EFS	x	x	x	-	x
CGA	x	x	x	x	x

FI-CGA = Frailty Index based on a Comprehensive Geriatric Assessment; CFS = Clinical Frailty Scale; CSHA-FI = Canadian Study of Health and Aging Frailty Index; EFS = Edmonton Frailty scale; CGA = Comprehensive Geriatric Evaluation.

4. Risk Assessment in the Frail Senior Patient with CCS

A frailty assessment using the Clinical Frailty Assessment Scale (CFS) was separately and closely linked to mortality at 6 months of all causes, including after full adjustment for the initial differences in other risk factors [43].

The advanced age segment, increased comorbidities, recurrence of decompensation and prolonged hospitalization (>10 days) and emergency readmission within 30 days of discharge were associated with a higher degree of frailty and, at the same time, with the mortality of any within 30 days of the date of admission. A higher degree of frailty, according to the CFS, is associated with a more reserved prognosis in terms of mortality or the development of complications [43].

Other data suggested a high probability of readmission to hospital and death in frail patients compared to those who are not frail but who are associated with heart failure or chronic coronary syndromes. Polypharmacy and the lack of individualization of treatment are also factors that affect mortality in senior patients with CCSs and explain some of the differences between mortality from any cause and that linked to cardiovascular disease [4].

In the frail old aged, aging accelerates physical and functional decline, which raise the risk of poor health outcomes. The occurrence of frailty is directly proportional to aging and is related to elevated rates of mortality, morbidity, disability and increased health care costs while also being a predictor of poor surgical and interventional outcomes [4]. One meta-analysis evaluating gender differences between frail seniors showed women were considerably more frail, while men had increased mortality. The same data showed that frail old women with CCSs have a higher death rate than frail men of similar age [4,44,45].

During the 6-year follow-up of the NHATS study, it was revealed that seniors with pre-frailty and frailty have higher incidences of all-cause mortality, mainly due to death, stroke and peripheral vascular disease. The means to include frailty evaluation into the care of seniors at risk for CCSs is limited due to low efficacy in the prevention of frailty, no fully efficient therapies of the frailty and limited access to comprehensive geriatric evaluation [46–48].

The battery of secondary prevention interventions in frail old people with CCS includes: training, management of risk factors (diet management, smoking abstinence), medical treatment and psychological intervention [1]. Because frailty is a predictor of adverse outcomes in patients with CCSs, both the American Heart Association and the European Society of Cardiology recommend frailty screening in seniors with CAD and the development of intervention plans [5,49].

A holistic evaluation of the high-risk old aged can aid to recognize the factors that determine the development of frailty. It has been shown that aging, limited financial resources, malnutrition and depression are key to the development of frailty in patients with CCSs. The results are significant in the identification of frail adults with CCSs and the emerging need to bring forth preventive interventions [49]. A comprehensive geriatric assessment to recognize frailty is fundamental prior to clinical treatment, as are interventions to limit or reverse frailty in old patients with CCSs [49,50].

5. Consequences of the Association of Frailty and CCSs in Senior Patients

The risk for developing CCSs has raised in frail and pre-frail people > 65 years of age. Both frailty and CCSs in the old aged leads to a higher risk of short-term mortality (3 months). As per the frailty phenotype model, the prevalence of CCSs has led to a two- or three-times growth in frail seniors and a tendency to precipitate pre-frailty [1,51].

In hospitalized seniors, malnutrition and hypoalbuminemia may show either a state of frailty or a complication of CCS. The explanation resides in the resemblance and overlap of biological and pathophysiological mechanisms, such as inflammation and age-related subclinical cardiovascular impairment that leads to both conditions [1,52].

In aging patients with CCSs, heart failure (HF) is widespread, and the risk of frailty is 3.4 times bigger, with a high prevalence of pre-frailty (46%) and frailty (40%) The ischemic cardiovascular state predisposes to HF development [53]. Pathophysiologically, it shares common mechanisms with sarcopenia, related especially to inflammation pathways. Thus, it seems that HF can negatively influence gait speed and precipitate malnourishment, resulting in anemia and negative outcomes [1].

The aging of the world's population is leading to an increase in the incidence and prevalence of geriatric syndromes, such as frailty and disability. The advanced age segment is associated with a series of worsened results related to the link between frailty and CCSs. On these grounds, all other comorbidities, such as sarcopenia, malnutrition, functional dependence, polypharmacy, bleeding risk and thromboembolic events, are precipitated [1,29].

6. Treatment Characteristics in the Fragile Senior Patient with CCS

6.1. Treatment Goals

The treatment goals in frail old patients, who are associated with CCSs, include increasing life expectancy, minimizing the risk of cardiovascular events, improving or remitting symptoms and returning to normal activities or a good quality of life [11,54].

In senior patients, improving the quality of life, maintaining independence in daily life and controlling symptoms are priorities. In most cases, these issues are more important than prolonging life [55].

6.2. Pharmacological Treatment

According to new standards, treatment interventions should take into consideration two ways of approaching frailty. The first one must concentrate on preventing or reducing the progress of frailty while the second will be concerned with the anticipation of side effects in frail seniors. Periodic physical exercise and an adequate diet bring known benefits in the prevention of frailty, but the efficacy of pharmacotherapy is still certain [28].

Concerns have persisted over the past few years that the development of pharmaceutical strategies, such as new lipid-lowering agents in the form of subtilizin/kexin-9 (protein PCSK-9) inhibitors of proprotein convertase, and the use of oral anticoagulants (e.g., Rivaroxaban in patients with increased risk) outshine the role of lifestyle changes. Beta-blockers and calcium channel blockers still are the primary drugs for controlling the symptoms of angina and should be administered depending on the patient's heart rate, blood pressure and left ventricular function. The utilization of other secondary prevention medications (e.g., angiotensin converting inhibitors and statins) also remains the same [56].

The pharmacological treatment in an old patient must be prescribed considering its particularities: pharmacological and pharmacokinetic changes due to aging, body composition which is different in the old aged compared to adult, pre-existing medication for other conditions, the coexisting comorbidities, the presence of impairments, life expectancy, quality of life, polypharmacy and even the financial aspect [57,58].

Compared to young adults, seniors tend not to adhere to medical regimens, including optimal medical therapy for CCSs. Based on the literature, higher medical treatment compliance improves the survivability rate, even for frail seniors with CCSs [59]. The efficiency of antithrombotic therapy in frail senior patients is comparable to that in young adults, but the first group has a higher risk of bleeding [60].

6.3. Interventional Treatment

In the context of worldwide aging and a life expectancy increase, there appeared to be more and more cases of seniors necessitating advanced cardiovascular procedures, such as coronary artery bypass grafting (CABG) and percutaneous coronary intervention (PCI). Increased comorbidity prevalence associated with CCSs predisposes this group to more revascularization complications and poor outcomes. Thus, there is need to preoperatively assess the physiological status of these patients to establish the eligibility for CABG, PCI or pharmacological treatment. In addition to conventional risk stratification, the assessment of frailty is increasingly recognized as an available indicator for predicting outcomes after cardiac surgery [61].

The treatment of chronic coronary syndromes in the old aged suffers from the impasse of vulnerabilities related to both conservative and invasive strategies, such as bleeding, kidney failure and neurological disorders. According to current guidelines, radial access is recommended to be used, when possible, to lower complications at the entry zone when considering an invasive approach for seniors management. It is indicated that diagnostic and revascularization arguments be based on clinical presentation, the rate of ischemia, frailty, life expectancy and other morbidities [5].

Data report that in old patients with isolated CABG, the Preoperative Clinical Frailty Scale (CFS) was a separate predictor of hospital mortality at 30 days. A slow gait has been reported to have an individual predictive role in poor outcomes, even after adjusting for the Thoracic Surgeons Society (STS) score [61]. Debate yet remains as to whether to consider PCI or CABG for senior patients with CCSs and frailty. The presence of asymptomatic myocardial ischemia can be a complication of the frailty status associated with CCSs. Thus, preoperative screening for the frailty of CCS patients remains crucial [61,62].

The frail senior patient with comorbidities has a higher risk of post-CABG mortality compared to young adults [63,64]. Moreover, data show that age over 65, female sex and the presence of comorbidities are associated with higher rates of rehospitalization after CABG [65,66]. CABG should be used cautiously in the frail senior patient.

A single-center cohort study of 3826 patients undergoing cardiac surgery found frailty to be associated with an increased risk of mortality in hospital (adjusted odds ratio, 1.8; 95% CI, 1.1–3.0) and at 2 years (adjusted HR, 1.5; 95% CI, 1.1–2.2) [67]. Another population-based, retrospective, cohort study included 40083 patients undergoing CABG. A total of 8803 (22%) were frail, with a prevalence of frailty higher in the older age groups. Frail patients had higher rates of 30-day mortality than those who were not frail, across all but the ≥85 years age group; at 30 days, 626 patients (1.6%) patients died, of whom 174 (27.8%) were frail. Moreover, at 4 years, there were lower probabilities of survival in patients who were frail at the time of surgery [68]. Frailty has a strong positive relationship with the risk of major adverse cardiac and cerebrovascular events in patients undergoing cardiac surgery; in patients undergoing traditional procedures, such as CABG and/or valve procedures, frailty was associated with an increased OR of mortality, ranging from 1.10 to 2.63 [69].

A PCI is associated with better outcomes in octogenarians compared to young adults, in a higher or at least equal measure. An increased quality of life is one such outcome, but the risks and benefits of the PCI must be considered [70]. However, the efficacy of a PCI is limited by the late addressability of the senior patient, as often they already have complications [60].

A metanalysis which included 2658 seniors identified that the prevalence of frailty ranged from 12.5 to 27.8%. Frailty was associated with increased in-hospital mortality (OR 3.59, 95% CI 2.01–6.42), short-term mortality (OR 6.61, 95% CI 2.89–15.16), as well as long-term mortality (HR 3.24, 95% CI 2.04–5.14) in patients undergoing a PCI. Moreover, prefrailty was a predictor of all-cause mortality in senior patients undergoing a PCI [71]. Frailty also has a negative impact not only on mortality in old patients undergoing a PCI but also in hospital stay and time interval from admission to the PCI. A prospective study including 745 patients undergoing a PCI observed that the time interval from admission to the PCI was longer for frail patients (2.9 ± 5.6 vs. 1.7 ± 3.1 days, $p < 0.001$). After the PCI, frail patients remained in hospital substantially longer than non-frail patients (14.1 ± 26.7 vs. 3.5 ± 8.8 days, $p < 0.001$), and frail patients were nearly five times more likely to die within 30 days after the PCI, compared with non-frail patients (HR 4.8, 95% CI 1.4 to 16.3, $p = 0.01$) [72].

There are scarce data regarding a comparison of an OMT, PCI and CABG in frail old patients. The few data are for old patients with coronary chronic total occlusion, regardless of their frailty status. In these patients, a complete revascularization is more frequently achieved with CABG rather than a PCI, quality of life could be elevated by CABG and the 30-day mortality and 1-year survival were similar between CABG and PCI. However, the authors stated that when patients have a higher surgical risk such as frailty, serious comorbidity or dementia, a PCI seems to be more appropriate [73]. The European Society of Cardiology recommends to adopt a conservative, a noninvasive or a less invasive strategy in frail old patients [72,74].

6.4. Monitoring and Rehabilitation Programs

A relationship of interdependence and mutual potentiation has been established between frailty and cardiovascular impairment. Therefore, it is plausible that some rehabilitation measures to reduce frailty, including resistance training or nutritional approach, which involve an increased intake of protein and amino acids, may benefit seniors with CVD and frailty [61].

Although there is much data regarding cardiac rehabilitation and its role in restoring functional capacity and the quality of life in the frail old aged, there are few data assessing the role of cardiac rehabilitation, by improving frailty, in improving the prognosis in patients with CVD, including CCSs. We also interpret this aspect based on the fact that resistance training is not advised in most patients with CVD, due to the fact that it raises the post-cardiac load [61,75].

Most frail old patients eligible for cardiac rehabilitation programs have limitations in accessing them: there is a need for resources in the use of mobile technologies and in the correct performance of physical therapy exercises. However, it is certain that these interventions, and especially those requiring high-intensity training, have not been fully explored in the senior population.

Telemedicine has also been shown to be an additional tool for frail seniors who are unable to participate in cardiovascular rehabilitation exercises in hospitals. New data and reviews have recently showed the advantages of hybrid programs, which use remote monitoring and telerehabilitation platforms. In old patients with HF, the improvement in distance after following these rehabilitation programs for 12 weeks was statistically significant [1,76,77].

Although no significant differences were identified in terms of increased quality of life, mortality and improved functional capacity between conventional and hybrid cardiac rehabilitation programs, greater compliance was shown with those who joined the latter.

Frail seniors with ACSs or CCSs are often excluded from multidisciplinary cardiac rehabilitation measures or programs based on exercise. Future studies will focus on identifying the best frailty assessment tool for developing individualized care models. Cardiac rehabilitation programs at home and telerehabilitation models imagined specifically for frail seniors are enthusiastically advised [1].

Cognitive-behavioral and psychological interventions, exercise-based cardiac rehabilitation, annual influenza vaccination and the holistic assessment of senior patients are the levers of an individualized therapeutic approach, with the chance to reduce disabilities, increase quality of life and increase life expectancy.

Author Contributions: Conceptualization, I.D.A. and A.C.I.; methodology A.C.I. and S.M.T.; validation: R.S. and A.I.P., investigation C.A.S.; resources, S.M.T., I.A.S. and A.-M.T.; data curation, I.D.A.; writing—original draft preparation, S.M.T.; writing—review and editing, A.C.I.; visualization, A.C.I. and R.S.; supervision, I.D.A. All authors have read and agreed to the published version of the manuscript.

Funding: This research received no external funding.

Institutional Review Board Statement: Not applicable.

Informed Consent Statement: Not applicable.

Conflicts of Interest: The authors declare no conflict of interest.

References

1. Giallauria, F.; Di Lorenzo, A.; Venturini, E.; Pacileo, M.; D'Andrea, A.; Garofalo, U.; Vigorito, C. Frailty in acute and chronic coronary syndrome patients entering cardiac rehabilitation. *J. Clin. Med.* **2021**, *10*, 1696. [CrossRef] [PubMed]
2. Dai, J.R.; Li, J.; He, X.; Huang, H.; Li, Y. A relationship among the blood serum levels of interleukin-6, albumin, and 25-hydroxyvitamin D and frailty in elderly patients with chronic coronary syndrome. *Aging Med.* **2022**, *5*, 17–29. [CrossRef]
3. Kleipool, E.E.; Hoogendijk, E.O.; Trappenburg, M.C.; Handoko, M.L.; Huisman, M.; Peters, M.J.; Muller, M. Frailty in Older Adults with Cardiovascular Disease: Cause, Effect or Both? *Aging Dis.* **2018**, *9*, 489–497. [CrossRef]
4. Davis-Ajami, M.L.; Chang, P.S.; Wu, J. Hospital readmission and mortality associations to frailty in hospitalized patients with coronary heart disease. *Aging Health Res.* **2021**, *1*, 100042. [CrossRef]
5. Knuuti, J.; Wijns, W.; Saraste, A.; Capodanno, D.; Barbato, E.; Funck-Brentano, C.; Prescott, E.; Storey, R.F.; Deaton, C.; Cuisset Agewall, S.; et al. ESC Scientific Document Group. 2019 ESC Guidelines for the diagnosis and management of chronic coronary syndromes. *Eur. Heart J.* **2020**, *41*, 407–477. [CrossRef]
6. Madhavan, M.; Gersh, B.; Alexander, K.; Granger, C.B.; Stone, G.W. Coronary Artery Disease in Patients ≥ 80 Years of Age. *J. Am. Coll. Cardiol.* **2018**, *71*, 2015–2040. [CrossRef]
7. Ozmen, C.; Deniz, A.; Günay, İ.; Ünal, İ.; Celik, A.I.; Çağlıyan, Ç.E.; Deveci, O.S.; Demir, M.; Kanadaşı, M.; Usal, A. Frailty Significantly Associated with a Risk for Mid-term Outcomes in Elderly Chronic Coronary Syndrome Patients: A Prospective Study. *Braz. J. Cardiovasc. Surg.* **2020**, *35*, 897–905. [CrossRef] [PubMed]
8. Ijaz, N.; Buta, B.; Xue, Q.L.; Mohess, D.T.; Bushan, A.; Tran, H.; Batchelor, W.; deFilippi, C.R.; Walston, J.D.; Bandeen-Roche, K.; et al. Interventions for Frailty Among Older Adults With Cardiovascular Disease: JACC State-of-the-Art Review. *J. Am. Coll. Cardiol.* **2022**, *79*, 482–503. [CrossRef] [PubMed]
9. Rockwood, K.; Mitnitski, A. Frailty defined by deficit accumulation and geriatric medicine defined by Frailty. *Clin. Geriatr. Med.* **2011**, *27*, 17–26. [CrossRef] [PubMed]
10. Fried, L.P.; Tangen, C.M.; Walston, J. Frailty in older adults: Evidence for a phenotype. *J. Gerontol. A Biol. Sci. Med. Sci.* **2001**, *56*, M146–M156. [CrossRef]
11. Qayyum, S.; Rossington, J.A.; Chelliah, R.; John, J.; Davidson, B.J.; Oliver, R.M.; Hoye, A. Prospective cohort study of elderly patients with coronary artery disease: Impact of frailty on quality of life and outcome. *Open Heart* **2020**, *7*, e001314. [CrossRef]
12. Barbalho, S.M.; Tofano, R.J.; Chagas, E.F.B.; Detregiachi, C.R.P.; de Alvares Goulart, R.; Flato, U.A.P. Benchside to the bedside of frailty and cardiovascular aging: Main shared cellular and molecular mechanisms. *Exp. Gerontol.* **2021**, *148*, 111302. [CrossRef] [PubMed]
13. Schnelle, M.; Sawyer, I.; Anilkumar, N.; Mohamed, B.; Richards, D.A.; Toischer, K.; Zhang, M.; Catibog, N.; Sawyer, G.; Mongue-Din, H.; et al. NADPH oxidase-4 promotes eccentric cardiac hypertrophy in response to volume overload. *Cardiovasc. Res.* **2021**, *117*, 178–187. [CrossRef] [PubMed]
14. Bechara, L.R.; Moreira, J.B.; Jannig, P.R.; Voltarelli, V.A.; Dourado, P.M.; Vasconcelos, A.R.; Scavone, C.; Ramires, P.R.; Brum, P.C. NADPH oxidase hyperactivity induces plantaris atrophy in heart failure rats. *Int. J. Cardiol.* **2014**, *175*, 499–507. [CrossRef]
15. Lee, H.; Jose, P.A. Coordinated Contribution of NADPH Oxidase- and Mitochondria-Derived Reactive Oxygen Species in Metabolic Syndrome and Its Implication in Renal Dysfunction. *Front. Pharmacol.* **2021**, *12*, 670076. [CrossRef]
16. Cui, L.; Cao, W.; Xia, Y.; Li, X. Ulinastatin alleviates cerebral ischemia-reperfusion injury in rats by activating the Nrf-2/HO-1 signaling pathway. *Ann. Transl. Med.* **2020**, *8*, 1136. [CrossRef]
17. Chen, J.; Zhang, J.; Wu, J.; Zhang, S.; Liang, Y.; Zhou, B.; Wu, P.; Wei, D. Low shear stress induced vascular endothelial cell pyroptosis by TET2/SDHB/ROS pathway. *Free Radic. Biol. Med.* **2020**, *162*, 582–591. [CrossRef]
18. Wehr, E.; Pilz, S.; Boehm, B.O.; Marz, W.; Grammer, T.; Obermayer-Pietsch, B. Low free testosterone is associated with heart failure mortality in older men referred for coronary angiography. *Eur. J. Heart Fail.* **2011**, *13*, 482–488. [CrossRef] [PubMed]
19. Berben, L.; Floris, G.; Kenis, C.; Dalmasso, B.; Smeets, A.; Vos, H.; Neven, P.; Antoranz Martinez, A.; Laenen, A.; Wildiers, H.; et al. Age-related remodelling of the blood immunological portrait and the local tumor immune response in patients with luminal breast cancer. *Clin. Transl. Immunol.* **2021**, *9*, e1184. [CrossRef] [PubMed]
20. Cho, J.; Choi, Y.; Sajgalik, P.; No, M.H.; Lee, S.H.; Kim, S.; Heo, J.W.; Cho, E.J.; Chang, E.; Kang, J.H.; et al. Exercise as a therapeutic strategy for sarcopenia in heart failure: Insights into underlying mechanisms. *Cells* **2021**, *9*, 2284. [CrossRef]
21. Kelley, N.; Jeltema, D.; Duan, Y.; He, Y. The NLRP3 Inflammasome: An Overview of Mechanisms of Activation and Regulation. *Int. J. Mol. Sci.* **2019**, *20*, 3328. [CrossRef]
22. Wang, X.; Chen, X.; Dobrev, D.; Li, N. The crosstalk between cardiomyocyte calcium and inflammasome signaling pathways in atrial fibrillation. *Pflug. Arch.* **2021**, *473*, 389–405. [CrossRef]
23. Yan, Z.; Qi, Z.; Yang, X.; Ji, N.; Wang, Y.; Shi, Q.; Li, M.; Zhang, J.; Zhu, Y. The NLRP3 inflammasome: Multiple activation pathways and its role in primary cells during ventricular remodeling. *J. Cell. Physiol.* **2021**, *236*, 5547–5563. [CrossRef]
24. Liang, Y.; Wang, B.; Huang, H.; Wang, M.; Wu, Q.; Zhao, Y.; He, Y. Silenced SOX2-OT alleviates ventricular arrhythmia associated with heart failure by inhibiting NLRP3 expression via regulating miR-2355-3p. *Immun. Inflamm. Dis.* **2021**, *9*, 255–264. [CrossRef]
25. Paneni, F.; Diaz Canestro, C.; Libby, P.; Luscher, T.F.; Camici, G.G. The aging cardiovascular system: Understanding it at the cellular and clinical levels. *J. Am. Coll. Cardiol.* **2017**, *69*, 1952–1967. [CrossRef]

26. Cybularz, M.; Wydra, S.; Berndt, K.; Poitz, D.M.; Barthel, P.; Alkouri, A.; Heidrich, F.M.; Ibrahim, K.; Jellinghaus, S.; Speiser, U.; et al. Frailty is associated with chronic inflammation and pro-inflammatory monocyte subpopulations. *Exp. Gerontol.* **2021**, *149*, 111317. [CrossRef] [PubMed]
27. Soysal, P.; Stubbs, B.; Lucato, P.; Luchini, C.; Solmi, M.; Peluso, R.; Sergi, G.; Isik, A.T.; Manzato, E.; Maggi, S.; et al. Inflammation and frailty in the elderly: A systematic review and meta-analysis. *Ageing Res. Rev.* **2016**, *31*, 1–8. [CrossRef]
28. Afilalo, J. Frailty in Patients with Cardiovascular Disease: Why, When, and How to Measure. *Curr. Cardiovasc. Risk Rep.* **2011**, *5*, 467–472. [CrossRef]
29. Walston, J.; McBurnie, M.A.; Newman, A.; Tracy, R.P.; Kop, W.J.; Hirsch, C.H.; Gottdiener, J.; Fried, L.P. Frailty and activation of the inflammation and coagulation systems with and without clinical comorbidities: Results from the Cardiovascular Health Study. *Arch. Intern. Med.* **2002**, *162*, 2333–2341. [CrossRef] [PubMed]
30. Johansen, K.L.; Dalrymple, L.S.; Delgado, C.; Chertow, G.M.; Segal, M.R.; Chiang, J.; Grimes, B.; Kaysen, G.A. Factors associated with frailty and its trajectory among patients on hemodialysis. *Clin. J. Am. Soc. Nephrol.* **2017**, *12*, 1100–1108. [CrossRef] [PubMed]
31. Schöttker, B.; Jorde, R.; Peasey, A.; Thorand, B.; Jansen, E.H.J.M.; de Groot, L.; Streppel, M.; Gardiner, J.; Ordóñez-Mena, J.M.; Perna, L.; et al. Vitamin D and mortality: Meta-analysis of individual participant data from a large consortium of cohort studies from Europe and the United States. *BMJ* **2014**, *348*, g3656. [CrossRef]
32. Knuuti, J.; Ballo, H.; Juarez-Orozco, L.E.; Saraste, A.; Kolh, P.; Rutjes, A.W.S.; Jüni, P.; Windecker, S.; Bax, J.J.; Wijns, W. The Performance of Non-Invasive Tests to Rule-in and Rule-out Significant Coronary Artery Stenosis in Patients with Stable Angina: A Meta-Analysis Focused on Post-Test Disease Probability. *Eur. Heart J.* **2018**, *39*, 3322–3330. [CrossRef] [PubMed]
33. NEWMAN, K.P.; PHILLIPS, J.H. Graded Exercise Testing for Diagnosis of Coronary Artery Disease in Elderly Patients. *South. Med. J.* **1988**, *81*, 430–432. [CrossRef] [PubMed]
34. Banerjee, A.; Newman, D.R.; Van den Bruel, A.; Heneghan, C. Diagnostic accuracy of exercise stress testing for coronary artery disease: A systematic review and meta-analysis of prospective studies. *Int. J. Clin. Pract.* **2012**, *66*, 477–492. [CrossRef]
35. Arruda, A.M.; Das, M.K.; Roger, V.L.; Klarich, K.W.; Mahoney, D.W.; Pellikka, P.A. Prognostic Value of Exercise Echocardiography in 2632 Patients ≥ 65 Years of Age. *J. Am. Coll. Cardiol.* **2001**, *37*, 1036–1041. [CrossRef]
36. Hiro, J.; Hiro, T.; Reid, C.L.; Ebrahimi, R.; Matsuzaki, M.; Gardin, J.M. Safety and Results of Dobutamine Stress Echocardiography in Women versus Men and in Patients Older and Younger than 75 Years of Age. *Am. J. Cardiol.* **1997**, *80*, 1014–1020. [CrossRef]
37. Lee, P.C.; Kini, A.S.; Ahsan, C. Anemia Is an Independent Predictor of Mortality after Percutaneous Coronary Intervention. *Am. J. Cardiol.* **2004**, *44*, 541–546. [CrossRef]
38. Esteban-Fernández, A.; Bastarrika, G.; Castanon, E.; Coma-Canella, I.; Barba-Cosials, J.; Jiménez-Martín, M.; Alpendurada, F.; Gavira, J.J.; Azcárate-Agüero, P.M. Prognostic Role of Stress Cardiac Magnetic Resonance in the Elderly. *Rev. Española Cardiol. (Engl. Ed.)* **2020**, *73*, 241–247. [CrossRef]
39. Jordan, A.; Green, P.; Lee, H.; Bull, R.; Radvan, J. Coronary CT Angiography: A Useful Diagnostic Modality in the Elderly? *Eur. Heart J.* **2013**, *34* (Suppl. S1), P5347. [CrossRef]
40. Rockwood, K.; Song, X.; Mac Knight, C.; Bergman, H.; Hogan, D.B.; McDowell, I.; Mitnitski, A. A global clinical measure of fitness and frailty in elderly people. *CMAJ* **2005**, *173*, 489–495. [CrossRef] [PubMed]
41. Liguori, I.; Russo, G.; Bulli, G.; Curcio, F.; Flocco, V.; Galizia, G.; Della-Morte, D.; Gargiulo, G.; Testa, G.; Cacciatore, F.; et al. Validation of "(fr)AGILE": A quick tool to identify multidimensional frailty in the elderly. *BMC Geriatr.* **2020**, *20*, 375. [CrossRef]
42. Jones, D.M.; Song, X.; Rockwood, K. Operationalizing a frailty index from a standardized comprehensive geriatric assessment. *J. Am. Geriatr. Soc.* **2004**, *52*, 1929–1933. [CrossRef]
43. Ekerstad, N.; Javadzadeh, D.; Alexander, K.P.; Bergström, O.; Eurenius, L.; Fredrikson, M.; Gudnadottir, G.; Held, C.; Ängerud, K.H.; Jahjah, R.; et al. Clinical Frailty Scale classes are independently associated with 6-month mortality for patients after acute myocardial infarction. *Eur. Heart J. Acute Cardiovasc. Care* **2022**, *11*, 89–98. [CrossRef]
44. Dou, Q.; Wang, W.; Wang, H.; Ma, Y.; Hai, S.; Lin, X.; Liu, Y.; Zhang, X.; Wu, J.; Dong, B. Prognostic value of frailty in elderly patients with acute coronary syndrome: A systematic review and meta-analysis. *BMC Geriatr.* **2019**, *19*, 222. [CrossRef]
45. Gordon, E.H.; Peel, N.M.; Samanta, M.; Theou, O.; Howlett, S.E.; Hubard, R.E. Sex difference in frailty: A systematic review and meta-analysis. *Exp. Gerontol.* **2017**, *89*, 30–40. [CrossRef] [PubMed]
46. Damluji, A.A.; Chung, S.E.; Xue, Q.L.; Hasan, R.K.; Moscucci, M.; Forman, D.E.; Bandeen-Roche, K.; Batchelor, W.; Walston, J.D.; Resar, J.R.; et al. Frailty and cardiovascular outcomes in the National Health and Aging Trends Study. *Eur. Heart J.* **2021**, *42*, 3856–3865. [CrossRef] [PubMed]
47. Qin, T.; Sheng, W.; Hu, G. To Analyze the Influencing Factors of Senile Coronary Heart Disease Patients Complicated with Frailty Syndrome. *J. Healthc. Eng.* **2022**, *2022*, 7619438. [CrossRef]
48. Roger, V.L.; Go, A.S.; Lloyd-Jones, D.M.; Adams, R.J.; Berry, J.D.; Brown, T.M.; Wylie-Rosett, J. Heart disease and stroke statistics—2011 update: A report from the American Heart Association. *Circulation* **2011**, *123*, e18–e209. [CrossRef]
49. Lyu, H.; Wang, C.; Jiang, H.; Wang, P.; Cui, J. Prevalence and determinants of frailty in older adult patients with chronic coronary syndrome: A cross-sectional study. *BMC Geriatr.* **2021**, *21*, 519. [CrossRef]
50. Rockwood, K.; Mitnitski, A. Frailty in relation to the accumulation of deficits. *J. Gerontol. A Biol. Sci. Med. Sci.* **2007**, *62*, 722–727. [CrossRef] [PubMed]
51. Rockwood, K.; Mitnitski, A.; Mac Knight, C. Some mathematical models of frailty and their clinical implications. *Rev. Clin. Gerontol.* **2002**, *12*, 109–117. [CrossRef]

52. Chen, L.; Huang, Z.; Lu, J.; Yang, Y.; Pan, Y.; Bao, K.; Wang, J.; Chen, W.; Liu, J.; Liu, Y.; et al. Impact of the Malnutrition on Mortality in Elderly Patients Undergoing Percutaneous Coronary Intervention. *Clin. Interv. Aging* **2021**, *16*, 1347–1356. [CrossRef]
53. Marengoni, A.; Zucchelli, A.; Vetrano, D.L.; Aloisi, G.; Brandi, V.; Ciutan, M.; Panait, C.L.; Bernabei, R.; Onder, G.; Palmer, K. Heart failure, frailty, and pre-frailty: A systematic review and meta-analysis of observational studies. *Int. J. Cardiol.* **2020**, *316*, 161–171. [CrossRef] [PubMed]
54. Dai, X.; Busby-Whitehead, J.; Forman, D.E.; Alexander, K.P. Stable ischemic heart disease in the older adults. *J. Geriatr. Cardiol.* **2016**, *13*, 109–114.
55. Singh, M.; Alexander, K.; Roger, V.L.; Rihal, C.S.; Whitson, H.E.; Lerman, A.; Jahangir, A.; Sreekumaran Nair, K. Frailty and its potential relevance to cardiovascular care. *Mayo Clin. Proc.* **2008**, *83*, 1146–1153. [CrossRef]
56. Kurdi, H. *Chronic Coronary Syndrome—A New Era for the Diagnosis and Management of Stable Coronary Artery Disease*; BCS Editorial: London, UK, 2020.
57. Zhao, M.; Song, J.X.; Zheng, F.F.; Huang, L.; Feng, Y.F. Potentially Inappropriate Medication and Associated Factors Among Older Patients with Chronic Coronary Syndrome at Hospital Discharge in Beijing, China. *Clin. Interv. Aging* **2021**, *16*, 1047–1056. [CrossRef] [PubMed]
58. Alexa, I.D.; Prada, G.I.; Donca, V.I.; Mos, L.M.; Alexa, O. Improving quality of life of elderly people aged 85 and older by improving treatment adherence. In Proceedings of the E-Health and Bioengineering Conference (EHB), Iasi, Romania, 21–23 November 2013; pp. 1–4.
59. Gnjidic, D.; Bennett, A.; Le Couteur, D.G.; Blyth, F.M.; Cumming, R.G.; Waite, L.; Handelsman, D.; Naganathan, V.; Matthews, S.; Hilmer, S.N. Ischemic heart disease, prescription of optimal medical therapy and geriatric syndromes in community-dwelling older men: A population-based study. *Int. J. Cardiol.* **2015**, *192*, 49–55. [CrossRef]
60. Kaehler, J.; Meinertz, T.; Hamm, C.W. Coronary interventions in the elderly. *Heart* **2006**, *92*, 1167–1171. [CrossRef]
61. Uchikado, Y.; Ikeda, Y.; Ohishi, M. Current understanding of the role of frailty in cardiovascular disease. *Circ. J.* **2020**, *84*, 1903–1908. [CrossRef]
62. Hubbard, R.E.; Eeles, E.M.; Rockwood, M.R.; Fallah, N.; Ross, E.; Mitnitski, A.; Rockwood, K. Assessing balance and mobility to track illness and recovery in older inpatients. *J. Gen. Intern. Med.* **2011**, *26*, 1471–1478. [CrossRef]
63. Chou, C.L.; Hsieh, T.C.; Wang, C.H.; Hung, T.H.; Lai, Y.H.; Chen, Y.Y.; Lin, Y.L.; Kuo, C.H.; Wu, Y.J.; Fang, T.C. Long-term outcomes of dialysis patients after coronary revascularization: A population-based cohort study in Taiwan. *Arch. Med. Res.* **2014**, *45*, 188–194. [CrossRef] [PubMed]
64. Carr, B.M.; Romeiser, J.; Ruan, J.; Gupta, S.; Seifert, F.C.; Zhu, W.; Shroyer, A.L. Long-Term Post-CABG Survival: Performance of Clinical Risk Models Versus Actuarial Predictions. *J. Card. Surg.* **2016**, *31*, 23–30. [CrossRef] [PubMed]
65. Shah, R.M.; Zhang, Q.; Chatterjee, S.; Cheema, F.; Loor, G.; Lemaire, S.A.; Wall, M.J., Jr.; Coselli, J.S.; Rosengart, T.K.; Ghanta, R.K. Incidence, Cost, and Risk Factors for Readmission After Coronary Artery Bypass Grafting. *Ann. Thorac. Surg.* **2019**, *107*, 1782–1789. [CrossRef] [PubMed]
66. Zea-Vera, R.; Zhang, Q.; Amin, A.; Shah, R.M.; Chatterjee, S.; Wall, M.J., Jr.; Rosengart, T.K.; Ghanta, R.K. Development of a Risk Score to Predict 90-Day Readmission After Coronary Artery Bypass Graft. *Ann. Thorac. Surg.* **2021**, *111*, 488–494. [CrossRef] [PubMed]
67. Lee, D.H.; Buth, K.J.; Martin, B.-J.; Yip, A.M.; Hirsch, G.M. Frail Patients Are at Increased Risk for Mortality and Prolonged Institutional Care After Cardiac Surgery. *Circulation* **2010**, *121*, 973–978. [CrossRef]
68. Tran, D.T.T.; Tu, J.V.; Dupuis, J.; Bader Eddeen, A.; Sun, L.Y. Association of Frailty and Long-Term Survival in Patients Undergoing Coronary Artery Bypass Grafting. *J. Am. Heart Assoc.* **2018**, *7*, e009882. [CrossRef]
69. Sepehri, A.; Beggs, T.; Hassan, A.; Rigatto, C.; Shaw-Daigle, C.; Tangri, N.; Arora, R.C. The Impact of Frailty on Outcomes after Cardiac Surgery: A Systematic Review. *J. Thorac. Cardiovasc. Surg.* **2014**, *148*, 3110–3117. [CrossRef]
70. Kähler, J.; Lütke, M.; Weckmüller, J.; Köster, R.; Meinertz, T.; Hamm, C.W. Coronary angioplasty in octogenarians. Quality of life and costs. *Eur. Heart J.* **1999**, *20*, 1791–1798. [CrossRef]
71. He, Y.-Y.; Chang, J.; Wang, X.-J. Frailty as a Predictor of All-Cause Mortality in Elderly Patients Undergoing Percutaneous Coronary Intervention: A Systematic Review and Meta-Analysis. *Arch. Gerontol. Geriatr.* **2022**, *98*, 104544. [CrossRef]
72. Murali-Krishnan, R.; Iqbal, J.; Rowe, R.; Hatem, E.; Parviz, Y.; Richardson, J.; Sultan, A.; Gunn, J. Impact of Frailty on Outcomes after Percutaneous Coronary Intervention: A Prospective Cohort Study. *Open Heart* **2015**, *2*, e000294. [CrossRef]
73. Guo, L.; Lv, H.-C.; Huang, R.-C. Percutaneous Coronary Intervention in Elderly Patients with Coronary Chronic Total Occlusions: Current Evidence and Future Perspectives. *Clin. Interv. Aging* **2020**, *15*, 771–781. [CrossRef]
74. Neumann, F.-J.; Sousa-Uva, M.; Ahlsson, A.; Alfonso, F.; Banning, A.P.; Benedetto, U.; Byrne, R.A.; Collet, J.; Falk, V.; Head, S.J.; et al. 2018 ESC/EACTS Guidelines on Myocardial Revascularization. *Eur. Heart J.* **2019**, *40*, 87–165. [CrossRef] [PubMed]
75. Taylor, H.L.; Jacobs, D.R., Jr.; Schucker, B.; Knudsen, J.; Leon, A.S.; Debacker, G.A. questionnaire for the assessment of leisure time physical activities. *J. Chronic Dis.* **1978**, *31*, 741–755. [CrossRef]
76. Kobulnik, J.; Wang, I.Y.; Bell, C.; Moayedi, Y.; Truong, N.; Sinha, S. Management of Frail and Older Homebound Patients With Heart Failure: A Contemporary Virtual Ambulatory Model. *CJC Open* **2021**, *4*, 47–55. [CrossRef] [PubMed]
77. Zulfiqar, A.A.; Hajjam, A.; Gény, B.; Talha, S.; Hajjam, M.; Hajjam, J.; Ervé, S.; Andrès, E. Telemedicine and Cardiology in the Elderly in France: Inventory of Experiments. *Adv. Prev. Med.* **2019**, *2019*, 2102156. [CrossRef]

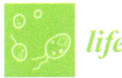

Review

Left Ventricular Remodeling after Myocardial Infarction: From Physiopathology to Treatment

Sabina Andreea Leancă [1], Daniela Crișu [1,*], Antoniu Octavian Petriș [1,2], Irina Afrăsânie [1], Antonia Genes [1], Alexandru Dan Costache [2,3], Dan Nicolae Tesloianu [1] and Irina Iuliana Costache [1,2]

[1] Department of Cardiology, Emergency Clinical Hospital "Sf. Spiridon", Bd. Independentei nr. 1, 700111 Iasi, Romania; sabinaandreea-leanca@email.umfiasi.ro (S.A.L.); antoniu.petris@umfiasi.ro (A.O.P.); irina-demsa@email.umfiasi.ro (I.A.); antonia.bobric@yahoo.com (A.G.); dan.tesloianu@umfiasi.ro (D.N.T.); irina.costache@umfiasi.ro (I.I.C.)
[2] Department of Internal Medicine, "Grigore T. Popa" University of Medicine and Pharmacy, Str. University nr. 16, 700083 Iasi, Romania; adcostache@yahoo.com
[3] Department of Cardiovascular Rehabilitation, Clinical Rehabilitation Hospital, 700661 Iasi, Romania
* Correspondence: daniela.crisu@umfiasi.ro; Tel.: +40-745-264-550

Abstract: Myocardial infarction (MI) is the leading cause of death and morbidity worldwide, with an incidence relatively high in developed countries and rapidly growing in developing countries. The most common cause of MI is the rupture of an atherosclerotic plaque with subsequent thrombotic occlusion in the coronary circulation. This causes cardiomyocyte death and myocardial necrosis, with subsequent inflammation and fibrosis. Current therapies aim to restore coronary flow by thrombus dissolution with pharmaceutical treatment and/or intravascular stent implantation and to counteract neurohormonal activation. Despite these therapies, the injury caused by myocardial ischemia leads to left ventricular remodeling; this process involves changes in cardiac geometry, dimension and function and eventually progression to heart failure (HF). This review describes the pathophysiological mechanism that leads to cardiac remodeling and the therapeutic strategies with a role in slowing the progression of remodeling and improving cardiac structure and function.

Keywords: left ventricular remodeling; myocardial infarction; wall stress; inflammation; neurohormonal activation; heart failure

1. Introduction

Postinfarct ventricular remodeling represents a prevailing cause of heart failure (HF), and it occurs in almost 30% of patients with a previous anterior myocardial infarction (MI) and in only approximately 17% of patients with non-anterior infarct [1].

Left ventricular (LV) adverse remodeling is a maladaptive process caused by cardiac injury characterized by morphological changes of LV structure and shape, with subsequent alteration of the cardiac function [2,3]. The term post-MI remodeling was first used in 1982 by Hockman and Buckey to describe the replacement of infarcted myocardium with scar tissue [4]. In 1990, Pfeffer and Braunwald published a review on ventricular remodeling after MI, showing that this process can affect the function of the ventricle and the prognosis of survival [5]. In the following years, the term cardiac remodeling was used to describe morphological and geometric changes in the LV after MI [6]. A consensus paper defines cardiac remodeling as a group of molecular, cellular and interstitial changes, which determine alterations in size, shape and function of the heart after cardiac injury [6].

In this narrative review, we have focused on the pathophysiological mechanisms and the assessment of cardiac remodeling post-myocardial infarction, as well as therapeutic approaches with proven or possible reverse remodeling effects. A comprehensive analysis of the current literature was made by searching Google Scholar and PubMed, using the keywords "cardiac remodeling", "myocardial infarction", "myocardial ischemia",

Citation: Leancă, S.A.; Crișu, D.; Petriș, A.O.; Afrăsânie, I.; Genes, A.; Costache, A.D.; Tesloianu, D.N.; Costache, I.I. Left Ventricular Remodeling after Myocardial Infarction: From Physiopathology to Treatment. *Life* 2022, *12*, 1111. https://doi.org/10.3390/life12081111

Academic Editor: Gopal J. Babu

Received: 16 June 2022
Accepted: 21 July 2022
Published: 24 July 2022

Publisher's Note: MDPI stays neutral with regard to jurisdictional claims in published maps and institutional affiliations.

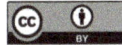

Copyright: © 2022 by the authors. Licensee MDPI, Basel, Switzerland. This article is an open access article distributed under the terms and conditions of the Creative Commons Attribution (CC BY) license (https://creativecommons.org/licenses/by/4.0/).

"cardiomyocyte metabolism", "neurohormonal activation". The results included original papers, prospective and retrospective studies, systematic reviews and meta-analysis, which underlined the pathophysiology of ventricular remodeling after myocardial infarction, as well as potential therapeutic strategies.

2. Pathophysiology of Adverse Remodeling

MI typically occurs consequently to the obstruction of epicardial coronary arteries. In an ischemic environment, cardiac myocytes develop an anaerobic metabolism with destabilization of the cell membrane and cell death through apoptosis, autophagy and necrosis [7–9]. Compared to other forms of myocardial injury, ischemic necrosis induces the death of millions of myocytes simultaneously, leading to an immune response and an influx of inflammatory cells into the infarcted area. Neutrophils and macrophages cause the destruction of the extracellular collagen matrix (ECM) and the expansion of the infarcted area, which consequently alter the ventricular shape, with thinning and dilatation of the infarcted myocardium. After reaching the maximum inflammatory response, fibroblasts are directed to the infarcted area where they create a new collagen matrix, and scar tissue is formed [3,10–15]. The inflammation may persist for a variable period of time after the ischemic event due to the continuous exposure of the myocardial wall to parietal stress. The compensatory activation of two major neurohormonal systems, the renin-angiotensin-aldosterone system (RAAS) and the sympathetic nervous system (SNS), in turn induces fibrosis and substantially intensifies the apoptotic changes. All of these processes lead to changes in the cardiac architecture and geometry, which are referred as adverse ventricular remodeling and are associated with a higher likelihood of HF and mortality [9,16].

Whereas ischemia caused by ST-segment elevation myocardial infarction (STEMI) in the absence of reperfusion therapy is more frequently associated with extensive scar formation and HF with reduced or mildly reduced ejection fraction (EF), in the case of non-ST-segment elevation myocardial infarction (NSTEMI), the adverse remodeling is rather associated with HF with preserved EF than with reduced EF. However, in terms of prognosis and mortality, there are no substantial differences between the two pathologies [16].

Furthermore, myocardial infarction can occur in the absence of obstructive coronary artery disease (MINOCA), and it is caused by various conditions, which create an imbalance between oxygen supply and demand, such as coronary vasospasm, coronary embolism, plaque disruption, microvascular dysfunction, tachyarrhythmias or arterial hypotension. Adverse remodeling occurs to a lower extent in this group of patients, as demonstrated by a study that showed that in more than half of the patients with a diagnosis of type 2 myocardial infarction, there was no imaging evidence of any functional consequences of myocardial infarction, such as a regional wall motion abnormality or scar formation. However, it is a known fact that these patients have a prognosis similar to those with an atherothrombotic MI, with a similar rate of future cardiovascular events [17].

2.1. The Sequence of Adverse Ventricular Remodeling

Ventricular remodeling following MI involves both the ischemic and the remote nonischemic myocardium, and it encompasses two stages. *The early stage of remodeling* occurs at the site of the infarct, a few hours from the acute coronary occlusion, continuing for nearly a week. In this phase, initial myocardial deformation by the persistent stretching of the myocytes activates stretch-induced signaling pathways mediated by a stretch sensor integrin, which will cause the pathological transformation of myocardial tissue with myocyte hypertrophy, followed by apoptosis and extracellular collagen matrix (ECM) changes with fibrosis. The cardiomyocyte lengthening and hypertrophy appear as an early compensatory mechanism for maintaining stroke volume (SV) following contractile tissue loss [6,11,13]. *The second phase of remodeling*, also called the "late phase", develops one month after the ischemic event, and it is characterized by potentially reversible structural and biochemical changes. It develops at a site distant from the infarcted area and it implies myocytes, which are still viable. Therefore, remote non-infarcted myocardial tissue becomes hypertrophied and dilated, as an adaptive response to the increased wall stress. This phase does not necessarily appear after every MI, and it is not always progressive [18–21].

2.2. Mechanisms of Adverse Remodeling

The main determinants of adverse ventricular remodeling post-myocardial infarction are represented by *mechanical* triggers and *biochemical* mechanisms, as described in Figure 1.

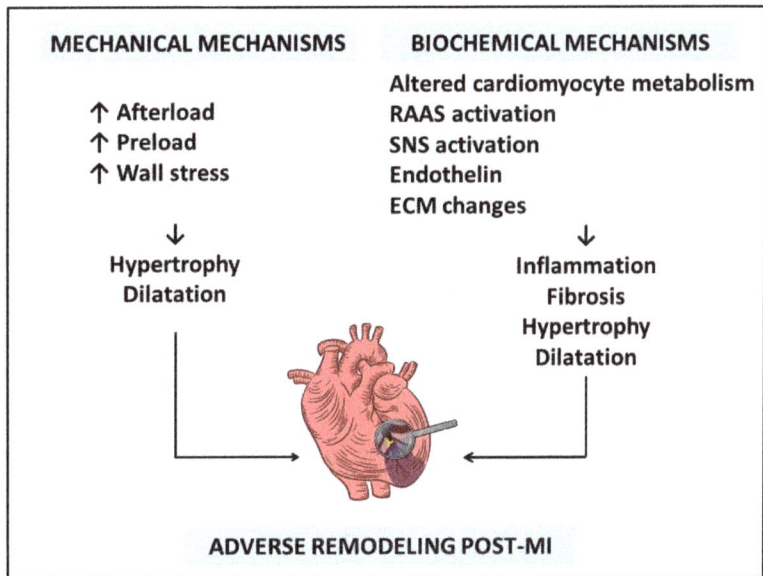

Figure 1. Mechanisms of adverse ventricular remodeling after myocardial infarction. RAAS: renin-angiotensin-aldosterone system; SNS: sympathetic nervous system; ECM: extracellular collagen matrix.

2.2.1. Mechanical Pathophysiology

The most important mechanical factors, which determine the ventricular remodeling after MI, are changes in *left ventricular geometry* and ventricular *wall stress* (WS), as shown in Figure 2 [22]. The progression of cardiac remodeling is simple to understand, according to Laplace's Law, which states that the LV WS is equal to the pressure in the chamber times the radius of the LV cavity, divided by the myocardial wall thickness. During the *early phase* of adverse remodeling, the infarcted segment is stretched due to a lack of counterbalance to the forces generated by the normally contracting myocardium. As a consequence, the increased wall tension from this level leads to a thinning of the infarcted wall and the expansion of the MI in the adjacent regions. Additionally, the stretched and dilated infarcted tissue increases the LV volume with a combined volume and pressure overload on the non-infarcted zones. During the *late phase* of remodeling, to maintain a normal stroke volume with a reduced number of properly functioning myocardial segments, in conditions of increased workload, the healthy cardiomyocytes will lengthen and progressively hypertrophy [23]. Finally, overstretching will cause the loss of the compensatory Frank–Starling mechanism and eventually lead to LV dilatation [20,22,24,25]. LV dilatation further increases WS, which in turn will accentuate chamber dilation and wall thinning, creating a vicious cycle [19,23,26].

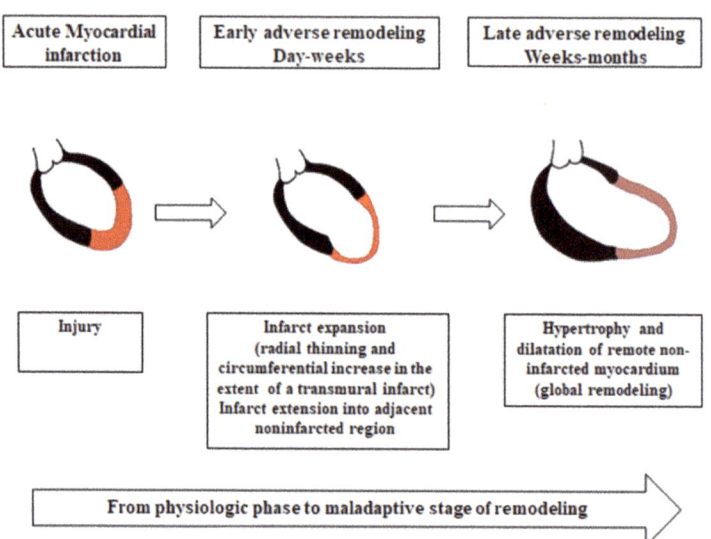

Figure 2. Mechanical mechanisms of adverse LV remodeling.

As a consequence of the adverse remodeling process, the left ventricle loses its ellipsoid shape and becomes more spherical, with increased end-diastolic and end-systolic volumes. The relaxation, as well as the radial, longitudinal contraction and torsion movement, is depressed, leading to diastolic and systolic dysfunction. The distorted left ventricle geometry causes secondary mitral regurgitation through tethering mechanism, which leads to increased intraventricular pressures and further promotes the adverse remodeling process [13].

2.2.2. Biochemical Pathophysiology

Adverse ventricular remodeling following myocardial infarction is the result of altered cardiomyocyte metabolism due to ischemic conditions, as well as the deleterious effects of several activated neurohormonal systems and molecular mechanisms.

Cardiomyocyte Metabolism

In the normally working myocardium, the energy required for myocyte contraction and relaxation results from the utilization of substrates, such as free fatty acids and carbohydrates by β-oxidation and glycolysis. The resulting metabolites will enter the tricarboxylic acid cycle (Krebbs cycle) in the mitochondria where energy will be produced by oxidative phosphorylation and stored in the form of high energy phosphates, mainly adenosine triphosphate (ATP). ATP production is significantly more efficient in the presence of oxygen, with more ATP being produced in the conditions of aerobiosis [27].

During ischemia, less oxygen and substrates are delivered to cardiac myocytes, which will lead to the less aerobic production of ATP. As a consequence of energy depletion, anaerobic glycolysis is triggered, and lactate is produced. Although initially lactate is utilized for the production of ATP, albeit with less metabolic efficiency, with prolonged ischemia it accumulates in the cells, decreasing the intracellular pH, which will further inhibit the glycolytic enzymes and lead to further energy depletion, calcium cellular overload and finally to altered cellular function and death [27,28].

While acute prolonged ischemia causes irreversible cellular damage, if reperfusion is established in time, the dysfunctional myocardium called "stunned myocardium" can potentially recover its function in hours or days after the normal coronary flow has been established. In the "stunned" myocytes, contractility is downregulated by the decrease in the intracellular pH, with significantly less ATP needed, thus making possible myocyte viability in conditions of reduced oxygen supply. However, myocardial reperfusion can itself produce further cellular damage and the extension of the infarcted area. The establishment of normal perfusion leads to rapid intracellular pH normalization, which will further lead to mitochondrial "re-energization", which will produce abundant ATP and reactive oxygen species (ROS). ROS damage the sarcoplasmic reticulum and cause a further increase in intracellular calcium. The result is cardiac myocyte hypercontracture and death. Furthermore, ROS act as chemoattractants for neutrophils, which further contribute to the local inflammation and damage [22,27,28].

During chronic ischemia, cardiac myocytes undergo metabolic and functional changes as an adaptive mechanism to decreased oxygen disponibility. The ischemic myocardium becomes hypocontractile, thus with a smaller consumption of ATP, being called "hibernating myocardium". Although free fatty acids are normally the main source of ATP, the hibernating tissue manifests a shift towards glucose substrate, as a protective mechanism to enable anaerobic metabolism during ischemic episodes. Although in "hibernating myocardium" dysfunction is reversible after reperfusion, it can progress to irreversible cellular damage and myocardium necrosis in the case of prolonged, severe ischemia and in the absence of reperfusion, finally leading to adverse ventricular remodeling [27,28].

Renin–Angiotensin–Aldosterone System (RAAS)

RAAS activation after MI leads to elevated circulating and tissue levels of angiotensin II (Ang II). By stimulating angiotensin type 1 (AT1) receptors, Ang II causes potent vasoconstriction and sodium and water retention, increasing cardiac preload and afterload, and subsequently increasing the WS. Additionally, Ang II directly affects the myocardium by causing cardiomyocyte hypertrophy and the hyperplasia of cardiac fibroblasts, promoting fibrosis. Furthermore, it promotes ECM deposition and the release of other growth factors and mediators, such as norepinephrine and endothelin, which will contribute to cardiac remodeling [29,30]. Aldosterone plays a major role in the adverse remodeling after MI, as it regulates and promotes LV collagen deposition, cardiomyocyte apoptosis, endothelial dysfunction and fibrosis. It also regulates sodium and potassium plasmatic concentrations, and it further activates the RAAS through feedback mechanisms [31–34].

Sympathetic Nervous System (SNS)

The SNS is activated immediately following acute MI. In the early phase of remodeling, sympathetic overdrive promotes neutrophil influx in the necrotic area and infarct expansion by activating apoptotic pathways [35]. Subsequently, the stimulation of β-1-adrenergic receptors (β1-ARs) activates signaling pathways, which promote cardiomyocyte hypertrophy. In the juxtaglomerular apparatus, activated β1-ARs induce renin release, which enhances the Ang II production of β-2-adrenergic receptors (β2-ARs) that may have cardioprotective effects, such as anti-apoptotic properties [30].

Endothelin

Endothelin is a potent vasoconstrictor peptide that is stimulated by hypoxia, ischemia, neurohormones (norepinephrine, Ang II) and inflammatory cytokines. Endothelin 1 (ET-1) contributes to adverse ventricular remodeling as it promotes inflammation, due to its ability to activate macrophages, release inflammatory cytokines (Tumor necrosis factor-alpha- TNF-α, Interleukin 6- IL-6, Interleukin 1 beta- IL-1β), increase adhesion molecule expression and stimulate neutrophil aggregation [36,37]. Moreover, ET-1 stimulates cardiomyocyte hypertrophy [36,38].

Natriuretic Peptides

The natriuretic peptide (NP) system includes three structurally homologous peptides, A-type NP (ANP), B-type NP (BNP) and C-type NP (CNP), that are secreted by the atrial and ventricular cardiomyocytes due to the increase in WS and stretching of the peri-MI tissue [22]. The NPs promote diuresis, natriuresis, vasodilation, as well as the inhibition of RAAS, endothelin production and SNS activation [39]. ANP inhibits apoptosis and cardiomyocyte hypertrophy, as well as collagen synthesis, which is the main driver of cardiac fibrosis [40]. NP concentrations might be used to stratify patients at risk for remodeling [22,41–45].

Extracellular Collagen Matrix (ECM) Changes

The cardiac ECM is a highly organized network of structural and functional proteins that surrounds the cardiomyocytes and produces a cellular scaffold that maintains the LV shape and geometry [12,46,47]. The ECM proteins are degraded by matrix metalloproteinases (MMPs), which in turn are inactivated by tissue metalloproteinase inhibitors (TIMPs) [48,49]. After MI, ECM undergoes significant changes. Initially, during the local inflammatory response from the infarct area, neutrophils degrade cellular debris and release MMPs, which cause aberrant degradation of the ECM and can lead to infarct expansion. At around day 3 after the MI, neutrophils are followed by macrophages, which will promote fibroblast differentiation to myofibroblasts, causing the synthesis of large amounts of ECM to form the infarct scar [3,47,50–52]. At the same time, TIMPs are activated, leading to collagen accumulation and scar formation. After around 2 weeks, the scar begins to mature, as the deposition of collagen increases and leukocytes and fibroblasts are cleared, most probably through apoptosis [53–58].

3. Biomarkers of Adverse Cardiac Remodeling

The role of biomarkers in the diagnosis, prediction, stratification and prevention of LV remodeling is not clearly stated. Several new biomarkers have been introduced in recent years, as summarized in Table 1.

Table 1. Biomarkers of adverse cardiac remodeling.

Biomarkers of cardiac injury and necrosis	hFABP IMA cMyC
Inflammatory biomarkers	TNF-α, IL-1β, IL-6 sST2 GDF-15 MPO
Biomarkers of cardiac fibrosis	Galectin-3
Biomarkers of collagen turnover	Carboxyterminal telopeptide of collagen type I Amino-terminal propeptide of type III procollagen MMPs TIMPs
Biomarkers of biomechanical myocardial stress	BNP, NT-proBNP Copeptin MR-proADM
Circulating ribonucleic acids	miR-1 miR-133a/b miR-208b miR-499

hFABP: heart-type fatty acid binding protein; IMA: ischemia-modified albumin; cMyC: sarcomeric cardiac myosin-binding protein C; TNF-α: tumor necrosis factor alpha; IL-1β: interleukin 1 beta; IL-6: interleukin 6; sST2: soluble suppression of tumorigenicity-2; GDF-15: growth differentiation factor-15; MPO: myeloperoxidase; MMPs: matrix metalloproteinases; TIMPs: tissue metalloproteinase inhibitors; BNP: B-type natriuretic peptide; NT-proBNP: N-terminal pro-brain natriuretic peptide; MR-proADM: mid-regional proadrenomedullin.

3.1. Biomarkers of Cardiac Injury and Necrosis

The classical biomarkers of myocardial necrosis have recently been supplemented with several new biomarkers, including the heart-type fatty acid binding protein (hFABP), the ischemia-modified albumin (IMA) and the sarcomeric cardiac myosin-binding protein C (cMyC).

hFABP is a low-molecular-weight, non-enzymatic protein involved in the intracellular buffering and transport of long-chain fatty acids. It is released into the circulation within an hour from the onset of the ischemic event, with levels returning to baseline in 12–24 h. Because it is relatively tissue-specific for the heart, hFABP has good specificity for myocardial necrosis [59,60]. Moreover, hFABP is a potential prognostic biomarker for long-term mortality. Matsumoto et al. showed that during the recovery stage, the hFABP levels in patients with prior MI could predict long-term mortality and the probability of readmission due to potential HF, even after discharge [61].

Acute myocardial ischemia causes significant protein changes, including alterations of the N-terminus of albumin, which lead to the formation of ***IMA***. IMA levels increase within 3 h following acute MI onset, but with reduced specificity for ischemia, since it also increases in a wide range of other medical conditions [62].

Sarcomeric cMyC is a myosin-binding protein isoform expressed only in the heart and it is one of the most promising new myocardial necrosis biomarkers. It is a specific marker of myocardial injury that is released into the bloodstream more quickly than troponin, allowing the earlier detection of myocardial injury [63,64].

3.2. Inflammatory Biomarkers

Inflammatory cytokines, such as TNF-α, IL-1β and IL-6 are significantly associated with LV adverse remodeling. These cytokines are released shortly after the ischemic injury and can acutely regulate myocyte survival or apoptosis, as well as initiate subsequent cellular inflammatory response [65,66]. Furthermore, cytokine secretion promotes gradual myocyte apoptosis or hypertrophy, and has effects on ECM by activating MMPs and collagen formation, mediating tissue repair and cardiac remodeling [16,67–70].

Soluble Suppression of Tumorigenicity-2 (ST2) is a member of the IL-1 receptor family that is expressed on endotheliocytes and secreted by cardiomyocytes and fibroblasts when under mechanical stress. It has a membrane-bound form (ST2 ligand- ST2L), as well as a soluble form (soluble ST2-sST2). IL-33 is a functional ligand of the ST2L receptor. The binding of IL-33 and ST2L on the inflammatory cell membrane activates intracellular signaling pathways and triggers the inflammatory response. On the other hand, the binding of IL-33 and ST2L on the cardiomyocyte membrane has a protective effect against the Ang II adverse remodeling effects, preventing myocardial fibrosis and maladaptive hypertrophy. However, sST, which increases in MI, acts as a decoy receptor for IL-33, decreasing the levels of IL-33 available to interact with ST2L. Therefore, the cardioprotective effects of IL-33/ST2L are attenuated when the levels of sST2 are increased. The sST2 secretion is associated with increased myocardial fibrosis, LV remodeling and unfavorable cardiovascular outcomes after MI [71–76].

Growth Differentiation Factor-15 (GDF-15) is a member of the transforming growth factor-β (TGF-β) superfamily, and it is highly expressed in the myocardium and endothelial cells in patients with cardiovascular disease. GDF-15 is an inflammatory and oxidative stress biomarker and recent research suggests a possible role of GDF-15 in myocardial fibrosis, hypertrophy and endothelial dysfunction [77]. GDF-15 might be an independent marker of LV remodeling after MI and an integrative biomarker of HF in patients with acute MI [78,79].

Myeloperoxidase (MPO) is an enzyme contained in neutrophils and monocytes, that is deployed in the extracellular environment by degranulation when inflammation is triggered. It is a promising, novel inflammatory biomarker as recent studies have shown that it is not only an excellent biomarker for diagnosing acute MI but also for identifying patients with vulnerable plaques, with an increased risk of plaque rupture [80–83].

3.3. Biomarkers of Cardiac Fibrosis

Galectin-3 is a β-galactoside-binding lectin that is mainly synthesized by macrophages from the infarcted tissue [84,85]. Apparently, in the early phase of MI, galectin-3 is involved in a reparative process in the infarcted area, which is critical for maintaining the LV geometry and function [86]. However, in the late phase of post-MI remodeling, galectin-3 stimulates tissue fibrosis and scar formation, therefore, being associated with cardiac remodeling. According to experimental studies, myocardial galectin-3 expression increases after MI, while several clinical studies indicate a relationship between elevated circulating levels of galectin-3 and a phenotype prone to HF after MI [16,87,88].

3.4. Biomarkers of Collagen Turnover

Excessive ECM protein production and accumulation, along with dysregulated turnover, promote post-MI remodeling and progression to HF. Targeting either protease-mediated fragmentation products (indicative of protein degradation) or the pro-peptide that is cleaved off the molecule during its maturation (indicative of protein formation) could offer information on ECM turnover. Circulating peptides released during collagen syntheses, such as *carboxyterminal telopeptide of collagen type I*, *amino-terminal propeptide of type III procollagen*, as well as *MMPs*, and *TIMPs*, may be helpful for risk stratification of the remodeling process [47,89,90]. Using multiple biomarkers, including the traditional biomarkers and indicators of ECM turnover, may increase the sensitivity and specificity of clinical outcomes in patients with post-MI remodeling [16].

3.5. Biomarkers of Biomechanical Myocardial Stress

NPs, as previously mentioned, promote vasodilatation AND natriuresis and have antiproliferative and antifibrotic effects, preventing adverse ventricular remodeling [16,91,92]. Therefore, NPs are excellent prognostic biomarkers of remodeling after acute MI. According to the 2020 European Society of Cardiology (ESC) guidelines for the management of acute coronary syndromes in patients presenting without persistent ST-segment elevation, BNP and N-terminal pro-brain natriuretic peptide (NT-proBNP) plasma concentrations should be considered when assessing patient's prognosis [93].

Copeptin is a stable glycopeptide derived from the C-terminal fragment of the vasopressin prohormone, which is an essential regulator of water homeostasis and plasma osmolality, with increased secretion in conditions of stress. Copeptin is released in an equimolar ratio to arginine vasopressin within the first 4 h following an acute MI. Therefore, copeptin might be an excellent surrogate marker of arginine vasopressin secretion, which has a relatively short half-life. However, copeptin is not a specific cardiac marker, as the circulating levels are also influenced by other conditions, including kidney disease or sepsis [16,94–96].

Midregional Proadrenomedullin (MR-ProADM) is a stable peptide fragment that serves as a precursor for adrenomedullin (ADM). ADM is a peptide hormone synthesized by the endothelial and vascular smooth muscle cells [16]. By binding to specific receptors, ADM increases nitric oxide and cyclic guanosine monophosphate synthesis, promoting vasodilation. It also mediates natriuresis, and it has a positive inotropic effect. Therefore, ADM exerts cardiac protection through several mechanisms: coronary vasodilation with subsequent increased myocardial blood flow and impaired maladaptive cardiac remodeling due to its antioxidant, antiapoptotic and antifibrotic effects [97]. In a study by Yoshitomi that evaluated plasmatic ADM in MI, the level of plasmatic ADM increased in the early stages of acute MI proportionately to the clinical severity, and it was further increased in patients with congestive HF [98]. In the LAMP Study, a significant increase in plasmatic MR-proADM after MI correlated with poor cardiac outcomes [99–101]. Furthermore, the increased levels of MR-proADM in acute MI patients, particularly in those developing HF, are associated with high rates of short and long-term mortality and hospitalization for HF [102,103].

3.6. Circulating Ribonucleic Acids

Non-coding ribonucleic acids (RNAs) are strong tissue- and cell-specific epigenetic regulators of cardiac gene expression and cell function. They are promising biomarkers in a broad spectrum of cardiovascular diseases and are widely investigated. **MicroRNAs** (miRNAs) are a class of tissue-specific or cell-specific small non-coding RNAs that regulate cell growth, proliferation, differentiation and apoptosis. Therefore, miRNA are extensively involved in cardiac remodeling in HF and after MI. Four miRNAs: *miR-1, miR-133a/b, miR-208b* and *miR-499* have increased circulating levels in acute MI, the last two being expressed exclusively in the cardiomyocytes [104,105]. MiRNAs are not only prognostic biomarkers in HF and ventricular remodeling but also targets for personalized intervention and translational therapy, with demonstrated effects in preventing maladaptive myocyte growth and improving ventricular function [22,106].

4. Imaging Techniques of Adverse Remodeling

Ventricular remodeling evaluation relies on assessing ventricular geometry and function, which can be performed with echocardiography or CMR (cardiac magnetic resonance).

Two-dimensional (D) echocardiography is widely accessible, and it is the first imaging technique to be used when evaluating ventricular remodeling. Left ventricular volumes, ventricular contractility and left ventricular ejection fraction calculated by the biplane summation of disks method are the main parameters that characterize ventricular remodeling. It can also evaluate valvulopathies and their mechanism, such as tethering in secondary mitral regurgitation, which is indicative of adverse remodeling. However, ***3D echocardiography*** offers more reproducible information when assessing ventricular volumes and function, especially when using contrast for the best delineation of the endocardial borders. Furthermore, it provides supplementary information compared to 2D echocardiography when assessing valvulopathies. ***Strain echocardiography*** is a newer echocardiographic technique and it offers a more comprehensive evaluation of myocardial contractility, being able to detect the subclinical disease as well. In addition, it is an excellent tool to assess the prognosis of patients with HF [22,107].

CMR is the gold standard imaging technique for the evaluation of ventricular volumes and function. However, the most valuable information derives from its ability to characterize the myocardial tissue. T2 mapping can identify myocardial edema, and, therefore, guide the diagnosis towards a cause of acute inflammation, such as acute myocarditis. Fibrosis is evaluated with T1 mapping, while the ventricular scar is assessed with late gadolinium enhancement imaging (LGE). Ventricular scar transmural extension determines the viability and subsequently guides potential coronary revascularization or cardiac resynchronization therapy (CRT). Scar localization offers further insight into the etiology of myocardial dysfunction, since it is mainly subendocardial in ischemic heart disease and mid-wall in dilated cardiomyopathy [108]. Furthermore, LGE can identify microvascular obstruction after MI, by visualizing the no-reflow phenomenon [22]. Finally, CMR is extremely useful in evaluating the etiology of MINOCA, and novel CMR techniques will bring further insight into ventricular remodeling after MI [17,22,107,108].

5. Therapeutic Implications in Adverse Cardiac Remodeling

The treatment in MI aims to prevent or attenuate left ventricular remodeling by reducing the size of the infarction and targeting the neurohormonal systems [12,13]. Reverse remodeling is the result of myocardial recovery in response to therapy, and it has been defined in previous studies as a decrease in LV end-systolic volume of 12% by CMR, while echocardiographic parameters include a reduction in end-systolic and end-diastolic volumes and an increase in LV EF of 12% to 15% [107,109]. It appears that in ischemic cardiomyopathy, there is no difference in the incidence of adverse remodeling between sexes. However, women have a lower predisposition to develop spherical distortion of the left ventricle, but a higher risk than men of developing HF [58]. In contrast, in non-ischemic cardiomyopathy, the rate of reverse remodeling is similar between sexes, but women have better outcomes [110]. The different response to therapy in adverse remodeling might be due to the fact that women develop less inflammation and apoptosis, with a less extended infarct area; sex hormones contribute to these processes [58]. Recent studies demonstrated that guideline-directed medical therapy, including angiotensin receptor neprilysin inhibitors promoting reverse remodeling both in ischemic and non-ischemic cardiomyopathy, improve the mortality and hospitalizations for HF. However, ischemic heart disease was associated with a lower probability of reverse remodeling and smaller improvements in ventricular diameters [111,112].

The main therapeutic strategies to prevent or reduce adverse remodeling are summarized in Figure 3.

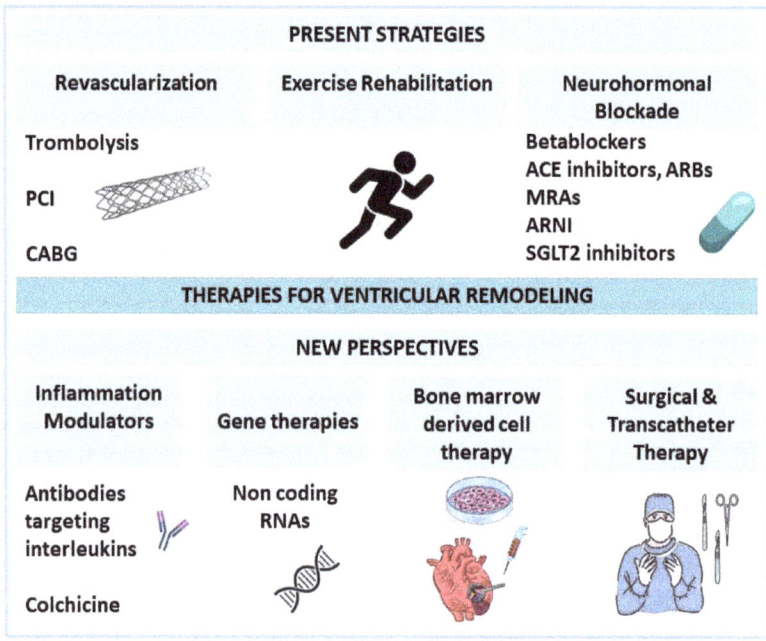

Figure 3. Therapies for ventricular remodeling. ACE: angiotensin-converting enzyme; ARBs: Ang II receptor blockers; MRAs: mineralocorticoid receptor antagonists; ARNI: angiotensin receptor neprilysin inhibitor; SGLT2: sodium-glucose cotransporter 2; RNAs: ribonucleic acids; PCI: percutaneous coronary intervention; CABG: coronary artery bypass graft.

5.1. Myocardial Revascularization

The main goal of treatment in acute MI is to restore myocardial perfusion and prevent necrosis through thrombolysis, percutaneous coronary intervention (PCI) or coronary artery bypass graft (CABG) surgery, with a significant reduction in mortality. The benefit of revascularization on cardiac remodeling is the reduction in the size of the infarction, with the consequent improvement of regional and global ventricular function [13,113,114].

The restoration of coronary flow by PCI is the standard of care for patients presenting in the first 12 h from symptom onset. In a prospective observational study, Marek Grabka et al. demonstrated a high rate of reverse cardiac remodeling in individuals diagnosed with the first anterior-wall STEMI and treated with primary PCI [115]. In the absence of PCI, early thrombolysis should be considered, and various studies have shown that early onset thrombolysis has reduced the extent of ventricular wall kinetic abnormalities. Current European and American guidelines recommend starting fibrinolysis in up to 30 min from the first medical contact in all eligible patients with STEMI when PCI is not possible [12,116,117]. Despite the evolution and success rate of PCI myocardial revascularization, cardiac remodeling continues to occur in one-third of patients with AMI [118].

5.2. Exercise-Based Cardiac Rehabilitation

Exercise-based cardiac rehabilitation is recommended, in addition to drug therapy, after an MI in order to prevent the progression of cardiac remodeling. The beneficial cardiac effects are caused by a decrease in Ang II secretion, sympathetic activity and circulating catecholamine levels, as well as an improvement in the balance between MMP-1 and TIMP-1 [12,119]. These results in reverse remodeling, with a reduction in the LV diameters and an improvement in LV contractility. In addition, Zhang et al. showed that changes in left ventricular remodeling were more significant when exercise training programs were initiated in the acute phase after MI. According to the 2020 ESC Guidelines on sports cardiology and exercise in patients with cardiovascular disease, patients should be referred to an early exercise training program for 8–12 weeks after an acute coronary syndrome (ACS) in order to reduce cardiac mortality and rehospitalization [120–122].

5.3. Neurohormonal Inhibition

5.3.1. Sympathetic Nervous System Blockade

SNS blockade plays a major role in the therapeutic strategy after MI. American and European guidelines support the use of beta-blockers after MI as a Class I recommendation. Long-term efficacy on morbidity and mortality was demonstrated by the CAPRICORN trial in which carvedilol was compared with a placebo in post-MI patients and with a LV EF $\leq$ 40% [123–125]. The benefit of beta-blockers is given by the inhibition of the effects of circulating catecholamines and reduction in heart rate and myocardial contractility, thus decreasing the oxygen demand. This prevents long-term interstitial fibrosis and significantly improves left ventricular remodeling [22,124,126–128]. In the CAPRICORN Echo substudy, carvedilol had a beneficial effect on ventricular remodeling: in the group of patients treated with carvedilol, there was a smaller increase in left ventricular end-systolic volume and a higher EF at 6 months after MI compared to controls [12,129]. In another study, Lee et al. compared the effects of propranolol and carvedilol on the volume and function of LV in patients benefiting from PCI after acute MI. Similar changes in LV end-diastolic volume in both groups were observed, proving that propranolol may be as beneficial as carvedilol [130,131].

5.3.2. RAAS Blockade

RAAS blockade has clearly demonstrated, in the landmark trials, beneficial effects on mortality and cardiovascular events in patients with MI, especially with low EF.

Angiotensin-converting enzyme inhibitors (ACEIs) prevent the formation of Ang II, and, therefore, block all its deleterious effects, improve LV remodeling and ameliorate the progression to HF. Current guidelines include treatment with ACEIs as Class I recommendations, based on numerous clinical trials that demonstrated ACEIs benefits on mortality and left ventricular systolic function after acute MI [3,13,132–134]. Trials, such as ISIS-4, GISSI-3, CCS-1, CONSENSUS-2 and SMILE, focused on the administration of ACEIs in the first 24 h, while in more recent trials (TRACE, AIRE), treatment was initiated 48 h after the acute event. In all studies, mortality after MI was significantly reduced. A meta-analysis of all major studies supports the benefit of ACEIs in the early and later management of MI [135,136].

Angiotensin II receptor blockers (ARBs) are recommended as an alternative when patients do not tolerate or have contraindications to ACEIs. By blocking the AT1 receptors, ARBs improve sodium and water retention, and prevent cardiac hypertrophy and fibrosis, thereby improving post-infarction ventricular remodeling [3,137–140]. Studies have shown a similar efficacy of ARBs compared to ACEIs post-MI. The OPTIMAAL clinical trial compared the efficacy of captopril with losartan, while in the VALIANT study captopril was compared with valsartan. Both ARBs showed similar efficacy with captopril on mortality. Regarding ventricular remodeling, the VALIANT Echo substudy showed that treatment with captopril or valsartan resulted in similar changes in ventricular size and function after MI [12,22,141]. The advantage of ARBs compared to ACEIs is given by fewer adverse effects, thus having a better tolerability profile. Moreover, the absence of degradation of bradykinin by ARBs appears to have beneficial effects on the cardiovascular system, as demonstrated by current research [140,142].

Mineralocorticoid receptor antagonists (MRAs) are currently recommended in the treatment of STEMI in patients with ventricular systolic dysfunction (EF < 40%) and HF or diabetes, who are already on treatment with ACEIs and beta-blockers. This recommendation of ESC guidelines is based on the results of the EPHESUS study, which compared the administration of eplerenone vs. placebo in addition to standard therapy in post-MI patients with LV dysfunction and HF or diabetes. After an average follow-up of 16 months, a reduction in all-cause mortality, cardiovascular mortality and sudden cardiac death by 15%, 17% and 21%, respectively, was observed [12,137,143–145]. The REMINDER study evaluated the effect of MRAs initiated in the first 24 h in STEMI patients without a history of HF, with a composite primary endpoint of cardiovascular mortality, re-hospitalization or extended initial hospital stay, due to diagnosis of heart failure, sustained ventricular arrhythmias, EF < 40%, or elevated BNP/NT-proBNP at 1 month or more after randomization. After 13 months of follow-up, the results showed good tolerance of eplerenone and a reduction in the primary endpoint, mainly due to significantly decreased natriuretic peptide levels. In contrast, ALBATROSS trial included patients with STEMI and non-STEMI and assessed the benefit of early MRA initiation in acute MI in addition to standard therapy (versus standard therapy alone), regardless of the presence of HF or LV dysfunction. The primary outcome was a composite of death, resuscitated cardiac arrest, ventricular arrhythmias, indication for implantable defibrillator or new or worsening HF at 6 months follow-up. However, the ALBATROSS trial failed to show benefits from early MRAs administration in addition to standard therapy in patients with MI. Experts consider that both trials were underpowered individually to validly evaluate the hard endpoints. The discrepancies might arise also from the fact that the ALBATROSS trial included both STEMI and NSTEMI patients. Furthermore, a pooled analysis of the REMINDER group and the ALBATROSS STEMI subgroup showed that mortality was significantly lower in patients treated with MRAs versus placebo [137,146,147].

5.3.3. Angiotensin Receptor Neprilysin Inhibitor (ARNI)

ARNI (sacubitril/valsartan) is a novel therapy that simultaneously inhibits the activation of RAAS by blocking AT1 receptors, and the degradation of bradykinin and natriuretic peptides by inhibiting neprilysin [148–150]. It is now considered one of the main pillars in the treatment of HF with reduced EF, since it demonstrated a significant reduction in mortality and hospitalization, greater than ACEIs, as shown by the PARADIGM–HF trial [151].

The effects of ARNI in patients with acute MI were studied in the PARADISE–MI study, which compared sacubitril/valsartan with ramipril in patients with acute MI and with an LV EF < 40% and/or signs of pulmonary congestion. The results of this study showed that sacubitril/valsartan did not reduce cardiovascular death or first HF hospitalization, compared to ramipril, however, it had a clear benefit in all HF events [152,153]. Moreover, in a recent meta-analysis, Zhang et al. showed that sacubitril/valsartan therapy after MI prevents adverse ventricular remodeling, thus improving cardiac function and reducing the rate of adverse cardiovascular events [149].

5.4. Sodium–Glucose Cotransporter 2 Inhibitors (SGLT2-I)

SGLT2-I, also called gliflozins (empagliflozin, canagliflozin and dapagliflozin), is another novel therapy that nowadays represents a cornerstone in the management of HF, given the outstanding results firstly showed by the landmark cardiovascular outcome trials

EMPA-REG, CANVAS and DECLARE-TIMI, in which SGLT2-I significantly reduced cardiovascular mortality, all-cause mortality and HF hospitalization [154–156]. Empagliflozin and dapagliflozin reduced the incidence of recurrent MI, which may be related to the gliflozins capacity to reduce the ischemic-reperfusion injury [157,158].

In MI, SGLT2 inhibitors switch the myocardial substrate utilization from glucose towards ketone bodies, free fatty acids and branched-chain amino acids, thereby improving myocardial energetics. Experimental evidence shows that SGLT2 inhibitors exert cardioprotective effects in animal models with acute MI by improving cardiac function during ischemia, reducing infarction size and subsequently attenuating HF development [159]. The early initiation and continuation of SGLT2 inhibition after acute MI could be beneficial to prevent ventricular remodeling and progression to chronic HF [160–167]. Patients with acute MI have been relatively understudied in SGLT2 inhibitor outcome trials to date. Currently, there are three trials ongoing, EMPACT-MI, EMMY and DAPA-MI, which will evaluate the efficacy and safety of the early initiation of SGLT2 inhibitors within days of an acute MI [168].

5.5. Statins

The use of statins is recommended by international guidelines for the secondary prevention of cardiovascular and cerebrovascular events. New evidence suggests that statins also manifest beneficial effects against cardiac remodeling by inhibiting the proliferation of cardiac fibroblasts and ECM turnover. Experimental studies have shown that statins improved LV dilation after MI, thus limiting cardiac remodeling [137,169–172].

5.6. Inflammation Modulators

Since inflammation plays a major role in ventricular remodeling post-MI, several cytokines could be therapeutic targets in modulating myocardial inflammation. Blocking IL-1β signaling improves heart remodeling and the possible progression to HF. Canakinumab, a human monoclonal antibody that inhibits IL-1β, was evaluated in the CANTOS study. Canakinumab, compared to a placebo in patients with prior MI, increased C-reactive protein (CRP), reduced circulating CRP levels and decreased the incidence of recurrent cardiovascular events [3,173–186]. Several studies have shown that the inhibition in mice of the NLR family pyrin domain containing 3 (NLPR3), the macromolecule involved in regulating IL-1β and IL-18 activation, preserves cardiac systolic function following in vivo ischemic and non-ischemic damage. The administration of colchicine, a non-specific inhibitor of NLPR3, resulted in a significantly reduced infarct size in mice and improved cardiac function after acute MI [3,177–180].

5.7. Gene Therapy

Gene therapy is an emerging therapeutic tool with significant implications in adverse remodeling post-MI. Angiotensin-(1-9) is a novel peptide that regulates the RAAS. A study by Fattah et al. using in vivo gene transfer in a murine model of MI showed that Angiotensin-(1-9) gene therapy preserved LV systolic function after MI, restoring cardiac function [181]. Non-coding RNAs are major regulators of adverse remodeling after MI, in chronic HF and when the ventricular WS is increased. Silencing microRNAs in vivo using specific antisense inhibitors prevents maladaptive remodeling and improves cardiac function [182,183]. In a study by Danielson et al., extracellular plasma RNAs after MI were associated with phenotypes of left ventricular remodeling [183]. Another study found that up-regulation of miR-17 in diabetic mice improved left ventricular function after acute MI and reduced the size of the infarction [22,184–186].

5.8. Cell-Based Therapy in Cardiac Remodeling

Bone marrow-derived cell (BMC) therapy enables the repair of the damaged myocardial tissue after MI by promoting transdifferentiation of progenitor cells into healthy cardiomyocytes. The REPAIR–AMI trial evaluated the effect of intracoronary transplantation of BMCs on post-MI remodeling and showed that the intracoronary infusion of enriched BMCs is certainly linked with the improvement of the LV global function in patients with acute MI. At 12 months post-transplantation of BMCs, transplanted patients had a significantly reduced incidence of death, re-infarction and revascularization [22,187,188]. However, other studies showed neutral results of BMC therapy in patients with MI, and further research is needed [189–191].

5.9. Surgical and Transcatheter Interventions

Surgical procedures aimed to correct the distorted LV geometry with large areas of akinesia and aneurysms did not prove to be superior when compared with reperfusion therapy alone. Therefore, surgical procedures that restore the ventricular shape are indicated for selected HF patients who have refractory symptoms or malignant ventricular arrhythmias [22]. Minimally invasive transcatheter procedures can be performed in patients with chronic anteroseptal infarction, with the exclusion of the anterior scarred myocardium from viable tissue by plicating the anterior and LV free wall scar against the right ventricle septal scar [22]. This technique reduces the LV volume and restores conical LV morphology, potentially improving the LV systolic function [192].

6. Conclusions

LV adverse remodeling after MI is a process of major importance as it leads invariably to HF, increased mortality and a high economic burden. Understanding the pathophysiology and implementing the potential biomarkers that predict adverse remodeling make possible an integrative therapeutic approach and a better estimation of prognosis. Novel imaging techniques offer a more detailed evaluation of adverse remodeling, as well as the response to therapies that target the maladaptive process. Advances have been made in the therapeutic field, and timely coronary reperfusion in associations with novel therapies, such as ARNI and SGLT2-I, along with MRAs and beta blockers, counteract adverse ventricular remodeling and promote reverse ventricular remodeling, decreasing progression to HF and mortality. Future therapeutic perspectives, such as microRNAs, bone marrow derived-cells, and molecules targeting inflammation are currently under research, with promising results.

Author Contributions: Conceptualization, S.A.L., D.C. and I.I.C.; methodology, I.I.C., A.O.P. and D.C.; investigation, data curation, S.A.L., I.A., A.G. and A.D.C.; writing—original draft preparation, S.A.L.; writing—review and editing, I.A., D.C., A.D.C. and A.G.; visualization, D.C., A.O.P., I.I.C. and D.N.T.; supervision, D.C., A.O.P., D.N.T. and I.I.C. All authors contributed equally to the study. All authors have read and agreed to the published version of the manuscript.

Funding: This research received no external funding.

Institutional Review Board Statement: Not applicable.

Informed Consent Statement: Not applicable.

Data Availability Statement: Not applicable.

Conflicts of Interest: The authors declare no conflict of interest.

Abbreviations

MI: myocardial infarction; HF: heart failure; LV: left ventricle; RAAS: renin-angiotensin-aldosterone system; SNS: sympathetic nervous system; ECM: extracellular collagen matrix; SV: stroke volume; WS: wall stress; ATP: adenosine triphosphate; ROS: reactive oxygen species; Ang II: angiotensin II; AT1: angiotensin type 1 receptor; β1-ARs: β-1-adrenergic receptors; β2-ARs: β-2-adrenergic receptors; ET-1: endothelin 1; TNF-α: tumor necrosis factor alpha; IL-6: interleukin 6; IL-1β: interleukin 1 beta; NP: natriuretic peptide; ANP: A-type natriuretic peptide; BNP: B-type natriuretic peptide; CNP: C-type natriuretic peptide; MMPs: matrix metalloproteinases; TIMPs: tissue metalloproteinase inhibitors; hFABP: heart-type fatty acid binding protein; IMA: ischemia-modified albumin; cMyC: sarcomeric cardiac myosin-binding protein C; sST2: soluble suppression of tumorigenicity-2;

GDF-15: growth differentiation factor-15; TGF-β: transforming growth factor-β; MPO: myeloperoxidase; ESC: European Society of Cardiology; NT-proBNP: N-terminal pro-brain natriuretic peptide; MR-proADM: mid-regional proadrenomedullin; ADM: adrenomedullin; RNAs: ribonucleic acids; miRNAs: microRNAs; CMR: cardiac magnetic resonance; LGE: late gadolinium enhancement; CRT: cardiac resynchronization therapy; PCI: percutaneous coronary intervention; CABG: coronary artery bypass graft; ACS: acute coronary syndrome; EF: ejection fraction; ACEIs: angiotensin-converting enzyme inhibitors; ARBs: Ang II receptor blockers; MRAs: mineralocorticoid receptor antagonists; ARNI: angiotensin receptor neprilysin inhibitor; SGLT2: sodium-glucose cotransporter 2; T2D: type 2 diabetes; CRP: C-reactive protein; NLPR3: NLR family pyrin domain containing 3; BMC: bone marrow-derived cell.

References

1. Masci, P.G.; Ganame, J.; Francone, M.; Desmet, W.; Lorenzoni, V.; Iacucci, I.; Barison, A.; Carbone, I.; Lombardi, M.; Agati, L.; et al. Relationship between location and size of myocardial infarction and their reciprocal influences on post-infarction left ventricular remodelling. *Eur. Heart J.* **2011**, *32*, 1640–1648. [CrossRef] [PubMed]
2. Reindl, M.; Reinstadler, S.J.; Tiller, C.; Feistritzer, H.-J.; Kofler, M.; Brix, A.; Mayr, A.; Klug, G.; Metzler, B. Prognosis-based definition of left ventricular remodeling after ST-elevation myocardial infarction. *Eur. Radiol.* **2019**, *29*, 2330–2339. [CrossRef] [PubMed]
3. Zhao, W.; Zhao, J.; Rong, J. Pharmacological Modulation of Cardiac Remodeling after Myocardial Infarction. *Oxidative Med. Cell. Longev.* **2020**, *2020*, 8815269. [CrossRef]
4. Hochman, J.S.; Bulkley, B.H. Expansion of acute myocardial infarction: An experimental study. *Circulation* **1982**, *65*, 1446–1450. [CrossRef] [PubMed]
5. Pfeffer, M.A.; Braunwald, E. Ventricular remodeling after myocardial infarction. Experimental observations and clinical implications. *Circulation* **1990**, *81*, 1161–1172. [CrossRef]
6. Cohn, J.N.; Ferrari, R.; Sharpe, N. Cardiac remodeling—Concepts and clinical implications: A consensus paper from an international forum on cardiac remodeling. Behalf of an International Forum on Cardiac Remodeling. *J. Am. Coll. Cardiol.* **2000**, *35*, 569–582. [CrossRef]
7. Fu, Z.; Jiao, Y.; Wang, J.; Zhang, Y.; Shen, M.; Reiter, R.J.; Xi, Q.; Chen, Y. Cardioprotective Role of Melatonin in Acute Myocardial Infarction. *Front. Physiol.* **2020**, *11*, 366. [CrossRef]
8. Heusch, G.; Gersh, B.J. The pathophysiology of acute myocardial infarction and strategies of protection beyond reperfusion: A continual challenge. *Eur. Heart J.* **2017**, *38*, 774–784. [CrossRef]
9. Curley, D.; Lavin Plaza, B.; Shah, A.M.; Botnar, R.M. Molecular imaging of cardiac remodelling after myocardial infarction. *Basic Res. Cardiol.* **2018**, *113*, 10. [CrossRef]
10. Kingma, J.G. Acute Myocardial Infarction: Perspectives on Physiopathology of Myocardial Injury and Protective Interventions. In *Cardiac Diseases-Novel Aspects of Cardiac Risk, Cardiorenal Pathology and Cardiac Interventions*; Gaze, D.C., Kibel, A., Eds.; IntechOpen: London, UK, 2021; ISBN 978-1-83968-162-2.
11. Ferrari, R.; Malagù, M.; Biscaglia, S.; Fucili, A.; Rizzo, P. Remodelling after an Infarct: Crosstalk between Life and Death. *Cardiology* **2016**, *135*, 68–76. [CrossRef]
12. Bhatt, A.S.; Ambrosy, A.P.; Velazquez, E.J. Adverse Remodeling and Reverse Remodeling After Myocardial Infarction. *Curr. Cardiol. Rep.* **2017**, *19*, 71. [CrossRef] [PubMed]
13. Sutton, M.G.S.J.; Sharpe, N. Left ventricular remodeling after myocardial infarction: Pathophysiology and therapy. *Circulation* **2000**, *101*, 2981–2988. [CrossRef] [PubMed]
14. Xie, M.; Burchfield, J.S.; Hill, J.A. Pathological ventricular remodeling: Mechanisms: Part 1 of 2. *Circulation* **2013**, *128*, 388. [CrossRef] [PubMed]
15. Gabriel-Costa, D. The pathophysiology of myocardial infarction-induced heart failure. *Pathophysiology* **2018**, *25*, 277–284. [CrossRef] [PubMed]
16. Berezin, A.E.; Berezin, A.A. Adverse Cardiac Remodelling after Acute Myocardial Infarction: Old and New Biomarkers. *Dis. Markers* **2020**, *2020*, 1215802. [CrossRef]
17. Bularga, A.; Hung, J.; Daghem, M.; Stewart, S.; Taggart, C.; Wereski, R.; Singh, T.; Meah, M.N.; Fujisawa, T.; Ferry, A.V.; et al. Coronary Artery and Cardiac Disease in Patients With Type 2 Myocardial Infarction: A Prospective Cohort Study. *Circulation* **2022**, *145*, 1188–1200. [CrossRef]
18. Yalta, K.; Yilmaz, M.B.; Yalta, T.; Palabiyik, O.; Taylan, G.; Zorkun, C. Late Versus Early Myocardial Remodeling After Acute Myocardial Infarction: A Comparative Review on Mechanistic Insights and Clinical Implications. *J. Cardiovasc. Pharmacol. Ther.* **2020**, *25*, 15–26. [CrossRef]
19. Tsuda, T. Clinical Assessment of Ventricular Wall Stress in Understanding Compensatory Hypertrophic Response and Maladaptive Ventricular Remodeling. *J. Cardiovasc. Dev. Dis.* **2021**, *8*, 122. [CrossRef]
20. Zouein, F.A.; Zgheib, C.; Liechty, K.W.; Booz, G.W. Post-infarct biomaterials, left ventricular remodeling, and heart failure: Is good good enough? *Congest. Heart Fail.* **2012**, *18*, 284–290. [CrossRef]

21. Weber, K.T.; Clark, W.A.; Janicki, J.S.; Shroff, S.G. Physiologic versus pathologic hypertrophy and the pressure-overloaded myocardium. *J. Cardiovasc. Pharmacol.* **1987**, *10*, S37–S50. [CrossRef]
22. Frantz, S.; Hundertmark, M.J.; Schulz-Menger, J.; Bengel, F.M.; Bauersachs, J. Left ventricular remodelling post-myocardial infarction: Pathophysiology, imaging, and novel therapies. *Eur. Heart J.* **2022**, ehac223. [CrossRef] [PubMed]
23. Zhang, Y.; Chan, A.K.Y.; Yu, C.-M.; Lam, W.W.M.; Yip, G.W.K.; Fung, W.-H.; So, N.M.C.; Wang, M.; Sanderson, J.E. Left ventricular systolic asynchrony after acute myocardial infarction in patients with narrow QRS complexes. *Am. Heart J.* **2005**, *149*, 497–503. [CrossRef] [PubMed]
24. Grossman, W.; Jones, D.; McLaurin, L.P. Wall stress and patterns of hypertrophy in the human left ventricle. *J. Clin. Investig.* **1975**, *56*, 56–64. [CrossRef] [PubMed]
25. Opie, L.H.; Commerford, P.J.; Gersh, B.J.; Pfeffer, M.A. Controversies in ventricular remodelling. *Lancet* **2006**, *367*, 356–367. [CrossRef]
26. Zhong, L.; Su, Y.; Yeo, S.-Y.; Tan, R.S.; Ghista, D.N.; Kassab, G. Left ventricular regional wall curvedness and wall stress in patients with ischemic dilated cardiomyopathy. *Am. J. Physiol. Circ. Physiol.* **2009**, *296*, H573–H584. [CrossRef]
27. Rosano, G.; Fini, M.; Caminiti, G.; Barbaro, G. Cardiac Metabolism in Myocardial Ischemia. *Curr. Pharm. Des.* **2008**, *14*, 2551–2562. [CrossRef]
28. Jiang, M.; Xie, X.; Cao, F.; Wang, Y. Mitochondrial Metabolism in Myocardial Remodeling and Mechanical Unloading: Implications for Ischemic Heart Disease. *Front. Cardiovasc. Med.* **2021**, *8*, 789267. [CrossRef]
29. Williams, B. Angiotensin II and the pathophysiology of cardiovascular remodeling. *Am. J. Cardiol.* **2001**, *87*, 10–17. [CrossRef]
30. Gajarsa, J.J.; Kloner, R.A. Left ventricular remodeling in the post-infarction heart: A review of cellular, molecular mechanisms, and therapeutic modalities. *Heart Fail. Rev.* **2011**, *16*, 13–21. [CrossRef]
31. Delcayre, C.; Silvestre, J.S.; Garnier, A.; Oubenaissa, A.; Cailmail, S.; Tatara, E.; Swynghedauw, B.; Robert, V. Cardiac aldos-terone production and ventricular remodeling. *Kidney Int.* **2000**, *57*, 1346–1351. [CrossRef]
32. Cohn, J.N.; Colucci, W. Cardiovascular Effects of Aldosterone and Post–Acute Myocardial Infarction Pathophysiology. *Am. J. Cardiol.* **2006**, *97*, 4–12. [CrossRef]
33. Mizuno, Y.; Yoshimura, M.; Yasue, H.; Sakamoto, T.; Ogawa, H.; Kugiyama, K.; Harada, E.; Nakayama, M.; Nakamura, S.; Ito, T.; et al. Aldosterone Production Is Activated in Failing Ventricle in Humans. *Circulation* **2001**, *103*, 72–77. [CrossRef] [PubMed]
34. Iraqi, W.; Rossignol, P.; Angioi, M.; Fay, R.; Nuée, J.; Ketelslegers, J.M.; Vincent, J.; Pitt, B.; Zannad, F. Extracellular cardiac matrix biomarkers in patients with acute myocardial infarction complicated by left ventricular dysfunction and heart failure: Insights from the Eplerenone Post-Acute Myocardial Infarction Heart Failure Efficacy and Survival Study (EPHESUS) study. *Circulation* **2009**, *119*, 2471–2479.
35. Amin, P.; Singh, M.; Singh, K. β-Adrenergic Receptor-Stimulated Cardiac Myocyte Apoptosis: Role of 1 Integrins. *J. Signal Transduct.* **2011**, *2011*, 179057. [CrossRef] [PubMed]
36. Zhang, J.; Wang, Y.-J.; Wang, X.; Xu, L.; Yang, X.-C.; Zhao, W.-S. PKC-Mediated Endothelin-1 Expression in Endothelial Cell Promotes Macrophage Activation in Atherogenesis. *Am. J. Hypertens.* **2019**, *32*, 880–889. [CrossRef] [PubMed]
37. Haryono, A.; Ramadhiani, R.; Ryanto, G.R.T.; Emoto, N. Endothelin and the Cardiovascular System: The Long Journey and Where We Are Going. *Biology* **2022**, *11*, 759. [CrossRef] [PubMed]
38. Olivier, A.; Girerd, N.; Michel, J.B.; Ketelslegers, J.M.; Fay, R.; Vincent, J.; Bramlage, P.; Pitt, B.; Zannad, F.; Rossignol, P.; et al. Combined baseline and one-month changes in big endothelin-1 and brain natriuretic peptide plasma concentrations predict clinical outcomes in patients with left ventricular dysfunction after acute myocardial infarction: Insights from the Eplerenone Post-Acute Myocardial Infarction Heart Failure Efficacy and Survival Study (EPHESUS) study. *Int. J. Cardiol.* **2017**, *241*, 344–350. [CrossRef]
39. Soeki, T.; Kishimoto, I.; Okumura, H.; Tokudome, T.; Horio, T.; Mori, K.; Kangawa, K. C-type natriuretic peptide, a novel antifibrotic and antihypertrophic agent, prevents cardiac remodeling after myocardial infarction. *J. Am. Coll. Cardiol.* **2005**, *45*, 608–616. [CrossRef]
40. Kasama, S.; Furuya, M.; Toyama, T.; Ichikawa, S.; Kurabayashi, M. Effect of atrial natriuretic peptide on left ventricular re-modelling in patients with acute myocardial infarction. *Eur. Heart J.* **2008**, *29*, 1485–1494. [CrossRef]
41. Chen, H.H.; Redfield, M.M.; Nordstrom, L.J.; Horton, D.P.; Burnett Jr, J.C. Subcutaneous administration of the cardiac hormone BNP in symptomatic human heart failure. *J. Card. Fail.* **2004**, *10*, 115–119. [CrossRef]
42. Wright, G.A.; Struthers, A.D. Natriuretic peptides as a prognostic marker and therapeutic target in heart failure. *Heart* **2006**, *92*, 149–151. [CrossRef]
43. Goetze, J.P.; Bruneau, B.G.; Ramos, H.R.; Ogawa, T.; de Bold, M.K.; de Bold, A.J. Cardiac natriuretic peptides. *Nat. Rev. Cardiol.* **2020**, *17*, 698–717. [CrossRef]
44. Chen, Y.; Burnett, J.C., Jr. Biochemistry, Therapeutics, and Biomarker Implications of Neprilysin in Cardiorenal Disease. *Clin. Chem.* **2017**, *63*, 108–115. [CrossRef] [PubMed]
45. Horio, T.; Nishikimi, T.; Yoshihara, F.; Matsuo, H.; Takishita, S.; Kangawa, K. Inhibitory regulation of hypertrophy by endogenous atrial natriuretic peptide in cultured cardiac myocytes. *Hypertension* **2000**, *35*, 19–24. [CrossRef]
46. Rienks, M.; Papageorgiou, A.P.; Frangogiannis, N.G.; Heymans, S. Myocardial extracellular matrix: An ever-changing and diverse entity. *Circ. Res.* **2014**, *114*, 872–888. [CrossRef]

47. Iyer, R.P.; de Castro Brás, L.E.; Jin, Y.F.; Lindsey, M.L. Translating Koch's postulates to identify matrix metalloproteinase roles in postmyocardial infarction remodeling: Cardiac metalloproteinase actions (CarMA) postulates. *Circ. Res.* **2014**, *114*, 860–871. [CrossRef]
48. Nielsen, S.H.; Mouton, A.J.; DeLeon-Pennell, K.Y.; Genovese, F.; Karsdal, M.; Lindsey, M.L. Understanding cardiac extra-cellular matrix remodeling to develop biomarkers of myocardial infarction outcomes. *Matrix Biol.* **2019**, *75*, 43–57. [CrossRef] [PubMed]
49. Jourdan-LeSaux, C.; Zhang, J.; Lindsey, M.L. Extracellular matrix roles during cardiac repair. *Life Sci.* **2010**, *87*, 391–400. [CrossRef]
50. van Amerongen, M.J.; Harmsen, M.C.; van Rooijen, N.; Petersen, A.H.; van Luyn, M.J. Macrophage depletion impairs wound healing and increases left ventricular remodeling after myocardial injury in mice. *Am. J. Pathol.* **2007**, *170*, 818–829. [CrossRef] [PubMed]
51. Van Amerongen, M.J.; Bou-Gharios, G.; Popa, E.; Van Ark, J.; Petersen, A.H.; Van Dam, G.M.; Van Luyn, M.J.; Harmsen, M.C. Bone marrow-derived myofibroblasts contribute functionally to scar formation after myocardial infarction. *J. Pathol.* **2008**, *214*, 377–386. [CrossRef] [PubMed]
52. Daskalopoulos, E.P.; Janssen, B.J.; Blankesteijn, W.M. Myofibroblasts in the Infarct Area: Concepts and Challenges. *Microsc. Microanal.* **2012**, *18*, 35–49. [CrossRef] [PubMed]
53. Mann, D.L.; Spinale, F.G. Activation of matrix metalloproteinases in the failing human heart: Breaking the tie that binds. *Circulation* **1998**, *98*, 1699–1702. [CrossRef] [PubMed]
54. Cleutjens, J.P.; Kandala, J.C.; Guarda, E.; Guntaka, R.V.; Weber, K.T. Regulation of collagen degradation in the rat myocardium after infarction. *J. Mol. Cell. Cardiol.* **1995**, *27*, 1281–1292. [CrossRef]
55. Shamhart, P.E.; Meszaros, J.G. Non-fibrillar collagens: Key mediators of post-infarction cardiac remodeling? *J. Mol. Cell. Cardiol.* **2010**, *48*, 530–537. [CrossRef]
56. Luther, D.J.; Thodeti, C.K.; Shamhart, P.E.; Adapala, R.K.; Hodnichak, C.; Weihrauch, D.; Bonaldo, P.; Chilian, W.M.; Meszaros, J.G. Absence of Type VI Collagen Paradoxically Improves Cardiac Function, Structure, and Remodeling After Myocardial Infarction. *Circ. Res.* **2012**, *110*, 851–856. [CrossRef]
57. Altara, R.; Manca, M.; Sabra, R.; Eid, A.A.; Booz, G.W.; Zouein, F.A. Temporal cardiac remodeling post-myocardial infarction: Dynamics and prognostic implications in personalized medicine. *Heart Fail. Rev.* **2016**, *21*, 25–47. [CrossRef]
58. Aimo, A.; Panichella, G.; Barison, A.; Maffei, S.; Cameli, M.; Coiro, S.; D'Ascenzi, F.; Di Mario, C.; Liga, R.; Marcucci, R.; et al. Sex-related differences in ventricular remodeling after myocardial infarction. *Int. J. Cardiol.* **2021**, *339*, 62–69. [CrossRef] [PubMed]
59. Kim, Y.; Kim, H.; Kim, S.Y.; Lee, H.K.; Kwon, H.J.; Kim, Y.G.; Lee, J.; Kim, H.M.; So, B.H. Automated heart-type fatty acid-binding protein assay for the early diagnosis of acute myocardial infarction. *Am. J. Clin. Pathol.* **2010**, *134*, 157–162. [CrossRef] [PubMed]
60. Dupuy, A.M.; Cristol, J.P.; Kuster, N.; Reynier, F.; Lefebvre, S.; Badiou, S.; Jreige, R.; Kailey, R.; Sebbane, M. Performances of the heart fatty acid protein assay for the rapid diagnosis of acute myocardial infarction in ED patients. *Am. J. Emerg. Med.* **2015**, *33*, 326–330. [CrossRef]
61. Matsumoto, S.; Nakatani, D.; Sakata, Y.; Suna, S.; Shimizu, M.; Usami, M.; Hara, M.; Sumitsuji, S.; Nanto, S.; Sasaki, T.; et al. Elevated serum heart-type fatty acid-binding protein in the convalescent stage predicts long-term outcome in patients sur-viving acute myocardial infarction. *Circ. J.* **2013**, *77*, 1026–1032. [CrossRef]
62. Manini, A.F.; Ilgen, J.; Noble, V.E.; Bamberg, F.; Koenig, W.; Bohan, J.S.; Hoffmann, U. Derivation and validation of a sensitive IMA cutpoint to predict cardiac events in patients with chest pain. *Emerg. Med. J.* **2009**, *26*, 791–796. [CrossRef] [PubMed]
63. Baker, J.O.; Tyther, R.; Liebetrau, C.; Clark, J.; Howarth, R.; Patterson, T.; Möllmann, H.; Nef, H.; Sicard, P.; Kailey, R.; et al. Cardiac myosin-binding protein C: A potential early biomarker of myocardial injury. *Basic Res. Cardiol.* **2015**, *110*, 23. [CrossRef] [PubMed]
64. Kaier, T.E.; Stengaard, C.; Marjot, J.; Sørensen, J.T.; Alaour, B.; Stavropoulou-Tatla, S.; Terkelsen, C.J.; Williams, L.; Thygesen, K.; Weber, E.; et al. Cardiac Myosin-Binding Protein C to Diagnose Acute Myocardial Infarction in the Pre-Hospital Setting. *J. Am. Heart Assoc.* **2019**, *8*, e013152. [CrossRef]
65. Nian, M.; Lee, P.; Khaper, N.; Liu, P. Inflammatory Cytokines and Postmyocardial Infarction Remodeling. *Circ. Res.* **2004**, *94*, 1543–1553. [CrossRef]
66. Gwechenberger, M.; Mendoza, L.H.; Youker, K.A.; Frangogiannis, N.G.; Smith, C.W.; Michael, L.H.; Entman, M.L. Cardiac myocytes produce interleukin-6 in culture and in viable border zone of reperfused infarctions. *Circulation* **1999**, *99*, 546–551. [CrossRef]
67. Pascual-Figal, D.A.; Bayes-Genis, A.; Asensio-Lopez, M.C.; Hernández-Vicente, A.; Garrido-Bravo, I.; Pastor-Perez, F.; Díez, J.; Ibáñez, B.; Lax, A. The Interleukin-1 Axis and Risk of Death in Patients With Acutely Decompensated Heart Failure. *J. Am. Coll. Cardiol.* **2019**, *73*, 1016–1025. [CrossRef] [PubMed]
68. Cao, Y.; Li, R.; Zhang, F.; Guo, Z.; Tuo, S.; Li, Y. Correlation between angiopoietin-like proteins in inflammatory mediators in peripheral blood and severity of coronary arterial lesion in patients with acute myocardial infarction. *Exp. Ther. Med.* **2019**, *17*, 3495–3500. [CrossRef] [PubMed]
69. Palojoki, E.; Saraste, A.; Eriksson, A.; Pulkki, K.; Kallajoki, M.; Voipio-Pulkki, L.-M.; Tikkanen, I. Cardiomyocyte apoptosis and ventricular remodeling after myocardial infarction in rats. *Am. J. Physiol. Circ. Physiol.* **2001**, *280*, H2726–H2731. [CrossRef]
70. Krown, K.A.; Page, M.T.; Nguyen, C.; Zechner, D.; Gutierrez, V.; Comstock, K.L.; Glembotski, C.C.; Quintana, P.J.; Sabbadini, R.A. Tumor necrosis factor alpha-induced apoptosis in cardiac myocytes. Involvement of the sphingolipid signaling cascade in cardiac cell death. *J. Clin. Investig.* **1996**, *98*, 2854–2865. [CrossRef] [PubMed]

71. Marino, R.; Magrini, L.; Orsini, F.; Russo, V.; Cardelli, P.; Salerno, G.; Hur, M.; Di Somma, S.; Great Network. Comparison Between Soluble ST2 and High-Sensitivity Troponin I in Predicting Short-Term Mortality for Patients Presenting to the Emergency Department with Chest Pain. *Ann. Lab. Med.* **2017**, *37*, 137–146. [CrossRef] [PubMed]
72. Sabatine, M.S.; Morrow, D.A.; Higgins, L.J.; MacGillivray, C.; Guo, W.; Bode, C.; Rifai, N.; Cannon, C.P.; Gerszten, R.E.; Lee, R.T. Complementary Roles for Biomarkers of Biomechanical Strain ST2 and N-Terminal Prohormone B-Type Natriuretic Peptide in Patients with ST-Elevation Myocardial Infarction. *Circulation* **2008**, *117*, 1936–1944. [CrossRef] [PubMed]
73. Bayes-Genis, A.; De Antonio, M.; Galán, A.; Sanz, H.; Urrutia, A.; Cabanes, R.; Cano, L.; González, B.; Diez-Quevedo, C.; Pascual, T.; et al. Combined use of high-sensitivity ST2 and NTproBNP to improve the prediction of death in heart failure. *Eur. J. Heart Fail.* **2012**, *14*, 32–38. [CrossRef] [PubMed]
74. Jenkins, W.S.; Roger, V.L.; Jaffe, A.S.; Weston, S.A.; AbouEzzeddine, O.F.; Jiang, R.; Manemann, S.M.; Enriquez-Sarano, M. Prognostic Value of Soluble ST2 After Myocardial Infarction: A Community Perspective. *Am. J. Med.* **2017**, *130*, 1112.e9–1112.e15. [CrossRef] [PubMed]
75. Weir, R.A.; Miller, A.M.; Murphy, G.E.; Clements, S.; Steedman, T.; Connell, J.M.; McInnes, I.B.; Dargie, H.J.; McMurray, J. Serum Soluble ST2: A Potential Novel Mediator in Left Ventricular and Infarct Remodeling After Acute Myocardial Infarction. *J. Am. Coll. Cardiol.* **2010**, *55*, 223–250. [CrossRef] [PubMed]
76. Ip, C.; Luk, K.S.; Yuen, V.L.C.; Chiang, L.; Chan, C.K.; Ho, K.; Gong, M.; Lee, T.T.L.; Leung, K.S.K.; Roever, L.; et al. Soluble suppression of tumorigenicity 2 (sST2) for predicting disease severity or mortality outcomes in cardiovascular diseases: A systematic review and meta-analysis. *IJC Heart Vasc.* **2021**, *37*, 100887. [CrossRef]
77. Wesseling, M.; de Poel, J.; de Jager, S. Growth differentiation factor 15 in adverse cardiac remodelling: From biomarker to causal player. *ESC Heart Fail.* **2020**, *7*, 1488–1501. [CrossRef]
78. Dominguez-Rodriguez, A.; Abreu-Gonzalez, P.; Avanzas, P. Relation of Growth-Differentiation Factor 15 to Left Ventricular Remodeling in ST-Segment Elevation Myocardial Infarction. *Am. J. Cardiol.* **2011**, *108*, 955–958. [CrossRef] [PubMed]
79. Rochette, L.; Maza, M.; Bichat, F.; Beer, J.C.; Chagué, F.; Cottin, Y.; Zeller, M.; Vergely-Vandriesse, C. Growth differentiation factor 15 as an integrative biomarker of heart failure in patients with acute myocardial infarction. *Arch. Cardiovasc. Dis.* **2019**, *11*, 45.
80. Hochholzer, W.; Morrow, D.A.; Giugliano, R.P. Novel biomarkers in cardiovascular disease: Update 2010. *Am. Heart J.* **2010**, *160*, 583–594. [CrossRef]
81. Malasky, B.R.; Alpert, J.S. Diagnosis of Myocardial Injury by Biochemical Markers: Problems and Promises. *Cardiol. Rev.* **2002**, *10*, 306–317. [CrossRef]
82. Aydin, S.; Ugur, K.; Aydin, S.; Sahin, İ.; Yardim, M. Biomarkers in acute myocardial infarction: Current perspectives. *Vasc. Health Risk Manag.* **2019**, *15*, 1–10. [CrossRef]
83. Teng, N.; Maghzal, G.J.; Talib, J.; Rashid, I.; Lau, A.K.; Stocker, R. The roles of myeloperoxidase in coronary artery disease and its potential implication in plaque rupture. *Redox Rep.* **2017**, *22*, 51–73. [CrossRef]
84. Dumic, J.; Dabelic, S.; Flögel, M. Galectin-3: An open-ended story. *Biochim. Et Biophys. Acta (BBA)-Gen. Subj.* **2006**, *1760*, 616–635. [CrossRef] [PubMed]
85. Yu, L.; Ruifrok, W.P.; Meissner, M.; Bos, E.M.; van Goor, H.; Sanjabi, B.; van der Harst, P.; Pitt, B.; Goldstein, I.J.; Koerts, J.A.; et al. Genetic and Pharmacological Inhibition of Galectin-3 Prevents Cardiac Remodeling by Interfering with Myocardial Fibrogenesis. *Circ. Heart Fail.* **2013**, *6*, 107–117. [CrossRef] [PubMed]
86. González, G.E.; Cassaglia, P.; Truant, S.N.; Fernández, M.M.; Wilensky, L.; Volberg, V.; Malchiodi, E.L.; Morales, C.; Gelpi, R.J. Galectin-3 is essential for early wound healing and ventricular remodeling after myocardial infarction in mice. *Int. J. Cardiol.* **2014**, *176*, 1423–1425. [CrossRef] [PubMed]
87. Weir, R.A.; Petrie, C.J.; Murphy, C.A.; Clements, S.; Steedman, T.; Miller, A.M.; McInnes, I.B.; Squire, I.B.; Ng, L.L.; Dargie, H.J.; et al. Galectin-3 and Cardiac Function in Survivors of Acute Myocardial Infarction. *Circ. Heart Fail.* **2013**, *6*, 492–498. [CrossRef] [PubMed]
88. van der Velde, A.R.; Lexis, C.P.H.; Meijers, W.C.; van der Horst, I.C.; Lipsic, E.; Dokter, M.M.; van Veldhuisen, D.J.; van der Harst, P.; de Boer, R.A. Galectin-3 Predicts Left Ventricular Ejection Fraction After Myocardial Infarction. *Circulation* **2018**, *130*, A18665.
89. Meijers, W.C.; van der Velde, A.R.; Figal, D.A.P.; de Boer, R.A. Galectin-3 and post-myocardial infarction cardiac remodeling. *Eur. J. Pharmacol.* **2015**, *763*, 115–121. [CrossRef]
90. Lindsey, M.L.; Iyer, R.P.; Jung, M.; DeLeon-Pennell, K.Y.; Ma, Y. Matrix metalloproteinases as input and output signals for post-myocardial infarction remodeling. *J. Mol. Cell. Cardiol.* **2016**, *91*, 134–140. [CrossRef]
91. Volpe, M.; Carnovali, M.; Mastromarino, V. The natriuretic peptides system in the pathophysiology of heart failure: From molecular basis to treatment. *Clin. Sci.* **2016**, *130*, 57–77. [CrossRef]
92. Drewniak, W.; Szybka, W.; Bielecki, D.; Malinowski, M.; Kotlarska, J.; Krol-Jaskulska, A.; Popielarz-Grygalewicz, A.; Kon-wicka, A.; Dąbrowski, M. Prognostic Significance of NT-proBNP Levels in Patients over 65 Presenting Acute Myocardial Infarction Treated Invasively or Conservatively. *Biomed Res. Int.* **2015**, *2015*, 782026. [CrossRef]
93. Collet, J.-P.; Thiele, H.; Barbato, E.; Barthélémy, O.; Bauersachs, J.; Bhatt, D.L.; Dendale, P.; Dorobantu, M.; Edvardsen, T.; Folliguet, T.; et al. 2020 ESC Guidelines for the management of acute coronary syndromes in patients presenting without persistent ST-segment elevation. *Eur. Heart J.* **2021**, *42*, 1289–1367. [CrossRef]
94. Morgenthaler, N.G.; Struck, J.; Alonso, C.; Bergmann, A. Assay for the Measurement of Copeptin, a Stable Peptide Derived from the Precursor of Vasopressin. *Clin. Chem.* **2006**, *52*, 112–119. [CrossRef]

95. Dobsa, L.; Edozien, K.C. Copeptin and its potential role in diagnosis and prognosis of various diseases. *Biochem. Med.* **2013**, *23*, 172–190. [CrossRef] [PubMed]
96. Jeong, J.H.; Seo, Y.H.; Ahn, J.Y.; Kim, K.H.; Seo, J.Y.; Chun, K.Y.; Lim, Y.S.; Park, P.W. Performance of Copeptin for Early Diagnosis of Acute Myocardial Infarction in an Emergency Department Setting. *Ann. Lab. Med.* **2020**, *40*, 7–14. [CrossRef] [PubMed]
97. Czajkowska, K.; Zbroch, E.; Bielach-Bazyluk, A.; Mitrosz, K.; Bujno, E.; Kakareko, K.; Rydzewska-Rosolowska, A.; Hryszko, T. Mid-Regional Proadrenomedullin as a New Biomarker of Kidney and Cardiovascular Diseases—Is It the Future? *J. Clin. Med.* **2021**, *10*, 524. [CrossRef] [PubMed]
98. Yoshitomi, Y.; Nishikimi, T.; Kojima, S.; Kuramochi, M.; Takishita, S.; Matsuoka, H.; Miyata, A.; Matsuo, H.; Kangawa, K. Plasma Levels of Adrenomedullin in Patients with Acute Myocardial Infarction. *Clin. Sci.* **1998**, *94*, 135–139. [CrossRef] [PubMed]
99. Khan, S.Q.; O'Brien, R.J.; Struck, J.; Quinn, P.; Morgenthaler, N.; Squire, I.; Davies, J.; Bergmann, A.; Ng, L.L. Prognostic value of midregional pro-adrenomedullin in patients with acute myocardial infarction: The LAMP (Leicester Acute Myocardial Infarction Peptide) study. *J. Am. Coll. Cardiol.* **2007**, *49*, 1525–1532. [CrossRef]
100. Arrigo, M.; Parenica, J.; Ganovska, E.; Pavlusova, M.; Mebazaa, A. Plasma bio-adrenomedullin is a marker of acute heart failure severity in patients with acute coronary syndrome. *IJC Heart Vasc.* **2019**, *22*, 174–176. [CrossRef]
101. Walter, T.; Brueckmann, M.; Lang, S.; Sauer, T.; Fiedler, E.; Papassotiriou, J.; Behnes, M.; Elmas, E.; Borggrefe, M.; Bertsch, T. Comparison of long-term prognostic value of N-terminal-proBNP and midregional-pro-adrenomedullin in patients with acute myocardial infarction. *Clin. Lab.* **2010**, *56*, 303–309.
102. Miyao, Y.; Nishikimi, T.; Goto, Y.; Miyazaki, S.; Daikoku, S.; Morii, I.; Matsumoto, T.; Takishita, S.; Miyata, A.; Matsuo, H.; et al. Increased plasma adrenomedullin levels in patients with acute myocardial infarction in proportion to the clinical severity. *Heart* **1998**, *79*, 39–44. [CrossRef] [PubMed]
103. Falkentoft, A.C.; Rørth, R.; Iversen, K.; Høfsten, D.E.; Kelbæk, H.; Holmvang, L.; Frydland, M.; Schoos, M.M.; Helqvist, S.; Axelsson, A.; et al. MR-proADM as a Prognostic Marker in Patients With ST-Segment-Elevation Myocardial Infarction-DANAMI-3 (a Danish Study of Optimal Acute Treatment of Patients With STEMI) Substudy. *J. Am. Heart Assoc.* **2018**, *7*, e008123. [CrossRef] [PubMed]
104. Bartel, D.P. MicroRNAs: Genomics, biogenesis, mechanism, and function. *Cell* **2004**, *116*, 281–297. [CrossRef]
105. Kloosterman, W.P.; Plasterk, R.H. The Diverse Functions of MicroRNAs in Animal Development and Disease. *Dev. Cell* **2006**, *11*, 441–450. [CrossRef]
106. Shah, P.; Bristow, M.R.; Port, J.D. MicroRNAs in Heart Failure, Cardiac Transplantation, and Myocardial Recovery: Biomarkers with Therapeutic Potential. *Curr. Heart Fail. Rep.* **2017**, *14*, 454–464. [CrossRef] [PubMed]
107. Boulet, J.; Mehra, M.R. Left Ventricular Reverse Remodeling in Heart Failure: Remission to Recovery. *Struct. Heart* **2021**, *5*, 466–481. [CrossRef]
108. McDonagh, T.A.; Metra, M.; Adamo, M.; Gardner, R.S.; Baumbach, A.; Böhm, M.; Burri, H.; Butler, J.; Čelutkienė, J.; Chioncel, O.; et al. 2021 ESC Guidelines for the diagnosis and treatment of acute and chronic heart failure: Developed by the Task Force for the diagnosis and treatment of acute and chronic heart failure of the European Society of Cardiology (ESC) With the special contribution of the Heart Failure Association (HFA) of the ESC. *Eur. Heart J.* **2021**, *42*, 3599–3726. [CrossRef]
109. Bulluck, H.; Carberry, J.; Carrick, D.; McEntegart, M.; Petrie, M.C.; Eteiba, H.; Hood, S.; Watkins, S.; Lindsay, M.; Mahrous, A.; et al. Redefining Adverse and Reverse Left Ventricular Remodeling by Cardiovascular Magnetic Resonance Following ST-Segment–Elevation Myocardial Infarction and Their Implications on Long-Term Prognosis. *Circ. Cardiovasc. Imaging* **2020**, *13*, e009937. [CrossRef]
110. Cannata, A.; Manca, P.; Nuzzi, V.; Gregorio, C.; Artico, J.; Gentile, P.; Loco, C.P.; Ramani, F.; Barbati, G.; Merlo, M.; et al. Sex-Specific Prognostic Implications in Dilated Cardiomyopathy after Left Ventricular Reverse Remodeling. *J. Clin. Med.* **2020**, *9*, 2426. [CrossRef]
111. Safdar, O.; Ervin, A.; Cozzi, S.; Danelich, I.; Shah, M.; Vishnevsky, A.; Alvarez, R.; Pirlamarla, P. Impact of Sacubitril/Valsartan in Cardiac Reverse Remodeling in Ischemic vs. Nonischemic Cardiomyopathy. *J. Heart Lung Transplant.* **2020**, *39*, S239–S240. [CrossRef]
112. Díez-Villanueva, P.; Vicent, L.; de la Cuerda, F.; Esteban-Fernández, A.; Gómez-Bueno, M.; de Juan-Bagudá, J.; Iniesta, A.M.; Ayesta, A.; Rojas-González, A.; Bocer-Freire, R.; et al. Left ventricular ejection fraction recovery in patients with heart failure and reduced ejection fraction treated with sacubitril/valsartan. *Cardiology* **2020**, *145*, 275–282. [CrossRef]
113. Peng, X.; Zhou, J.; Wu, X.-S. New Strategies for Myocardial Infarction Treatment. *J. Cardiol. Ther.* **2017**, *4*, 664–670. [CrossRef]
114. Aylward, P. Acute myocardial infarction: Early treatment. *Aust. Prescr.* **1996**, *19*, 52–54. [CrossRef]
115. McCartney, P.J.; Berry, C. Redefining successful primary PCI. *Eur. Heart J. Cardiovasc. Imaging* **2019**, *20*, 133–135. [CrossRef] [PubMed]
116. Grabka, M.; Kocierz-Woźnowska, M.; Wybraniec, M.; Turski, M.; Wita, M.; Wita, K.; Mizia-Stec, K. Left ventricular reverse remodeling in patients with anterior wall ST-segment elevation acute myocardial infarction treated with primary percutaneous coronary intervention. *Postepy Kardiol. Interwencyjnej* **2018**, *14*, 373–382. [CrossRef]
117. Cokkinos, D.V.; Belogiannes, C. Left Ventricular Remodelling: A Problem in Search of Solutions. *Eur. Cardiol. Rev.* **2016**, *11*, 29–35. [CrossRef]
118. Solhpour, A.; Yusuf, S.W. Fibrinolytic therapy in patients with ST-elevation myocardial infarction. *Expert Rev. Cardiovasc. Ther.* **2014**, *12*, 201–215. [CrossRef] [PubMed]

119. Huttin, O.; Coiro, S.; Selton-Suty, C.; Juillière, Y.; Donal, E.; Magne, J.; Sadoul, N.; Zannad, F.; Rossignol, P.; Girerd, N. Pre-diction of Left Ventricular Remodeling after a Myocardial Infarction: Role of Myocardial Deformation: A Systematic Review and Meta-Analysis. *PLoS ONE* **2016**, *11*, e0168349. [CrossRef] [PubMed]
120. Liu, S.; Meng, X.; Li, G.; Gokulnath, P.; Wang, J.; Xiao, J. Exercise Training after Myocardial Infarction Attenuates Dysfunc-tional Ventricular Remodeling and Promotes Cardiac Recovery. *Rev. Cardiovasc. Med.* **2022**, *23*, 148. [CrossRef]
121. Al Shahi, H.; Kadoguchi, T.; Shimada, K.; Fukao, K.; Matsushita, S.; Aikawa, T.; Ouchi, S.; Shiozawa, T.; Takahashi, S.; Sato-Okabayashi, Y.; et al. Voluntary exercise and cardiac remodeling in a myocardial infarction model. *Open Med.* **2020**, *15*, 545–555. [CrossRef]
122. Zhang, Y.M.; Lu, Y.; Tang, Y.; Yang, D.; Wu, H.F.; Bian, Z.P.; Xu, J.D.; Gu, C.R.; Wang, L.S.; Chen, X.J. The effects of different initiation time of exercise training on left ventricular remodeling and cardiopulmonary rehabilitation in patients with left ventricular dysfunction after myocardial infarction. *Disabil. Rehabil.* **2016**, *38*, 268–276. [CrossRef] [PubMed]
123. Pelliccia, A.; Sharma, S.; Gati, S.; Bäck, M.; Börjesson, M.; Caselli, S.; Collet, J.-P.; Corrado, D.; Drezner, J.A.; Halle, M.; et al. 2020 ESC Guidelines on sports cardiology and exercise in patients with cardiovascular disease. *Eur. Heart J.* **2021**, *42*, 17–96. [CrossRef] [PubMed]
124. Moreira, J.I. Beta-blocker therapy after myocardial infarction or acute coronary syndrome: What we don't know. *Rev. Port. Cardiol. (Engl. Ed.)* **2021**, *40*, 291–292. [CrossRef]
125. Noble, S.; Roffi, M. Routine beta-blocker administration following acute myocardial infarction: Why still an unsolved issue? *J. Thorac. Dis.* **2017**, *9*, 4191–4194. [CrossRef]
126. Bahit, M.C.; Kochar, A.; Granger, C.B. Post-Myocardial Infarction Heart Failure. *JACC Heart Fail.* **2018**, *6*, 179–186. [CrossRef]
127. Hwang, D.; Lee, J.M.; Kim, H.K.; Choi, K.H.; Rhee, T.-M.; Park, J.; Park, T.K.; Yang, J.H.; Song, Y.B.; Choi, J.-H.; et al. Prognostic Impact of β-Blocker Dose After Acute Myocardial Infarction. *Circ. J.* **2019**, *83*, 410–417. [CrossRef] [PubMed]
128. Sutton, M.S.J.; Ferrari, V.A. Prevention of Left Ventricular Remodeling after Myocardial Infarction. *Curr. Treat. Options Cardiovasc. Med.* **2002**, *4*, 97–108. [CrossRef]
129. O'Connell, J.L.; Borges, G.C.; de Almeida, R.P.; Lisboa da Silva, R.M.F.; Roerver-Borges, A.S.; Resende, E.S.; Penha-Silva, N.; Roever, L.; Tse, G.; Liu, T.; et al. Beta blockers: Effects Beyond Heart Rate Control. *Int. J. Clin. Cardiol. Res.* **2018**, *2*, 53–57.
130. Doughty, R.N.; Whalley, G.A.; Walsh, H.A.; Gamble, G.D.; López-Sendón, J.; Sharpe, N.; CAPRICORN Echo Substudy Investiga-tors. Effects of carvedilol on left ventricular remodeling after acute myocardial infarction: The CAPRICORN Echo Substudy. *Circulation* **2004**, *109*, 201–206. [CrossRef]
131. Lee, S.H.; Yoon, S.B.; Cho, J.R.; Choi, S.; Jung, J.H.; Lee, N. The effects of different beta-blockers on left-ventricular volume and function after primary coronary stenting in acute myocardial infarction. *Angiology* **2008**, *59*, 676–681. [CrossRef]
132. Srinivasan, A.V. Propranolol: A 50-Year Historical Perspective. *Ann. Indian Acad. Neurol.* **2019**, *22*, 21–26. [CrossRef]
133. Park, H.; Kim, H.K.; Jeong, M.H.; Cho, J.Y.; Lee, K.H.; Sim, D.S.; Yoon, N.S.; Yoon, H.J.; Hong, Y.J.; Kim, K.H.; et al. Clinical impacts of inhibition of renin-angiotensin system in patients with acute ST-segment elevation myocardial infarction who underwent successful late percutaneous coronary intervention. *J. Cardiol.* **2017**, *69*, 216–221. [CrossRef]
134. Park, K.; Kim, Y.-D.; Kim, K.-S.; Lee, S.-H.; Park, T.-H.; Lee, S.-G.; Kim, B.-S.; Hur, S.-H.; Yang, T.-H.; Oh, J.-H.; et al. The impact of a dose of the angiotensin receptor blocker valsartan on post-myocardial infarction ventricular remodelling. *ESC Heart Fail.* **2018**, *5*, 354–363. [CrossRef] [PubMed]
135. Reed, G.W.; Rossi, J.E.; Cannon, C.P. Acute myocardial infarction. *Lancet* **2017**, *389*, 197–210. [CrossRef]
136. Chua, D.; Ignaszewski, A.; Schwenger, E. Angiotensin-converting enzyme inhibitors: An ACE in the hole for everyone? *BC Med. J.* **2011**, *53*, 220–223.
137. Kim, K.-H.; Choi, B.G.; Rha, S.-W.; Choi, C.U.; Jeong, M.-H.; Other KAMIR-NIH investigators. Impact of renin angiotensin system inhibitor on 3-year clinical outcomes in acute myocardial infarction patients with preserved left ventricular systolic function: A prospective cohort study from Korea Acute Myocardial Infarction Registry (KAMIR). *BMC Cardiovasc. Disord.* **2021**, *21*, 1–13. [CrossRef]
138. Ibanez, B.; James, S.; Agewall, S.; Antunes, M.J.; Bucciarelli-Ducci, C.; Bueno, H.; Caforio, A.; Crea, F.; Goudevenos, J.A.; Halvorsen, S.; et al. 2017 ESC Guidelines for the management of acute myocardial infarction in patients presenting with ST-segment elevation: The Task Force for the management of acute myocardial infarction in patients presenting with ST-segment elevation of the European Society of Cardiology (ESC). *Eur. Heart J.* **2018**, *39*, 119–177.
139. Ko, D.; Azizi, P.; Koh, M.; Chong, A.; Austin, P.; Stukel, T.; Jackevicius, C. Comparative effectiveness of ACE inhibitors and angiotensin receptor blockers in patients with prior myocardial infarction. *Open Heart* **2019**, *6*, e001010. [CrossRef] [PubMed]
140. Winkelmayer, W.C.; Bucsics, A.E.; Schautzer, A.; Wieninger, P.; Pogantsch, M.; Pharmacoeconomics Advisory Council of the Austrian Sickness Funds. Use of recommended medications after myocardial infarction in Austria. *Eur. J. Epidemiol.* **2008**, *23*, 153–162. [CrossRef] [PubMed]
141. Rincon-Choles, H. ACE inhibitor and ARB therapy: Practical recommendations. *Clevel. Clin. J. Med.* **2019**, *86*, 608–611. [CrossRef] [PubMed]
142. Solomon, S.D.; Skali, H.; Anavekar, N.S.; Bourgoun, M.; Barvik, S.; Ghali, J.K.; Warnica, J.W.; Khrakovskaya, M.; Arnold, J.M.O.; Schwartz, Y.; et al. Changes in Ventricular Size and Function in Patients Treated With Valsartan, Captopril, or Both After Myocardial Infarction. *Circulation* **2005**, *111*, 3411–3419. [CrossRef]
143. Gulec, S. Valsartan after myocardial infarction. *Anatol. J. Cardiol.* **2014**, *14*, 9–13. [CrossRef]

144. Zwadlo, C.; Bauersachs, J. Mineralocorticoid receptor antagonists for therapy of coronary artery disease and related compli-cations. *Curr. Opin. Pharmacol.* **2013**, *13*, 280–286. [CrossRef] [PubMed]
145. Bossard, M.; Binbraik, Y.; Beygui, F.; Pitt, B.; Zannad, F.; Montalescot, G.; Jolly, S.S. Mineralocorticoid receptor antagonists in patients with acute myocardial infarction—A systematic review and meta-analysis of randomized trials. *Am. Heart J.* **2018**, *195*, 60–69. [CrossRef] [PubMed]
146. Montalescot, G.; Pitt, B.; Lopez de Sa, E.; Hamm, C.W.; Flather, M.; Verheugt, F.; Shi, H.; Turgonyi, E.; Orri, M.; Vincent, J.; et al. Early eplerenone treatment in patients with acute ST-elevation myocardial infarction without heart failure: The Random-ized Double-Blind Reminder Study. *Eur. Heart J.* **2014**, *35*, 2295–2302. [CrossRef] [PubMed]
147. Beygui, F.; Cayla, G.; Roule, V.; Roubille, F.; Delarche, N.; Silvain, J.; Van Belle, E.; Belle, L.; Galinier, M.; Motreff, P.; et al. Early Aldosterone Blockade in Acute Myocardial Infarction: The ALBATROSS Randomized Clinical Trial. *J. Am. Coll. Cardiol.* **2016**, *67*, 1917–1927. [CrossRef] [PubMed]
148. Zhang, L.; Yan, K.; Zhao, H.; Shou, Y.; Chen, T.; Chen, J. Therapeutic effects and safety of early use of sacubitril/valsartan after acute myocardial infarction: A systematic review and meta-analysis. *Ann. Palliat. Med.* **2022**, *11*, 1017–1027. [CrossRef]
149. Jering, K.S.; Claggett, B.; Pfeffer, M.A.; Granger, C.; Køber, L.; Lewis, E.F.; Maggioni, A.P.; Mann, D.; McMurray, J.J.V.; Rouleau, J.L.; et al. Prospective ARNI vs. ACE inhibitor trial to DetermIne Superiority in reducing heart failure Events after Myocardial Infarction (PARADISE-MI): Design and baseline characteristics. *Eur. J. Heart Fail.* **2021**, *23*, 1040–1048. [CrossRef]
150. Liu, S.; Yin, B.; Wu, B.; Fan, Z. Protective effect of sacubitril/valsartan in patients with acute myocardial infarction: A meta-analysis. *Exp. Ther. Med.* **2022**, *23*, 1–9. [CrossRef]
151. Mcmurray, J.J.V.; Packer, M.; Desai, A.S.; Gong, J.; Lefkowitz, M.P.; Rizkala, A.R.; Rouleau, J.L.; Shi, V.C.; Solomon, S.D.; Swedberg, K.; et al. Angiotensin–Neprilysin Inhibition versus Enalapril in Heart Failure. *N. Engl. J. Med.* **2014**, *371*, 993–1004. [CrossRef] [PubMed]
152. Pfeffer, M.A.; Claggett, B.; Lewis, E.F.; Granger, C.B.; Køber, L.; Maggioni, A.P.; Mann, D.L.; McMurray, J.J.; Rouleau, J.-L.; Solomon, S.D.; et al. Angiotensin Receptor–Neprilysin Inhibition in Acute Myocardial Infarction. *N. Engl. J. Med.* **2021**, *385*, 1845–1855. [CrossRef] [PubMed]
153. Gatto, L. Does sacubitril/valsartan work in acute myocardial infarction? The PARADISE-AMI study. *Eur. Heart J. Suppl.* **2021**, *23*, E87–E90. [CrossRef]
154. Zinman, B.; Lachin, J.M.; Inzucchi, S.E. Empagliflozin, Cardiovascular Outcomes, and Mortality in Type 2 Diabetes. *NEJM* **2016**, *374*, 1094. [CrossRef] [PubMed]
155. Neuen, B.L.; Ohkuma, T.; Neal, B.; Matthews, D.R.; de Zeeuw, D.; Mahaffey, K.W.; Fulcher, G.; Desai, M.; Li, Q.; Deng, H.; et al. Cardiovascular and Renal Outcomes With Canagliflozin According to Baseline Kidney Function. *Circulation* **2018**, *138*, 1537–1550. [CrossRef]
156. Wiviott, S.D.; Raz, I.; Bonaca, M.P.; Mosenzon, O.; Kato, E.T.; Cahn, A.; Silverman, M.G.; Zelniker, T.A.; Kuder, J.F.; Murphy, S.A.; et al. Dapagliflozin and Cardiovascular Outcomes in Type 2 Diabetes. *N. Engl. J. Med.* **2019**, *380*, 347–357. [CrossRef] [PubMed]
157. McGuire, D.K.; Zinman, B.; Inzucchi, S.E.; Anker, S.D.; Wanner, C.; Kaspers, S.; George, J.T.; Elsasser, U.; Woerle, H.J.; Lund, S.S.; et al. P5334 Effect of empagliflozin on cardiovascular events including recurrent events in the EMPA-REG OUT-COME trial. *Eur. Heart J.* **2018**, *39* (Suppl. S1), ehy566-P5334. [CrossRef]
158. Andreadou, I.; Bell, R.M.; Bøtker, H.E.; Zuurbier, C.J. SGLT2 inhibitors reduce infarct size in reperfused ischemic heart and improve cardiac function during ischemic episodes in preclinical models. *Biochim. Et Biophys. Acta (BBA)-Mol. Basis Dis.* **2020**, *1866*, 165770. [CrossRef]
159. Lee, S.Y.; Lee, T.W.; Park, G.T.; Kim, J.H.; Lee, H.C.; Han, J.H.; Yoon, A.; Yoon, D.; Kim, S.; Jung, S.M.; et al. Sodium/glucose Co-Transporter 2 Inhibitor, Empagliflozin, Alleviated Transient Expression of SGLT2 after Myocardial Infarction. *Korean Circ. J.* **2021**, *51*, 251–262. [CrossRef]
160. Liu, Y.; Wu, M.; Xu, J.; Xu, B.; Kang, L. Empagliflozin prevents from early cardiac injury post myocardial infarction in non-diabetic mice. *Eur. J. Pharm. Sci.* **2021**, *161*, 105788. [CrossRef]
161. Lim, V.G.; Bell, R.M.; Arjun, S.; Kolatsi-Joannou, M.; Long, D.A.; Yellon, D.M. SGLT2 Inhibitor, Canagliflozin, Attenuates Myocardial Infarction in the Diabetic and Nondiabetic Heart. *JACC Basic Transl. Sci.* **2019**, *4*, 15–26. [CrossRef]
162. Santos-Gallego, C.G.; Requena-Ibanez, J.A.; Antonio, R.S.; Ishikawa, K.; Watanabe, S.; Picatoste, B.; Flores, E.; Garcia-Ropero, A.; Sanz, J.; Hajjar, R.J.; et al. Empagliflozin Ameliorates Adverse Left Ventricular Remodeling in Nondiabetic Heart Failure by Enhancing Myocardial Energetics. *J. Am. Coll. Cardiol.* **2019**, *73*, 1931–1944. [CrossRef] [PubMed]
163. Griffin, M.; Rao, V.S.; Ivey-Miranda, J.; Fleming, J.; Mahoney, D.; Maulion, C.; Suda, N.; Siwakoti, K.; Ahmad, T.; Jacoby, D.; et al. Empagliflozin in Heart Failure: Diuretic and Cardiorenal Effects. *Circulation* **2020**, *142*, 1028–1039. [CrossRef]
164. Shimizu, W.; Kubota, Y.; Hoshika, Y.; Mozawa, K.; Tara, S.; Tokita, Y.; Yodogawa, K.; Iwasaki, Y.-K.; Yamamoto, T.; Takano, H.; et al. Effects of empagliflozin versus placebo on cardiac sympathetic activity in acute myocardial infarction patients with type 2 diabetes mellitus: The EMBODY trial. *Cardiovasc. Diabetol.* **2020**, *19*, 1–12. [CrossRef] [PubMed]
165. Batzias, K.; Antonopoulos, A.S.; Oikonomou, E.; Siasos, G.; Bletsa, E.; Stampouloglou, P.K.; Mistakidi, C.V.; Noutsou, M.; Katsiki, N.; Karopoulos, P.; et al. Effects of Newer Antidiabetic Drugs on Endothelial Function and Arterial Stiffness: A Sys-tematic Review and Meta-Analysis. *J. Diabetes Res.* **2018**, *2018*, 1232583. [CrossRef] [PubMed]

166. Oshima, H.; Miki, T.; Kuno, A.; Mizuno, M.; Sato, T.; Tanno, M.; Yano, T.; Nakata, K.; Kimura, Y.; Abe, K.; et al. Empagliflozin, an SGLT2 Inhibitor, Reduced the Mortality Rate after Acute Myocardial Infarction with Modification of Cardiac Metabolomes and Antioxidants in Diabetic Rats. *J. Pharmacol. Exp. Ther.* **2019**, *368*, 524–534. [CrossRef] [PubMed]
167. Udell, J.A.; Jones, W.S.; Petrie, M.C.; Harrington, J.; Anker, S.D.; Bhatt, D.L.; Hernandez, A.F.; Butler, J. Sodium Glucose Cotransporter-2 Inhibition for Acute Myocardial Infarction: JACC Review Topic of the Week. *J. Am. Coll. Cardiol.* **2022**, *79*, 2058–2068. [CrossRef]
168. Bauersachs, J.; Galuppo, P.; Fraccarollo, D.; Christ, M.; Ertl, G. Improvement of left ventricular remodeling and function by hydroxymethylglutaryl coenzyme a reductase inhibition with cerivastatin in rats with heart failure after myocardial infarction. *Circulation* **2001**, *104*, 982–985. [CrossRef]
169. Nahrendorf, M.; Hu, K.; Hiller, K.-H.; Galuppo, P.; Fraccarollo, D.; Schweizer, G.; Haase, A.; Ertl, G.; Bauer, W.R.; Bauersachs, J. Impact of hydroxymethylglutaryl coenzyme a reductase inhibition on left ventricular remodeling after myocardial infarction: An experimental serial cardiac magnetic resonance imaging study. *J. Am. Coll. Cardiol.* **2002**, *40*, 1695–1700. [CrossRef]
170. Toso, A.; Leoncini, M.; De Servi, S. Statins and myocardial infarction: From secondary 'prevention' to early 'treatment'. *J. Cardiovasc. Med.* **2019**, *20*, 220–222. [CrossRef]
171. Reichert, K.; Pereira do Carmo, H.R.; Galluce Torina, A.; Diógenes de Carvalho, D.; Carvalho Sposito, A.; de Souza Vilarinho, K.A.; da Mota Silveira-Filho, L.; Martins de Oliveira, P.P.; Petrucci, O. Atorvastatin Improves Ventricular Remodeling after Myocardial Infarction by Interfering with Collagen Metabolism. *PLoS ONE* **2016**, *11*, e0166845. [CrossRef]
172. Duncan, S.E.; Gao, S.; Sarhene, M.; Coffie, J.W.; Linhua, D.; Bao, X.; Jing, Z.; Li, S.; Guo, R.; Su, J.; et al. Macrophage Activities in Myocardial Infarction and Heart Failure. *Cardiol. Res. Pract.* **2020**, *2020*, 4375127. [CrossRef] [PubMed]
173. Mouton, A.J.; Rivera, O.J.; Lindsey, M.L. Myocardial infarction remodeling that progresses to heart failure: A signaling misunderstanding. *Am. J. Physiol. Circ. Physiol.* **2018**, *315*, H71–H79. [CrossRef] [PubMed]
174. Sager, H.B.; Heidt, T.; Hulsmans, M.; Dutta, P.; Courties, G.; Sebas, M.; Wojtkiewicz, G.R.; Tricot, B.; Iwamoto, Y.; Sun, Y.; et al. Targeting Interleukin-1β Reduces Leukocyte Production After Acute Myocardial Infarction. *Circulation* **2015**, *132*, 1880–1890. [CrossRef] [PubMed]
175. Ridker, P.M.; Everett, B.M.; Thuren, T.; MacFadyen, J.G.; Chang, W.H.; Ballantyne, C.; Fonseca, F.; Nicolau, J.; Koenig, W.; Anker, S.D.; et al. Antiinflammatory Therapy with Canakinumab for Atherosclerotic Disease. *N. Engl. J. Med.* **2017**, *377*, 1119–1131. [CrossRef] [PubMed]
176. Marchetti, C.; Toldo, S.; Chojnacki, J.; Mezzaroma, E.; Liu, K.; Salloum, F.N.; Nordio, A.; Carbone, S.; Mauro, A.G.; Das, A.; et al. Pharmacologic Inhibition of the NLRP3 Inflammasome Preserves Cardiac Function After Ischemic and Nonischemic Injury in the Mouse. *J. Cardiovasc. Pharmacol.* **2015**, *66*, 1–8. [CrossRef] [PubMed]
177. Mauro, A.G.; Bonaventura, A.; Mezzaroma, E.; Quader, M.; Toldo, S. NLRP3 Inflammasome in Acute Myocardial Infarction. *J. Cardiovasc. Pharmacol.* **2019**, *74*, 175–187. [CrossRef]
178. Fujisue, K.; Sugamura, K.; Kurokawa, H.; Matsubara, J.; Ishii, M.; Izumiya, Y.; Kaikita, K.; Sugiyama, S. Colchicine Improves Survival, Left Ventricular Remodeling, and Chronic Cardiac Function After Acute Myocardial Infarction. *Circ. J.* **2017**, *81*, 1174–1182. [CrossRef]
179. Akodad, M.; Fauconnier, J.; Sicard, P.; Huet, F.; Blandel, F.; Bourret, A.; de Santa Barbara, P.; Aguilhon, S.; LeGall, M.; Hugon, G.; et al. Interest of colchicine in the treatment of acute myocardial infarct responsible for heart failure in a mouse model. *Int. J. Cardiol.* **2017**, *240*, 347–353. [CrossRef]
180. Delbridge, L.M.; Bienvenu, L.A.; Mellor, K.M. Angiotensin-(1-9): New Promise for Post-Infarct Functional Therapy. *J. Am. Coll. Cardiol.* **2016**, *68*, 2667–2669. [CrossRef]
181. Thum, T.; Gross, C.; Fiedler, J.; Fischer, T.; Kissler, S.; Bussen, M.; Galuppo, P.; Just, S.; Rottbauer, W.; Frantz, S.; et al. Mi-croRNA-21 contributes to myocardial disease by stimulating MAP kinase signalling in fibroblasts. *Nature* **2008**, *456*, 980–984. [CrossRef]
182. Kumarswamy, R.; Thum, T. Non-coding RNAs in Cardiac Remodeling and Heart Failure. *Circ. Res.* **2013**, *113*, 676–689. [CrossRef] [PubMed]
183. Danielson, K.M.; Shah, R.; Yeri, A.; Liu, X.; Camacho Garcia, F.; Silverman, M.; Tanriverdi, K.; Das, A.; Xiao, C.; Jerosch-Herold, M.; et al. Plasma Circulating Extracellular RNAs in Left Ventricular Remodeling Post-Myocardial Infarction. *EBioMedicine* **2018**, *32*, 172–181. [CrossRef]
184. Kowara, M.; Borodzicz-Jazdzyk, S.; Rybak, K.; Kubik, M.; Cudnoch-Jedrzejewska, A. Therapies Targeted at Non-Coding RNAs in Prevention and Limitation of Myocardial Infarction and Subsequent Cardiac Remodeling—Current Experience and Perspectives. *Int. J. Mol. Sci.* **2021**, *22*, 5718. [CrossRef] [PubMed]
185. Yan, M.; Chen, K.; Sun, R.; Lin, K.; Qian, X.; Yuan, M.; Wang, Y.; Ma, J.; Qing, Y.; Xu, J.; et al. Glucose impairs angiogenesis and promotes ventricular remodelling following myocardial infarction via upregulation of microRNA-17. *Exp. Cell Res.* **2019**, *381*, 191–200. [CrossRef]
186. Schächinger, V.; Erbs, S.; Elsässer, A.; Haberbosch, W.; Hambrecht, R.; Hölschermann, H.; Yu, J.; Corti, R.; Mathey, D.G.; Hamm, C.W.; et al. Intracoronary Bone Marrow–Derived Progenitor Cells in Acute Myocardial Infarction. *N. Engl. J. Med.* **2006**, *355*, 1210–1221. [CrossRef]
187. Schächinger, V.; Erbs, S.; Elsässer, A.; Haberbosch, W.; Hambrecht, R.; Hölschermann, H.; Yu, J.; Corti, R.; Mathey, D.G.; Hamm, C.W.; et al. Improved clinical outcome after intracoronary administration of bone-marrow-derived progenitor cells in acute myocardial infarction: Final 1-year results of the REPAIR-AMI trial. *Eur. Heart J.* **2006**, *27*, 2775–2783. [CrossRef] [PubMed]

188. Dill, T.; Schächinger, V.; Rolf, A.; Möllmann, S.; Thiele, H.; Tillmanns, H.; Assmus, B.; Dimmeler, S.; Zeiher, A.M.; Hamm, C. Intracoronary administration of bone marrow-derived progenitor cells improves left ventricular function in patients at risk for adverse remodeling after acute ST-segment elevation myocardial infarction: Results of the Reinfusion of Enriched Pro-genitor cells And Infarct Remodeling in Acute Myocardial Infarction study (REPAIR-AMI) cardiac magnetic resonance imaging substudy. *Am. Heart J.* **2009**, *157*, 541–547.
189. Wollert, K.C.; Meyer, G.P.; Lotz, J.; Lichtenberg, S.R.; Lippolt, P.; Breidenbach, C.; Fichtner, S.; Korte, T.; Hornig, B.; Messinger, C.; et al. Intracoronary autologous bone-marrow cell transfer after myocardial infarction: The BOOST randomised controlled clinical trial. *Lancet* **2004**, *364*, 141–148. [CrossRef]
190. Makkar, R.R.; Kereiakes, D.J.; Aguirre, F.; Kowalchuk, G.; Chakravarty, T.; Malliaras, K.; Francis, G.S.; Povsic, T.J.; Schatz, R.; Traverse, J.H.; et al. Intracoronary ALLogeneic heart STem cells to Achieve myocardial Regeneration (ALLSTAR): A ran-domized, placebo-controlled, double-blinded trial. *Eur. Heart J.* **2020**, *41*, 3451–3458. [CrossRef]
191. Mathur, A.; Fernández-Avilés, F.; Bartunek, J.; Belmans, A.; Crea, F.; Dowlut, S.; Galiñanes, M.; Good, M.-C.; Hartikainen, J.; Hauskeller, C.; et al. The effect of intracoronary infusion of bone marrow-derived mononuclear cells on all-cause mortality in acute myocardial infarction: The BAMI trial. *Eur. Heart J.* **2020**, *41*, 3702–3710. [CrossRef]
192. Biffi, M.; Loforte, A.; Folesani, G.; Ziacchi, M.; Attinà, D.; Niro, F.; Pasquale, F.; Pacini, D. Hybrid transcatheter left ventricular reconstruction for the treatment of ischemic cardiomyopathy. *Cardiovasc. Diagn. Ther.* **2021**, *11*, 183–192. [CrossRef] [PubMed]

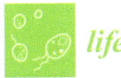

Review

Myocardial Ischemia Related to Common Cancer Therapy—Prevention Insights

Minerva Codruta Badescu [1,2], Oana Viola Badulescu [3,4,*,†], Dragos Viorel Scripcariu [5,6,*,†], Lăcrămioara Ionela Butnariu [7,*,†], Iris Bararu-Bojan [3], Diana Popescu [1], Manuela Ciocoiu [3], Eusebiu Vlad Gorduza [7], Irina Iuliana Costache [1,8], Elena Rezus [9,10] and Ciprian Rezus [1,2]

1. Department of Internal Medicine, "Grigore T. Popa" University of Medicine and Pharmacy, 16 University Street, 700115 Iasi, Romania; minerva.badescu@umfiasi.ro (M.C.B.); popescu.diana@umfiasi.ro (D.P.); irina.costache@umfiasi.ro (I.I.C.); ciprian.rezus@umfiasi.ro (C.R.)
2. III Internal Medicine Clinic, "St. Spiridon" County Emergency Clinical Hospital, 1 Independence Boulevard, 700111 Iasi, Romania
3. Department of Pathophysiology, "Grigore T. Popa" University of Medicine and Pharmacy, 16 University Street, 700115 Iasi, Romania; iris.bararu@umfiasi.ro (I.B.-B.); manuela.ciocoiu@umfiasi.ro (M.C.)
4. Hematology Clinic, "St. Spiridon" County Emergency Clinical Hospital, 1 Independence Boulevard, 700111 Iasi, Romania
5. Surgery Department, "Grigore T. Popa" University of Medicine and Pharmacy, 16 University Street, 700115 Iasi, Romania
6. 1st Surgical Oncology Unit, Regional Institute of Oncology, 2-4 General Henri Mathias Berthelot Street, 700483 Iasi, Romania
7. Department of Mother and Child Medicine, "Grigore T. Popa" University of Medicine and Pharmacy, 700115 Iasi, Romania; eusebiu.gorduza@umfiasi.ro
8. Cardiology Clinic, "St. Spiridon" County Emergency Clinical Hospital, 700111 Iasi, Romania
9. Department of Rheumatology and Physiotherapy, "Grigore T. Popa" University of Medicine and Pharmacy, 16 University Street, 700115 Iasi, Romania; elena.rezus@umfiasi.ro
10. I Rheumatology Clinic, Clinical Rehabilitation Hospital, 14 Pantelimon Halipa Street, 700661 Iasi, Romania
* Correspondence: oana.badulescu@umfiasi.ro (O.V.B.); dragos-viorel.scripcariu@umfiasi.ro (D.V.S.); ionela.butnariu@umfiasi.ro (L.I.B.)
† These authors contributed equally to this work.

Abstract: Modern antineoplastic therapy improves survival and quality of life in cancer patients, but its indisputable benefits are accompanied by multiple and major side effects, such as cardiovascular ones. Endothelial dysfunction, arterial spasm, intravascular thrombosis, and accelerated atherosclerosis affect the coronary arteries, leading to acute and chronic coronary syndromes that negatively interfere with the oncologic treatment. The cardiac toxicity of antineoplastic agents may be mitigated by using adequate prophylactic measures. In the absence of dedicated guidelines, our work provides the most comprehensive, systematized, structured, and up-to-date analyses of the available literature focusing on measures aiming to protect the coronary arteries from the toxicity of cancer therapy. Our work facilitates the implementation of these measures in daily practice. The ultimate goal is to offer clinicians the necessary data for a personalized therapeutic approach for cancer patients receiving evidence-based oncology treatments with potential cardiovascular toxicity.

Keywords: accelerated atherosclerosis; coronary spasm; coronary thrombosis; endothelial dysfunction; cancer; prevention; radiotherapy; chemotherapy

1. Introduction

Early diagnosis and modern therapies have significantly improved the survival and quality of life in cancer patients. The 5-year relative survival rate for all cancer sites combined has increased by 19% over the past 30 years in the USA [1], and its steady increase over the past 20 years was found in all European regions as well [2]. Still, cancer therapy has harmful effects on the cardiovascular system, which can diminish the benefits obtained. Cardiovascular disease increases morbidity and mortality not only by itself but also by limiting the use of anticancer therapies [3], and to date, it is the main cause of mortality in cancer survivors [4].

Cancer treatment is based on three major pillars, namely surgery, chemotherapy (CT), and radiation therapy (RT), that can be used in various combinations, reflecting the great complexity of modern oncologic therapy. Cardiovascular complications of cancer therapy are multiple and may affect all heart structures as well as blood vessels. The cardiovascular toxicities of antineoplastic agents manifest as myocardial dysfunction and heart failure, coronary artery disease (CAD), valvular disease, arrhythmias, arterial hypertension, peripheral vascular disease and stroke, thromboembolic disease, pulmonary hypertension, and pericardial complications [5]. RT induces endothelial dysfunction and fibrosis. All components of the heart can be affected, which leads to CAD, cardiomyopathy, valvulopathy, arrhythmias, and pericardial disease [6].

Cancer treatments act unfavorably on coronary arteries. The main mechanisms are endothelial dysfunction, vasospasm, thrombosis, and fibrosis. The process of atheroma plaque formation is more intense and takes place at a much faster rate. Toxic effects of the cancer treatments can destabilize a normal endothelium or a pre-existing atheroma plaque. Therefore, patients can develop acute coronary syndromes (ACSs) or accelerated atherosclerosis and early CAD while on oncologic treatment. This risk is enhanced by the presence of classical cardiovascular risk factors and varies with the type, dose, and duration of cancer therapy [7]. In patients receiving both CT and RT, the risk of CAD is the highest: two or even three times higher than in patients receiving only RT [8,9].

The scope of our review is to realize a comprehensive, systematized, structured, and up-to-date analyze of the available literature focusing on measures aiming to protect the coronary arteries from the toxicity of cancer therapy. Cardiac toxicity exhibited by anticancer drugs is based on multiple mechanisms; therefore, extensive search on the *Web of Science* database was performed in order to collect the necessary data. Starting from the pathophysiological mechanisms of coronary artery dysfunction induced by cancer treatment, we provided reliable data regarding modern approaches to prevention. The 2016 European Society of Cardiology position paper on cancer treatments and cardiovascular toxicity mainly focuses on RT and three categories of anticancer drugs, namely antimetabolites, platinum compounds, and vascular endothelial growth factor pathway inhibitors, as the most important toxic agents for the coronary arteries [5]. Our work is concordant with this guideline.

2. Antimetabolites (5-FU, Capecitabine, Gemcitabine)

Fluoropyrimidines (FP), namely 5-fluorouracil (5-FU) and its oral prodrug capecitabine, are commonly used for the treatment of various solid tumors, e.g., breast, gastric, colorectal, and head and neck cancers, due to their wide antitumor effect and their synergic activity with other anticancer drugs [10]. Despite the benefits, cardiac adverse effects are very common. Only the cardiac toxicity of anthracyclines exceeds that of FP [11]. The reported incidence of cardiovascular toxicity ranges from 1% to 19% [12] and mainly manifests as CAD. Myocardial ischemia usually has clinical expression, but the existence of asymptomatic forms leads to an underestimation of the prevalence of 5-FU-induced CAD [13,14]. Gemcitabine is preferred in old or fragile patients due to its lower toxicity profile compared to other anticancer drugs. Meta-analyzes reported an overall incidence of cardiovascular adverse effects of 1% and myocardial infarction (MI) of 0.5% [15].

The mechanism of FP-related cardiovascular toxicity is very complex and not fully elucidated despite the long-term use of these compounds. The coronary artery spasm in the first place and thrombosis in the second place were identified as major pathogenic substrates [16,17]. Vasoconstriction is triggered by two mechanisms, and both are the consequence of vascular endothelial cell injury. The first is endothelium-independent and a result of the activation of the protein kinase C pathway [18]. The second is endothelium-dependent and mediated by high levels of endothelin-1 [19]. Transient coronary vasospasm may cause an episode of chest pain or unstable angina pectoris, whereas persistent vasospasm may produce an acute MI. This mechanism is considered responsible for the onset of acute MI during intravenous administration of 5-FU. Moreover, coronary artery vasospasm can be directly visualized during coronary angiography [11]. Interestingly, the multivessel coronary spasm is uncommon although the distribution of the drug is systemic. Epicardial vasospasm was typically observed in a single vessel during coronary angiography, usually the vessel supplying the largest territory of the myocardium. Of note, the bolus therapy of 5-FU was associated with a much lower risk of cardiac toxicity (5%) than continuous infusion (10–18%) because the half-life of the drug is 15–20 min, so it is eliminated quickly when given as a bolus [11].

The coronary spasm usually occurs in the absence of classic cardiovascular risk factors and significant coronary stenosis on angiography [20]. Moreover, the angiography is typically normal without evidence of a thrombotic event [21]. However, microthrombotic occlusions have been identified by scanning electron microscopy in animal studies [22]. 5-FU produces endothelial dysfunction, endothelial cells cytolysis, and denudation of the underlying internal elastic lamina, followed by activation of platelets and coagulation cascade and thrombus formation [23]. Accelerated thrombosis of small vessels was noted in many studies [17,24–26].

Cytotoxic endothelial dysfunction was considered a contributing mechanism. 5-FU reduces the antioxidant capacity, enhancing the generation of free radicals and resulting in lipid peroxidation and early atherosclerosis [26,27]. Moreover, 5-FU induces changes in the morphology and metabolism of red blood cells and decreases their ability to transfer oxygen. All these changes impair the myocardial oxygenation and lead to cardiomyocyte ischemia [28].

Although initially considered less cardiotoxic than 5-FU, capecitabine was related to acute coronary events as well. The spasm of the coronary artery was considered the underlining substrate [29,30]. The incidence of cardiotoxicity of capecitabine varies between 3% and 9%, which is similar to that of continuous 5-FU infusion therapy [31]. Gemcitabine rarely induces ACSs, but when they do occur, they are the most acute MI. Patients receiving gemcitabine in combination with another anticancer drug are at the highest risk [20].

The timing from drug administration to acute coronary event onset is highly variable. Coronary artery spasm may manifest during infusion or hours or days after drug administration [20,32–34]. The explanation for this phenomenon is still elusive.

Coronary spasm is the main expression of the vascular damage caused by FP. Therefore, FP must be discontinued immediately, and the treatment with low-dose aspirin, calcium channel blockers (CCBs), and long-acting nitrates should be initiated. The efficacy of non-dihydropyridine CCB, such as diltiazem and verapamil, and of nitrates was reported in different clinical scenarios. One patient with transient ST-segment elevation ACS and ventricular tachycardia was temporarily treated with diltiazem 180 mg/day, while capecitabine was definitively withdrawn. Low-dose aspirin and an inhibitor of the renin-angiotensin system, telmisartan, were also recommended [35]. Another therapeutic option is to administer a bolus of diltiazem and an intravenous infusion of nitroglycerin, followed by isosorbide mononitrate 40 mg/day and diltiazem 90 mg/day [36]. In both cases the troponin and coronary angiography were normal, reinforcing the idea that coronary spasm was the underlining substrate. Antianginal therapy with nitrates and non-dihydropyridine CCB allowed symptoms control in up to 70% of patients [31].

However, the prevention of coronary spasm using CCB and/or nitrates showed mixed results. While diltiazem and nifedipine have accumulated positive evidence, verapamil failed to prevent 5-FU-induced vasospasm [37–39].

Cardiac ischemia related to the use of FP is associated with an 82 to 100% risk of symptom recurrence at the reintroduction of the drug and up to 13% risk of death; therefore, further treatment with these compounds should be discouraged [40]. If mandatory, i.e., the best chance for survival or lack of other therapeutic alternatives, CT may be restarted under protection from CCB and nitrates [35]. Drug re-challenge include short-acting diltiazem and sublingual nitroglycerin as needed during FP infusion and pre- and post-treatment with extended-release nifedipine and isosorbide mononitrate [41].

Endothelial damage leads to microthrombosis, and experimental studies suggested that the use of anticoagulants may partially mitigate this toxicity. The protective role of a low-molecular-weight heparin against the prothrombotic effect of 5-FU on the vascular endothelium was assessed in an animal model [25]. Dalteparin reduced the burden of thrombosis, but the reversibility of the endothelial damage was impaired. It was concluded that dalteparin offers protection from the thrombogenic effect of 5-FU, but this anticoagulant per se had a toxic effect on the endothelium, which was different from that of 5-FU.

The efficacy of probucol—a lipid-lowering drug with strong antioxidant properties—was assessed in the prevention of 5-FU toxicity on vascular endothelium, and it showed promising results. The damage to the endothelium was minimal and comparable to that of the control group [26].

3. Platinum Compounds (Cisplatin)

Cisplatin-based CT is widely used for the treatment of many solid-organ cancers. Still, its high efficiency is accompanied by multiple toxicities: ototoxicity, renal, digestive, cardiovascular, pulmonary toxicities, myelosuppression, and allergic reactions [42]. One of the manifestations of cardiovascular toxicity is arterial and venous thrombotic events. Although rare, any of the following have been reported: angina pectoris, acute MI, transient ischemic attack, stroke, and deep vein thrombosis. The overall incidence of thrombotic complications is 10% and less in the arterial system (1.6%) than in the venous system (8.4%) [43]. Acute cardiovascular complications usually occur during treatment, but cisplatin-based CT increases the risk of acute vascular events in the long term as well.

Cisplatin has direct and acute vascular toxicity. It inhibits the proliferation of endothelial cells, induces their apoptosis, and thereby reduces their survival [44]. Cisplatin increases the generation of reactive oxygen species and triggers an inflammatory response with cytokine release. The oxidative stress and inflammation intensify each other and lead to endothelial dysfunction. As a consequence, the nitric oxide (NO) levels decrease leading to a prolonged vasoconstrictor response. Moreover, a prothrombotic environment is created, characterized by increased platelet activation and high levels of von Willebrand factor, fibrinogen, and tissue-type plasminogen activator. The activity of natural anticoagulants is impaired, as evidenced by decreased functional protein C levels.

Cisplatin also indirectly contributes to increased cardiovascular risk. Its ability to generate reactive oxygen species leads to increased lipid peroxidation. It disrupts the lipid metabolism leading to proatherogenic dyslipidemia [45,46]. Total cholesterol, LDL-cholesterol, total cholesterol/HDL cholesterol ratio, and triglycerides were significantly higher in patients receiving CT compared with those treated only with surgery. In one study, the prevalence of hypercholesterolemia was as high as 80% [47]. Long-term observational studies showed that cisplatin can induce hypertension and insulin resistance. The overall prevalence of diabetes was 7.3% and was the highest in patients who received both RT and CT. It was four times higher than in patients treated with surgery alone. Moreover, metabolic syndrome was more common in patients who received CT than in those who did not [48].

The patients treated with cisplatin-based CT have a significantly increased risk of major coronary events, especially during and shortly after drug administration. Intravascular thrombosis is considered the main underlining substrate. Cisplatin may induce arterial thrombosis with subsequent myocardial and cerebrovascular ischemia in 2% of patients [49]. While in the general population, a complicated atherosclerotic plaque is responsible for the acute MI, in patients treated with cisplatin, arterial thrombosis occurs even in the absence of underlying atherosclerosis or classical cardiovascular risk factors. In a 71-year-old woman presenting with ACS, the coronary angiography showed a subtotal thrombotic occlusion of the proximal segment of anterior descending artery (ADA) and embolic occlusion of the distal segment of ADA but no significant coronary stenosis [50]. Similarly, in a 31-year-old man without cardiovascular risk factors presenting with ST-elevation myocardial infarction (STEMI) 24 h after CT, the coronary angiography performed the day after intravenous thrombolysis showed moderate mid-ADA disease with residual thrombosis [51]. In another young male presenting with STEMI, extensive left coronary thrombosis was identified, with the thrombotic load of the circumflex being more important than that of the ADA [52].

Vasoconstriction is considered an important contributor to the ACS, especially when the patients are very young, there are no cardiovascular risk factors, or the coronary angiography is normal [45,53]. In a 34-year-old man with no cardiovascular risk factors presenting with STEMI 5 days after CT, the coronary angiography revealed mild stenosis at the level of the right coronary artery with overlying thrombus and vasospasm and no other significant coronary lesions [54]. Two cases of vasospastic angina and one case of acute MI secondary to vasospasm have also been reported in connection with ongoing cisplatin CT [55,56]. Because 70–80% of patients treated with cisplatin develop hypomagnesaemia, and this can induce vasospasm, in the latter case, a possible role for this electrolyte imbalance has been considered as a stimulator of vasospasm.

Spontaneous coronary artery dissection during cisplatin therapy is extremely rare [57]. In a 33-year-old man who presented STEMI at the end of the first cycle of CT, coronary angiography revealed a circumscribed stenosis of the circumflex artery with intima dissection and associated thrombosis and no atherosclerotic plaque [58]. In another young patient, a chronic dissection of the right coronary artery was identified at the angiography.

In 5.7–6.7% of cisplatin-treated cancer survivors, CAD manifests more than a decade after CT [59]. The absolute risk of CAD is up to 8% over 20 years [9]. At 30-year follow-up, the same population had more CAD and was more frequently treated for hypertension and dyslipidemia than controls [60]. Data from a Norwegian study showed that the risk of CAD is 2.6 times higher in patients receiving cisplatin-based CT and 4.8 times higher in those receiving CT and RT than in patients treated only by surgery [9]. In an older study, the risk of CAD, reported as non-fatal MI and angina pectoris with proven myocardial ischemia, was 7 times higher in patients receiving cisplatin than in the general population [47]. Because these data come from studies that have enrolled patients with germ cell tumors, which most commonly affect men between the ages of 15 and 35, it can be concluded that cisplatin treatment induces accelerated atherosclerosis and premature CAD [61]. It was observed that intima-media thickness is higher than the estimated value for age, confirming that cisplatin triggers a degenerative process of the vessel walls, leading to occlusive vascular disease in the long term [62]. Moreover, cisplatin has the potential risk of delayed onset of vasospastic angina [63].

Cisplatin therapy is associated with oxidative stress and increased reactive oxygen species production. Moreover, an increase in oxygen free radicals also exists during the reperfusion of ischemic cardiac tissue. Therefore, inhibiting this pathway can be beneficial. In an animal model, the administration of N-Acetyl-l-cysteine—a free radical scavenger—ameliorated the coronary flow and alleviated the effects of cisplatin [64]. In preclinical studies, acetyl-carnitine, α-lipoic acid, and silymarin have also been shown to have antioxidant potential, limiting the cardiac toxic effects of cisplatin [65].

Coronary vasospasm during treatment may lead to decreased dose or discontinuation of cisplatin and a more unfavorable oncological prognosis for the patient. The decision to withdraw cisplatin after acute MI due to coronary spasm was reported [56]. The CCB and long-acting nitrates effectively prevent coronary spasm and currently constitute the treatment of choice of vasospastic angina in the general population [66]. A CCB was initiated in a patient with ACS and normal angiography, with cisplatin-induced coronary spasm as a substrate. Under this protection, the course of CT was without further events [53]. This strategy is in line with current guideline recommendations [66]. However, routine administration of low-dose aspirin or lipid-lowering treatment in patients with normal angiographic coronaries is not recommended [67].

Cisplatin-based CT is often followed by the onset of metabolic syndrome [48,68,69], which will further increase the risk of major coronary events. Therefore, aggressive therapeutic interventions aimed at correcting the components of the metabolic syndrome should be a priority. In the absence of specific recommendations, the therapeutic intervention consisting of lifestyle interventions and drug therapy mimics that in the general population [70]. One study explored the utility of tailored exercise interventions to ameliorate cardiovascular dysfunction in patients with a history of cisplatin CT, highlighting the favorable metabolic impact [71].

4. VEGF/VEGFR Inhibitors (Bevacizumab, Sorafenib, Sunitinib)

Vascular endothelial growth factor (VEGF) pathway inhibitors are drugs used to treat a wide variety of cancers due to their inhibitory effect on angiogenesis. The most extensive experience comes from advanced renal cell carcinoma patients in whom the treatment increased the overall survival rate [72]. VEGF pathway inhibitors have also been used successfully in treating non-small cell lung cancers, hepatocellular carcinomas, pancreatic neuroendocrine tumors, gastrointestinal stromal tumors, colorectal, breast, ovarian and thyroid cancers, and glioblastoma [73–80].

Bevacizumab is a recombinant humanized monoclonal antibody that binds to VEGF and blocks the interaction between VEGF and its receptor on the surface of endothelial cells. As a result, endothelial cell proliferation and the formation of new blood vessels are inhibited [81]. Sunitinib and sorafenib are tyrosine kinase inhibitors for VEGF receptor (VEGFR) and act by inhibiting the VEGF pathway.

While inhibiting angiogenesis is a therapeutic advantage, the decreased endothelial cell regeneration capacity leads to the formation of areas of endothelial discontinuity, where exposed subendothelial collagen interacts with tissue factor and initiates coagulation. VEGF inhibition diminished NO production as well, thus impairing vasodilation. Since NO prevents leukocyte and platelet adhesion to endothelial cells and platelet aggregation and stimulates disaggregation of preformed platelet aggregates, its decreased production leads to a prothrombotic state [82]. Moreover, bevacizumab increases the expression of proinflammatory cytokines, enhancing thrombosis.

Up to 4–5% of patients receiving bevacizumab will develop arterial thrombotic events during treatment, with the highest risk being recorded in patients with metastatic cancer and in the first 3 months of therapy [40,83]. Adding bevacizumab to CT will double the risk of stroke, MI, coronary heart disease, and cardiac death. When only coronary events were assessed, bevacizumab increased the incidence of MI/angina pectoris from 1% to 1.5% [84]. In clinical studies, the incidence of CAD ranged from 0.52% to 1.7%. A meta-analysis of seven studies evaluating the effect of bevacizumab on the occurrence of CAD in cancer patients showed that the risk was 2.5 higher compared to the general population. The risk was not evenly distributed between tumor types, with patients with colorectal cancer having the highest risk [81]. A larger meta-analysis showed that adding bevacizumab to standard CT increases the overall risk of cardiac ischemia by 2.47 times. In patients receiving a high dose of bevacizumab regimen, the risk was 4.4 times higher [85]. Age over 65 years and a positive history of CAD/atherosclerosis were identified as risk factors for arterial thrombosis [84].

The incidence of arterial thrombotic events is 1.7% for sorafenib and 1.4% for sunitinib [86]. In addition, the treatment with sorafenib or sunitinib increases three times the risk of arterial thrombotic events regardless of the drug used or the cancer type. In patients with advanced clear-cell renal-cell carcinoma, the treatment with sorafenib increased the incidence of cardiac ischemia or MI from less than 1% to 3% ($p = 0.01$) [87]. In one case acute MI was recurrent at four and five years after initiation of sorafenib [88].

A large meta-analysis of 23 trials showed that anti-VEGF agents significantly increased the risk of severe arterial thrombotic events [89]. Major arterial thrombotic events—mostly involving the coronary arteries—affected one in 27 patients receiving bevacizumab [90]. In general, 1–15% of patients treated with an inhibitor of the VEGF pathway will report chest pain episodes, ranging from stable angina to ACS [91]. Cardiac events are still underestimated in patients receiving either sorafenib or sunitinib. One study reported that 33.8% of patients experienced a cardiac event. Still, after adequate cardiovascular management, all patients continued the treatment with tyrosine kinase inhibitors [92].

Hypertension is the most frequent complication during bevacizumab treatment, occurring in one of three patients. The risk of hypertension is increased three times with a low dose and 7.5 times with a high dose of bevacizumab [93]. Sorafenib and sunitinib are associated with an increased risk of hypertension as well. One in four patients receiving sorafenib and one in five patients receiving sunitinib will develop abnormal blood pressure values [94,95]. Hypertension leads to endothelial dysfunction and may enhance the vascular toxicity of VEGF pathway inhibition.

Bevacizumab treatment is associated with an increased risk for bleeding, which is usually minor and not requiring intervention. Severe bleedings occur in less than 5% of cases [96]. When added to CT, sorafenib or sunitinib double the risk of bleeding, but the incidence of severe bleeding was raised only slightly, probably due to the limited sample size and events [97]. Therefore, in patients with cancer under CT that have an increased risk of both thrombosis and bleeding, thromboprophylaxis is a challenge.

Baseline cardiovascular risk assessment and optimal control of arterial hypertension are general measures aiming to reduce the risk for acute coronary events, especially when evidence-based oncology treatments have potential cardiovascular toxicity. Risk assessment provides the opportunity for early intervention on modifiable cardiovascular risk factors to properly diagnose and treat cardiovascular disease in order to reduce the risk of cardiovascular complications during and after cancer treatment. The risk scores for the general population do not fully reflect the cardiovascular risk of neoplastic, so baseline risk stratification proformas have been specifically developed for patients scheduled to receive medication known to be cardiotoxic, including VEGF pathway inhibitors [98].

Although hypertension has a multifactorial substrate, the role of NO depletion should be emphasized. NO regulates the renal blood flow and tubular sodium excretion. Low NO levels lead to impaired sodium excretion and consequently fluid retention and salt-dependent hypertension [99]. Therefore, diuretics and NO donors such as nitrates should be considered [100]. CCB are potent vasodilators. Only nifedipine and amlodipine are allowed because they do not have the adverse effect of increasing VEGF levels as do verapamil and diltiazem, which are therefore to be avoided [79]. Of beta-blockers, carvedilol is the best choice, as it has both vasodilatory and antiangiogenic effects. Although nebivolol has an appropriate mechanism of action, i.e., it increases endothelial NO production, it is not preferred, as it may counteract the inhibitory effect of anticancer drugs in tumor vessels [101]. The renin-angiotensin system is less important in the mechanism of hypertension induced by the treatment with VEGF pathway inhibitors [102]. Still, angiotensin system inhibitors added benefits to cancer treatment, leading to superior survival outcomes for patients with metastatic renal cell carcinoma. In light of this evidence, angiotensin system inhibitors—with or without amlodipine—are the first choice in patients without comorbidities that require the use of other pharmaceutical classes. Carvedilol is the third step, followed by diuretics. Long-acting nitrates are reserved for resistant hypertension [79]. Optimal blood pressure goals are not defined at present; therefore, those valid for the general population apply. Still, due to their high cardiovascular risk, some authors have proposed lower targets in cancer patients [79,103].

There is evidence for and against the use of statins. Statins have pleiotropic effects and can ameliorate endothelial dysfunction. However, by improving NO bioavailability and eNOS activity, they could reduce the efficacy of VEGF pathway inhibitors. Statins reduce VEGF expression in microvascular endothelial cells and enhance it in macrovascular endothelial cells. Moreover, statins are proangiogenic at low doses and antiangiogenic at high doses [104]. Due to this duality, when given to cancer patients, high doses of statins are recommended.

Because a large number of patients, in some studies up to 20–40%, experience bleeding during cancer treatment with VEGF pathway inhibitors, the use of antiplatelet and anticoagulant therapy is of major concern, especially when intended for primary prevention [96].

Low-dose aspirin use slightly reduced the rate of arterial thrombotic events in patients treated with bevacizumab. The effect was more important in the subgroup of patients over the age of 65 and with a history of arterial thromboembolism [84]. Still, no conclusion could be drawn due to the small number of events per risk factor subgroup. No significant differences in the risk of major bleeding were found between low-dose aspirin users and non-users among control and bevacizumab-treated patients. In a non-randomized study, the rate of arterial thrombotic events in patients treated with bevacizumab was 2.7% in non-low-dose aspirin users and 8.9% in low-dose aspirin users [90]. Once again, no definitive conclusions could be reached regarding any preventive effects associated with low-dose aspirin use. The interpretation of the data was hampered by a higher proportion of patients with cardiovascular risk factors or a previous arterial thrombotic event among the low-dose aspirin users.

The benefits of low-dose aspirin in CAD patients in the general population are undisputed [105]. Therefore, antiplatelet therapy should be continued during the treatment with VEGF pathway inhibitors in patients with a diagnosis of CAD because the potential benefits outweigh the risk of bleeding complications [106,107]. However, patients without CAD should not receive antiplatelet drugs as part of primary prevention. Moreover, it is recommended to discontinue bevacizumab for any arterial thrombotic event.

5. Radiotherapy

Chest RT is an essential part of the treatment of hematological malignancies and thoracic solid tumors, such as lung, esophageal, and breast cancers. Due to close proximity to the irradiated area, the heart and coronary arteries receive variable amount of radiation. Any of the heart structures can be affected, leading to constrictive pericarditis, CAD, myocardial disease, valvular heart disease, and conduction system dysfunction. Radiation-induced CAD (RICAD) is a late complication of RT. The most vulnerable patients are those with Hodgkin's lymphoma and women undergoing treatment for left-sided breast cancer [108–110]. RICAD is the second most common cause of morbidity and mortality in patients with RT for thoracic malignancies, especially breast cancer and Hodgkin's lymphoma, due to the favorable long-term prognosis and/or relatively young age of patients. The time between RT and RICAD onset may be short—a year or two—if the radiation dose was high, i.e., above 30–35 Gy, or traditional atherosclerotic risk factors were present, but more than a decade could elapse if lower doses were used [111–114]. RICAD occurs more than 10 years from the completion of treatment in patients with breast cancer [115] and after two or three decades post-therapy in patients with Hodgkin's lymphoma [116].

During the irradiation of the left breast and internal mammary chain, the heart receives a radiation dose of 0.9–14 Gy and 3–17 Gy, respectively. Lower doses of 0.4–6 Gy and 2–10 Gy, respectively, are received by the heart during the irradiation of the right breast and internal mammary chain [117]. This difference is important because it results in a higher prevalence of RICAD and MI in women receiving RT for left compared to the right breast cancer [118]. Moreover, RT increases the cardiac mortality in women with breast cancer [119]. Although cardiac irradiation is less intense with current modern techniques, the mean dose to which the heart is exposed varies between 1 and 5 Gy [113,120,121]. It must be emphasized that the radiation dose received by the ADA is greater than the whole heart dose; therefore, the risk of developing ischemic heart disease remains. The risk of a major coronary event, e.g., MI, coronary revascularization, or death from ischemic heart disease, increases linearly with the mean dose of radiation to the heart over several decades, with 7.4% per Gy, whether or not there are pre-existing cardiovascular risk factors [113]. There was no threshold below which there was no risk. The risk of major cardiovascular events doubles in the presence of cardiovascular risk factors and increases more than 6 times in the case of an ischemic heart disease history [113,122,123]. Up to 3- to 4-fold increase in the risk of MI due to CAD has been observed if mediastinal irradiation was combined with CT [124].

RICAD is highly prevalent in Hodgkin's disease survivors and brings significant morbidity and mortality. The most robust evidence of coronary damage due to RT comes from studies on pediatric population [125,126]. Mediastinal RT during childhood is significantly correlated with the presence of coronary artery abnormalities on computed tomography angiography (CTA) and is associated with a 4 to 6 times increase in the risk of CAD compared to the general population [108]. In asymptomatic patients, the risk of RICAD is 16% in the first 10 years, and it is dependent on the radiation dose, being 6.8 times higher in those who received more than 20 Gy compared to those who received lower doses [127]. The need for coronary artery bypass grafting (CABG) and percutaneous coronary intervention (PCI) is 3.2 times and 1.6 times higher, respectively, than in the general population [128], and MI is the most common cause of cardiac death in these patients. Severe fibrotic and calcified stenosis of the proximal part of the left main (LM) was identified during autopsy in a 12-year-old boy with MI six years after chest RT [129].

RT leads to both macrovascular and microvascular disease. The evolution of atheroma plaques in these patients mimics that of the general population, but the process is accelerated, and the amount of fibrosis is higher [115,130]. Radiation injures the endothelial cells and disrupts their membranes. It also triggers the activation of inflammatory pathways, platelets, and coagulation cascade, leading to thrombosis. The endothelium becomes porous, releases inflammatory mediators, and expresses adhesion molecules that facilitate the passage of low-density lipoproteins and monocytes in the subintimal space [131]. The formation of foam cells sustains chronic inflammation that ultimately leads to atherosclerotic plaque instability and rupture, diffuse fibrosis of all layers of the coronary artery wall, and intimal hyperplasia [116,132–134]. Endovascular thrombosis and capillary luminal stenosis determine a reduction in capillary density [135]. The endothelial dysfunction is responsible not only for impaired vascular reactivity, e.g., coronary spasm or persistent vasoconstriction, but also acts synergistically with sustained inflammation to maintain the prothrombotic environment [136].

Typical for RICAD are ostial stenoses and severe atherosclerotic lesions on the proximal segments of the epicardial coronary arteries. The LM trunk and the proximal segments of the ADA and right coronary artery are mainly affected. Due to their anterior and central position in the mediastinum, they receive higher doses of radiation compared to the lateral, posterior, and peripheral coronary vessels. The atherosclerotic plaques are long, smooth, fibrotic, and cause concentric and tubular narrowing of the vessel lumen. Negative remodeling is frequently encountered [116]. Long segments of diffuse disease and areas of stenosis from soft plaque were also found [126]. Microvascular fibrosis and reduction of capillary density lead to dysfunction in microcirculation, reduction of the coronary flow reserve, and, finally, to myocardial ischemia [3]. Acute coronary events may occur, as RT can trigger coronary spasm and atherosclerotic plaque rupture, followed by partially or totally obstructive thrombosis [137].

The deleterious effects of RT on heart structures are well-known, and over the last decades, continuous efforts have been made to limit them. Many improvements to RT protocols have been added, such as enhanced localization and gated techniques. Three- and four-dimensional planning models and those based on positron emission tomography/X-ray computed tomography are widely implemented in practice [135,138]. For patients with left-sided breast cancer, intensity-modulated RT and deep inspiration breath-hold (DIBH) technique are also used to reduce the harmful effect of radiation [139–142]. A reduction in the maximum and mean dose received by the ADA or by the whole heart was obtained in several studies evaluating the DIBH technique, but this did not apply to all patients, emphasizing the importance of individual anatomical chest features [140,143–146]. Nowadays, proton therapy—the most precise form of radiation treatment available—is gaining more and more ground in front of photon therapy [147].

Although the most important prophylaxis of IRCAD is to reduce the dose of radiation to the heart and coronary arteries—current RT protocols strive to achieve this—some exposure remains inevitable. Therefore, pharmacologic cardio-protective interventions have been considered as well, mainly focusing on limiting oxidative stress, inflammation, fibrosis, and thrombosis [147].

Statins are drugs with multiple effects. They have lipid-lowering properties, reducing cholesterol and lipoprotein density by inhibiting 3-hydroxy-3-methylglutaryl coenzyme A reductase. However, the mechanism of action of statins exceeds the metabolism of lipids. Their pleiotropic effects are numerous and encompass vascular tone improvement and anti-inflammatory, antithrombotic, antifibrotic, and oxidative stress-reducing properties [148]. The benefit of statin treatment on the atherosclerotic plaque is unquestionable. The inflammation within the atherosclerotic plaque is reduced [149], and the composition and volume are altered, leading to plaque stabilization [150] and even regression [151]. One of the strengths of statins is that they can prevent endothelial damage. Since this is the main trigger of the complex pathophysiological processes leading to both atherosclerosis and fibrosis, statin treatment can hinder the development and progression of atherosclerotic plaques, acting from the early phases of this process [152].

In animal and cell culture models, statins ameliorated radiation-induced inflammation and fibrosis in different tissues [153–155]. When their effect on the heart and blood vessels was specifically assessed, atorvastatin ameliorated radiation-induced cardiac fibrosis, prevented vascular damage, reduced endothelial cell apoptosis, and promoted the healing of the radioactive injuries [124,156,157]. Nevertheless, the association between atorvastatin and an anti-platelet drug, i.e., clopidogrel, failed to inhibit either age-related or radiation-induced atherosclerosis [158]. Lovastatin prevented endothelial cells from radiation-induced cell death [159]. Simvastatin partially mitigated the radiation-induced fibrosis of the penetrating coronary vessels, the severity of MI, and the increase in low-density lipoprotein levels [160]. Pravastatin had anti-inflammatory and antithrombotic effects on endothelial cells [161]. It has the potential to reduce radiation-induced endothelial dysfunction and limit the leukocyte and platelet's adhesion to endothelial cells [162].

Although there is abundant evidence of the beneficial effect of statins in reducing cancer-related and overall morbidity and mortality after RT for thorax, head, and neck cancers [135], the direct assessment of the radio-protective role of statins on the cardiovascular system is still very limited. The main data come from Boulet et al.'s study, which proved that statin treatment provided protection against vascular events by reducing the composite endpoint of stroke, MI, or death caused by stroke or MI [4]. It should be noted that the patients enrolled were over the age of 65, with a history of coronary angiography, ACS, or coronary revascularization, and therefore, the results may be blunted by the high-risk population included. Complementary data are provided by the study of Addison et al. that enrolled younger patients with fewer comorbidities undergoing RT for head and neck cancers [163]. Patients treated with statins during RT had a 60% reduction in the incidence of ischemic stroke or TIA, which confirmed the benefit of statin therapy in reducing the risk of cerebrovascular events. Since no randomized clinical trials offer to date an assessment of the clinical impact of statins on outcomes in radiation-induced vascular disease, this result allows us to only assume that statins could have a similar radio-protective effect on the coronary arteries.

Low-dose aspirin is a widely prescribed drug that can block platelet aggregation, reduce inflammation, and prevent thromboxane A2-induced vasoconstriction. In the general population, all the evidence supports the usefulness of low-dose aspirin in the secondary prevention of cardiovascular disease [105]. In individuals without atherosclerotic disease, more evidence is needed. Still, there is consensus that low-dose aspirin should not be given routinely but only in patients with high or very high cardiovascular disease risk, taking into consideration both ischemic and bleeding risks. In preclinical studies, aspirin showed a radioprotective effect in different tissues [135] but not on the vascular bed [164]. Both nitric oxide-releasing aspirin and aspirin attenuated age-related atherosclerosis but failed to reduce radiation-induced atherosclerosis. In clinical studies, low-dose aspirin registers the overwhelming evidence to reduce cancer mortality [165]. Still, there are no clinical trials to specifically evaluate the role of low-dose aspirin in the modulation and prevention of RICAD.

Angiotensin-converting enzyme inhibitors have multiple effects on endothelial cells. They reduce the endothelial production of angiotensin II and therefore limit vasoconstriction, reduce levels of adhesion molecules and growth factors, decrease oxidative stress, and prevent apoptosis. They also decrease the degradation of endothelial bradykinin, thus leading to vasodilation by stimulating the production of nitric oxide and other relaxing factors [166]. Angiotensin II receptor blockers limit vasoconstriction by selectively inhibiting the AT1 receptor and exert antiplatelet, anti-inflammatory, and antimitogenic effects independently of action on the AT1 receptor [167]. Angiotensin II levels increase locally after irradiation and contribute to inflammatory responses, vascular damage, and fibrosis [168], and as such, limiting these effects could be beneficial. Captopril is the angiotensin-converting enzyme inhibitor with the most evidence of reducing radiation damage in various tissues, most likely due to the sulfhydryl group with the activity of free radical scavenger. Angiotensin II may initiate cardiac perivascular fibrosis, but captopril administration was associated with reduced early radiation-induced cardiac fibrosis [169]. Moreover, captopril exerted inhibitory effects on the TGF-β1-mediated pathway leading from endothelial dysfunction to fibrosis [170]. Preclinical studies showed that AT1-receptor blockade mediated similar radioprotection as the ACE inhibitor [171–173], but there are no data from clinical trials.

Colchicine has anti-inflammatory properties with a mechanism of action independent of the arachidonic acid pathway and reduces thrombin-induced platelet aggregation [174]. It impairs leukocyte mobility and inhibits neutrophil infiltration into the intima. Hence, there are two major advantages: it decreases the risk of atherosclerotic plaque destabilization and mitigates the fibrotic process, as neutrophils are their major contributors [175]. In clinical trials, colchicine reduced the risk of MI in patients with CAD [176], and based on these encouraging results, low-dose colchicine may be considered in selected high-risk patients with the established atherosclerotic disease [105]. The possibility of using colchicine in the prevention of RICAD has been highlighted based on preclinical data and results from trials in patients with CAD in the general population [135,177,178]. However, there are no clinical trials specifically evaluating colchicine in the prevention of RICAD.

Despite the presence of data showing the association between RT and vascular disease, be it additive or multiplicative to traditional cardiovascular risk factors, no guidelines currently exist for the treatment or prevention of radiation-induced atherosclerosis. Risk factor modification appears to have the greatest potential for reducing RICHD risk though it has not been prospectively studied and should begin prior to RT.

6. Discussion

The burden of cancer incidence and cancer-related deaths is growing rapidly worldwide. The International Agency for Research on Cancer has announced that 19.3 million new cancer cases and 10.0 million cancer-related deaths occurred in 2020 [179]. Breast, lung, colorectal, prostate, and gastric cancers are the malignancies with the highest global incidence, accounting for 11.7, 11.4, 10, 7.3, and 5.6% of all newly diagnosed cancers, respectively. In men, lung cancer ranks first (14.3%), followed by prostate (14.1%), colorectal (10.6%), and gastric cancers (7.1%). Breast (24.5%), colorectal (9.4%), and lung cancers (8.4%) are the most common newly diagnosed malignancies in women. In the last decade, in many countries, the prevention and treatment of cardiovascular disease have intensified, leading to a marked decrease in the mortality rate caused by stroke and CAD relative to cancer, which has now positioned cancer as the leading cause of death in the world. Lung cancer is responsible for 18% of all cancer-related deaths. In terms of mortality, it ranks first in men and second in women after breast cancer [179].

In the last 30 years, more than 150 new molecules have been introduced into the treatment of cancer. Platinum-based anticancer drugs, anti-angiogenesis agents, and anthracyclines are among the most prescribed anticancer drugs today [180–182]. Moreover, platinum-based anticancer drugs are used as components of almost half of all cancer treatments. Among anti-angiogenesis agents, those targeting the VEGF pathway are by far the most commonly used. FPs are currently the third most commonly used anticancer drug in the treatment of solid cancers, such as colorectal and breast cancer [183]. RT is frequently used in combination with surgery or systemic CT, and more than half of patients receive RT as part of their cancer treatment.

Due to the high frequency of cancers globally and the widespread use of potentially cardiotoxic antineoplastic drugs, the possibility of cardiovascular adverse events during evidence-based oncological treatments should be considered. Many cancers are diagnosed after the age of 50, when cardiovascular risk factors such as high blood pressure, diabetes mellitus, dyslipidemia, obesity, and smoking may be present, which can exacerbate the cardiovascular toxicity of some anticancer drugs [184].

Cancer treatments induce endothelial dysfunction, spasm of the coronary arteries, thrombosis, and fibrosis. The effort to mitigate these harmful pathophysiological processes is hampered by the lack of randomized studies to provide robust and reliable data. Although unitary as a concept, all starting from the pathophysiological triad aforementioned, the therapeutic lines of prevention that have been outlined so far have a number of individual features determined by the mechanism of action of the anticancer drug (Table 1).

Vascular injury may have clinical expression during or shortly after treatment, as in the case of oncological therapy that induces vasospasm or thrombosis, or it may develop asymptomatically for a long time, as in the case of atheroma plaque formation and growth. The symptoms may occur months and sometimes years following the completion of CT. Factors attributable to the drug, such as type of drug, cumulative or total dose, and schedule, along with individual factors influence the incidence and severity of CT-induced adverse cardiac effects [20].

For other anticancer drugs, namely anthracyclines, the hypothesis of impaired coronary circulation as a contributor to their cardiac toxicity is gaining increasing interest. Although they have been in use for more than half a century and are the anticancer drugs the most associated with CT-induced cardiac toxicity, the exact mechanism by which heart damage occurs is not yet fully elucidated [182,185]. Anthracyclines' main adverse cardiac effect is overt heart failure or a drop in the left ventricular ejection fraction [186]. There is indirect evidence of the toxic effect of anthracyclines on coronary arteries. In cultured cells, doxorubicin and daunorubicin caused endothelial cell dysfunction by increasing oxidative stress in the vessel wall [187,188]. Moreover, anthracyclines induced apoptosis in smooth muscle cells [189] and increased the thickness of media, adventitia, and total coronary arteriolar wall [190]. Recently, in an animal model, it was shown that anthracyclines produced irreversibly damage to the coronary microcirculation [191], and in patients with lymphoma, defects were identified in myocardial perfusion by positron emission tomography after a single doxorubicin dose [192]. Therefore, in-depth research on the effect of oncological therapy on coronary arteries is expected to provide clear answers in the future for many of the current unknowns related to the cardiac toxic effects of anticancer drugs.

Several practical aspects must be retained. Firstly, the cardiovascular risk factors must be identified since they are important contributors to the progression of atherosclerosis and the onset of acute coronary events. This is of major concern since studies of cancer survivors beyond 5 years post-diagnosis have demonstrated a 1.7- to 18.5-times increased incidence of cardiovascular risk factors including hypertension, diabetes mellitus, and dyslipidemia when compared with age-matched counterparts without a history of cancer [193]. Lifestyle changes such as smoking cessation and exercise and pharmacological therapies are similar to those in the general population although some authors have proposed stricter targets [79,103]. Baseline risk stratification proformas are currently available and allow clinicians to stratify cancer patients into low-, medium-, high-, and very-high-risk categories of cardiovascular complications prior to starting treatment and whenever needed during treatment. The ultimate goal is to provide personalized approaches to minimize the risk of cardiovascular toxicity from cancer therapies [98].

Table 1. Mechanisms of CAD induced by cancer treatment and proposed interventions.

Drug	Mechanism	Intervention	References
Antimetabolites (5-FU, Capecitabine, Gemcitabine)	Coronary artery spasm Intravascular thrombosis Endothelial injury	Immediate discontinuation of the drug Calcium channel blockers Long-acting nitrates Short-acting nitrates (on demand) Low-dose aspirin Dalteparin [b] Probucol [b]	[25,26,31,35–39,41]
Platinum Compounds (Cisplatin)	Intravascular thrombosis Coronary artery spasm Coronary artery dissection Endothelial injury Accelerated atherosclerosis Proatherogenic dyslipidemia Hypertension Insulin resistance	Decreased dose or discontinuation of the drug Calcium channel blockers Long-acting nitrates Low-dose aspirin [a] Statins [a] N-Acetyl-l-cysteine [b] Acetyl-carnitine [b] α-lipoic acid [b] Silymarin [b]	[53,56,64,65,67]
VEGF/VEGFR inhibitors (Bevacizumab, Sorafenib, Sunitinib)	Intravascular thrombosis Endothelial injury Hypertension	RAS inhibitors Calcium channel blockers (only DHP) Beta-blockers (only carvedilol) Diuretics Long-acting nitrates Statins Low-dose aspirin [a]	[79,84,90,96,100–102,104,106,107]
Radiotherapy	Accelerated atherosclerosis Endothelial injury Plaque rupture Intravascular thrombosis	Radiation dose reduction Statins RAS inhibitors [b] Low-dose aspirin [a] Colchicine [b]	[135,138–147] [4,158–163] [135,164,165] [169–173] [135,177,178]

[a] selected cases; [b] non-human studies; 5-FU, 5-fluorouracil; VEGF, vascular endothelial growth factor; VEGFR, vascular endothelial growth factor receptor; DHP, dihydropyridines; RAS, renin-angiotensin system.

Secondly, there are no randomized clinical trials specifically dedicated to the study of prevention measures to support any specific strategy. The available data come from studies evaluating specific oncological therapies in specific types of cancers, so a general conclusion is far from drawn. However, there is a benefit the existence of a sufficient amount of evidence to allow some modulation and customization in cancer patients of the treatments indicated in the general population, including medical therapy, PCI, and CABG.

Although based on an extensive search, our study has several limitations. Firstly, there was no universal definition of the cardiovascular toxicities of anticancer drugs until earlier this year, when an international consensus statement defined the cardiovascular toxicities of cancer therapies [194]. In the already published literature, the term includes the myocardial, pericardial, endocardial, and conduction systems and CAD due to cancer treatments, which made it difficult to select only the information related to coronary arteries. Moreover, many studies reported acute thromboembolic events as a sum of coronary and cerebral arterial events. Secondly, there are many therapeutic agents used in the treatment of cancers and a huge amount of literature published so far, sometimes with conflicting data, which made it difficult to interpret them. Moreover, some drugs have recently been introduced in practice and therefore offer little or no data on the effects on the coronary arteries.

7. Conclusions

Antineoplastic therapy saves or at least prolongs life, but this is achieved at the cost of major side effects, such as cardiovascular ones. CAD and especially acute MI have the potential to limit the benefits of cancer treatment. Our work provides the most comprehensive, systematized, structured, and up-to-date analysis of the available literature, focusing on measures aiming to protect the coronary arteries from the toxicity of cancer therapy. This approach facilitates their implementation in daily practice.

Author Contributions: Conceptualization, M.C.B., O.V.B., D.V.S. and L.I.B.; methodology, I.B.-B. and D.P.; writing—original draft preparation, M.C.B., O.V.B., D.V.S. and L.I.B.; writing—review and editing, M.C., I.I.C. and E.R.; supervision, E.V.G. and C.R. All authors have read and agreed to the published version of the manuscript.

Funding: This research received no external funding.

Institutional Review Board Statement: Not applicable.

Informed Consent Statement: Not applicable.

Data Availability Statement: Not applicable.

Conflicts of Interest: The authors declare no conflict of interest.

References

1. Siegel, R.L.; Miller, K.D.; Jemal, A. Cancer statistics, 2015. *CA Cancer J. Clin.* **2015**, *65*, 5–29. [CrossRef] [PubMed]
2. De Angelis, R.; Sant, M.; Coleman, M.P.; Francisci, S.; Baili, P.; Pierannunzio, D.; Trama, A.; Visser, O.; Brenner, H.; Ardanaz, E.; et al. Cancer survival in Europe 1999–2007 by country and age: Results of EUROCARE–5-a population-based study. *Lancet Oncol.* **2014**, *15*, 23–34. [CrossRef]
3. Han, X.J.; Li, J.Q.; Khannanova, Z.; Li, Y. Optimal management of coronary artery disease in cancer patients. *Chronic Dis. Transl. Med.* **2019**, *5*, 221–233. [CrossRef] [PubMed]
4. Boulet, J.; Pena, J.; Hulten, E.A.; Neilan, T.G.; Dragomir, A.; Freeman, C.; Lambert, C.; Hijal, T.; Nadeau, L.; Brophy, J.M.; et al. Statin Use and Risk of Vascular Events Among Cancer Patients After Radiotherapy to the Thorax, Head, and Neck. *J. Am. Heart Assoc.* **2019**, *8*, e005996. [CrossRef] [PubMed]
5. Zamorano, J.L.; Lancellotti, P.; Rodriguez Munoz, D.; Aboyans, V.; Asteggiano, R.; Galderisi, M.; Habib, G.; Lenihan, D.J.; Lip, G.Y.H.; Lyon, A.R.; et al. 2016 ESC Position Paper on cancer treatments and cardiovascular toxicity developed under the auspices of the ESC Committee for Practice Guidelines: The Task Force for cancer treatments and cardiovascular toxicity of the European Society of Cardiology (ESC). *Eur. Heart J.* **2016**, *37*, 2768–2801. [CrossRef]
6. Belzile-Dugas, E.; Eisenberg, M.J. Radiation-Induced Cardiovascular Disease: Review of an Underrecognized Pathology. *J. Am. Heart Assoc.* **2021**, *10*, e021686. [CrossRef]
7. Min, S.S.; Wierzbicki, A.S. Radiotherapy, chemotherapy and atherosclerosis. *Curr. Opin. Cardiol.* **2017**, *32*, 441–447. [CrossRef]
8. Carlson, L.E.; Watt, G.P.; Tonorezos, E.S.; Chow, E.J.; Yu, A.F.; Woods, M.; Lynch, C.F.; John, E.M.; Mellemkjr, L.; Brooks, J.D.; et al. Coronary Artery Disease in Young Women After Radiation Therapy for Breast Cancer: The WECARE Study. *JACC Cardio Oncol.* **2021**, *3*, 381–392. [CrossRef]
9. Haugnes, H.S.; Wethal, T.; Aass, N.; Dahl, O.; Klepp, O.; Langberg, C.W.; Wilsgaard, T.; Bremnes, R.M.; Fossa, S.D. Cardiovascular risk factors and morbidity in long-term survivors of testicular cancer: A 20-year follow-up study. *J. Clin. Oncol.* **2010**, *28*, 4649–4657. [CrossRef]
10. Miura, K.; Kinouchi, M.; Ishida, K.; Fujibuchi, W.; Naitoh, T.; Ogawa, H.; Ando, T.; Yazaki, N.; Watanabe, K.; Haneda, S.; et al. 5-FU metabolism in cancer and orally-administrable 5-FU drugs. *Cancers* **2010**, *2*, 1717–1730. [CrossRef]
11. Sara, J.D.; Kaur, J.; Khodadadi, R.; Rehman, M.; Lobo, R.; Chakrabarti, S.; Herrmann, J.; Lerman, A.; Grothey, A. 5-fluorouracil and cardiotoxicity: A review. *Ther. Adv. Med. Oncol.* **2018**, *10*, 1758835918780140. [CrossRef] [PubMed]
12. Lestuzzi, C.; Vaccher, E.; Talamini, R.; Lleshi, A.; Meneguzzo, N.; Viel, E.; Scalone, S.; Tartuferi, L.; Buonadonna, A.; Ejiofor, L.; et al. Effort myocardial ischemia during chemotherapy with 5-fluorouracil: An underestimated risk. *Ann. Oncol.* **2014**, *25*, 1059–1064. [CrossRef]
13. Rezkalla, S.; Kloner, R.A.; Ensley, J.; al-Sarraf, M.; Revels, S.; Olivenstein, A.; Bhasin, S.; Kerpel-Fronious, S.; Turi, Z.G. Continuous ambulatory ECG monitoring during fluorouracil therapy: A prospective study. *J. Clin. Oncol.* **1989**, *7*, 509–514. [CrossRef]
14. Ng, M.; Cunningham, D.; Norman, A.R. The frequency and pattern of cardiotoxicity observed with capecitabine used in conjunction with oxaliplatin in patients treated for advanced colorectal cancer (CRC). *Eur. J. Cancer* **2005**, *41*, 1542–1546. [CrossRef] [PubMed]
15. Hilmi, M.; Ederhy, S.; Waintraub, X.; Funck-Brentano, C.; Cohen, A.; Vozy, A.; Lebrun-Vignes, B.; Moslehi, J.; Nguyen, L.S.; Salem, J.E. Cardiotoxicity Associated with Gemcitabine: Literature Review and a Pharmacovigilance Study. *Pharmaceuticals* **2020**, *13*, 325. [CrossRef]
16. Shiga, T.; Hiraide, M. Cardiotoxicities of 5-Fluorouracil and Other Fluoropyrimidines. *Curr. Treat Options Oncol.* **2020**, *21*, 27. [CrossRef] [PubMed]
17. Saif, M.W.; Shah, M.M.; Shah, A.R. Fluoropyrimidine-associated cardiotoxicity: Revisited. *Expert Opin. Drug Saf.* **2009**, *8*, 191–202. [CrossRef]

18. Mosseri, M.; Fingert, H.J.; Varticovski, L.; Chokshi, S.; Isner, J.M. In vitro evidence that myocardial ischemia resulting from 5-fluorouracil chemotherapy is due to protein kinase C-mediated vasoconstriction of vascular smooth muscle. *Cancer Res.* **1993**, *53*, 3028–3033.
19. Thyss, A.; Gaspard, M.H.; Marsault, R.; Milano, G.; Frelin, C.; Schneider, M. Very high endothelin plasma levels in patients with 5-FU cardiotoxicity. *Ann. Oncol.* **1992**, *3*, 88. [CrossRef]
20. Ozturk, B.; Tacoy, G.; Coskun, U.; Yaman, E.; Sahin, G.; Buyukberber, S.; Yildiz, R.; Kaya, A.O.; Topal, S.; Ozdemir, M.; et al. Gemcitabine-induced acute coronary syndrome: A case report. *Med. Princ. Pract.* **2009**, *18*, 76–80. [CrossRef]
21. Shoemaker, L.K.; Arora, U.; Rocha Lima, C.M. 5-fluorouracil-induced coronary vasospasm. *Cancer Control* **2004**, *11*, 46–49. [CrossRef] [PubMed]
22. Layoun, M.E.; Wickramasinghe, C.D.; Peralta, M.V.; Yang, E.H. Fluoropyrimidine-Induced Cardiotoxicity: Manifestations, Mechanisms, and Management. *Curr. Oncol. Rep.* **2016**, *18*, 35. [CrossRef] [PubMed]
23. Polk, A.; Vistisen, K.; Vaage-Nilsen, M.; Nielsen, D.L. A systematic review of the pathophysiology of 5-fluorouracil-induced cardiotoxicity. *BMC Pharmacol. Toxicol.* **2014**, *15*, 47. [CrossRef]
24. Jensen, S.A.; Sorensen, J.B. Risk factors and prevention of cardiotoxicity induced by 5-fluorouracil or capecitabine. *Cancer Chemother. Pharmacol.* **2006**, *58*, 487–493. [CrossRef] [PubMed]
25. Kinhult, S.; Albertsson, M.; Eskilsson, J.; Cwikiel, M. Antithrombotic treatment in protection against thrombogenic effects of 5-fluorouracil on vascular endothelium: A scanning microscopy evaluation. *Scanning* **2001**, *23*, 1–8. [CrossRef] [PubMed]
26. Kinhult, S.; Albertsson, M.; Eskilsson, J.; Cwikiel, M. Effects of probucol on endothelial damage by 5-fluorouracil. *Acta Oncol.* **2003**, *42*, 304–308. [CrossRef]
27. Focaccetti, C.; Bruno, A.; Magnani, E.; Bartolini, D.; Principi, E.; Dallaglio, K.; Bucci, E.O.; Finzi, G.; Sessa, F.; Noonan, D.M.; et al. Effects of 5-fluorouracil on morphology, cell cycle, proliferation, apoptosis, autophagy and ROS production in endothelial cells and cardiomyocytes. *PLoS ONE* **2015**, *10*, e0115686. [CrossRef]
28. Spasojevic, I.; Jelic, S.; Zakrzewska, J.; Bacic, G. Decreased oxygen transfer capacity of erythrocytes as a cause of 5-fluorouracil related ischemia. *Molecules* **2008**, *14*, 53–67. [CrossRef]
29. Karakulak, U.N.; Aladag, E.; Maharjan, N.; Ovunc, K. Capecitabine-induced coronary artery vasospasm in a patient who previously experienced a similar episode with fluorouracil therapy. *Turk Kardiyol Dern Ars* **2016**, *44*, 71–74. [CrossRef]
30. Wijesinghe, N.; Thompson, P.I.; McAlister, H. Acute coronary syndrome induced by capecitabine therapy. *Heart Lung Circ.* **2006**, *15*, 337–339. [CrossRef]
31. Yuan, C.; Parekh, H.; Allegra, C.; George, T.J.; Starr, J.S. 5-FU induced cardiotoxicity: Case series and review of the literature. *Cardiooncology* **2019**, *5*, 13. [CrossRef]
32. Bdair, F.M.; Graham, S.P.; Smith, P.F.; Javle, M.M. Gemcitabine and acute myocardial infarction–a case report. *Angiology* **2006**, *57*, 367–371. [CrossRef] [PubMed]
33. Dumontet, C.; Morschhauser, F.; Solal-Celigny, P.; Bouafia, F.; Bourgeois, E.; Thieblemont, C.; Leleu, X.; Hequet, O.; Salles, G.; Coiffier, B. Gemcitabine as a single agent in the treatment of relapsed or refractory low-grade non-Hodgkin's lymphoma. *Br. J. Haematol.* **2001**, *113*, 772–778. [CrossRef] [PubMed]
34. Kalapura, T.; Krishnamurthy, M.; Reddy, C.V. Acute myocardial infarction following gemcitabine therapy—A case report. *Angiology* **1999**, *50*, 1021–1025. [CrossRef] [PubMed]
35. Farina, A.; Malafronte, C.; Valsecchi, M.A.; Achilli, F. Capecitabine-induced cardiotoxicity: When to suspect? How to manage? A case report. *J. Cardiovasc. Med.* **2009**, *10*, 722–726. [CrossRef] [PubMed]
36. Senturk, T.; Kanat, O.; Evrensel, T.; Aydinlar, A. Capecitabine-induced cardiotoxicity mimicking myocardial infarction. *Neth. Heart J.* **2009**, *17*, 277–280. [CrossRef]
37. Eskilsson, J.; Albertsson, M. Failure of preventing 5-fluorouracil cardiotoxicity by prophylactic treatment with verapamil. *Acta Oncol.* **1990**, *29*, 1001–1003. [CrossRef]
38. Ambrosy, A.P.; Kunz, P.L.; Fisher, G.A.; Witteles, R.M. Capecitabine-induced chest pain relieved by diltiazem. *Am. J. Cardiol.* **2012**, *110*, 1623–1626. [CrossRef]
39. Oleksowicz, L.; Bruckner, H.W. Prophylaxis of 5-fluorouracil-induced coronary vasospasm with calcium channel blockers. *Am. J. Med.* **1988**, *85*, 750–751. [CrossRef]
40. Senkus, E.; Jassem, J. Cardiovascular effects of systemic cancer treatment. *Cancer Treat Rev.* **2011**, *37*, 300–311. [CrossRef]
41. Clasen, S.C.; Ky, B.; O'Quinn, R.; Giantonio, B.; Teitelbaum, U.; Carver, J.R. Fluoropyrimidine-induced cardiac toxicity: Challenging the current paradigm. *J. Gastrointest. Oncol.* **2017**, *8*, 970–979. [CrossRef] [PubMed]
42. Chovanec, M.; Abu Zaid, M.; Hanna, N.; El-Kouri, N.; Einhorn, L.H.; Albany, C. Long-term toxicity of cisplatin in germ-cell tumor survivors. *Ann. Oncol.* **2017**, *28*, 2670–2679. [CrossRef] [PubMed]
43. Weijl, N.I.; Rutten, M.F.; Zwinderman, A.H.; Keizer, H.J.; Nooy, M.A.; Rosendaal, F.R.; Cleton, F.J.; Osanto, S. Thromboembolic events during chemotherapy for germ cell cancer: A cohort study and review of the literature. *J. Clin. Oncol.* **2000**, *18*, 2169–2178. [CrossRef] [PubMed]
44. Soultati, A.; Mountzios, G.; Avgerinou, C.; Papaxoinis, G.; Pectasides, D.; Dimopoulos, M.A.; Papadimitriou, C. Endothelial vascular toxicity from chemotherapeutic agents: Preclinical evidence and clinical implications. *Cancer Treat Rev.* **2012**, *38*, 473–483. [CrossRef]

45. Hanchate, L.P.; Sharma, S.R.; Madyalkar, S. Cisplatin Induced Acute Myocardial Infarction and Dyslipidemia. *J. Clin. Diagn. Res.* 2017, *11*, OD05–OD07. [CrossRef]
46. Wang, G.; Su, C.; Yin, T. Paclitaxel and platinum-based chemotherapy results in transient dyslipidemia in cancer patients. *Mol. Clin. Oncol.* 2017, *6*, 261–265. [CrossRef]
47. Meinardi, M.T.; Gietema, J.A.; van der Graaf, W.T.; van Veldhuisen, D.J.; Runne, M.A.; Sluiter, W.J.; de Vries, E.G.; Willemse, P.B.; Mulder, N.H.; van den Berg, M.P.; et al. Cardiovascular morbidity in long-term survivors of metastatic testicular cancer. *J. Clin. Oncol.* 2000, *18*, 1725–1732. [CrossRef]
48. Haugnes, H.S.; Aass, N.; Fossa, S.D.; Dahl, O.; Klepp, O.; Wist, E.A.; Svartberg, J.; Wilsgaard, T.; Bremnes, R.M. Components of the metabolic syndrome in long-term survivors of testicular cancer. *Ann. Oncol.* 2007, *18*, 241–248. [CrossRef]
49. Moore, R.A.; Adel, N.; Riedel, E.; Bhutani, M.; Feldman, D.R.; Tabbara, N.E.; Soff, G.; Parameswaran, R.; Hassoun, H. High incidence of thromboembolic events in patients treated with cisplatin-based chemotherapy: A large retrospective analysis. *J. Clin. Oncol.* 2011, *29*, 3466–3473. [CrossRef]
50. Centola, M.; Lucreziotti, S.; Cazzaniga, S.; Salerno-Uriarte, D.; Sponzilli, C.; Carugo, S. A rare case of large intracoronary thrombosis in advanced breast cancer patient treated with epirubicin and cisplatin. *J. Cardiovasc. Med.* 2016, *17* (Suppl S2), e241–e243. [CrossRef]
51. Khalid, S.B.; Mahmood, J. Cisplatin induced coronary artery atherosclerosis leading to ST-elevation myocardial infarction: A case report. *Circulation* 2021, *144*, A17234. [CrossRef]
52. Karabay, K.O.; Yildiz, O.; Aytekin, V. Multiple coronary thrombi with cisplatin. *J. Invasive Cardiol.* 2014, *26*, E18–E20. [PubMed]
53. Berliner, S.; Rahima, M.; Sidi, Y.; Teplitsky, Y.; Zohar, Y.; Nussbaum, B.; Pinkhas, J. Acute coronary events following cisplatin-based chemotherapy. *Cancer Investig.* 1990, *8*, 583–586. [CrossRef] [PubMed]
54. Scafa-Udriste, A.; Popa-Fotea, N.M.; Bataila, V.; Calmac, L.; Dorobantu, M. Acute inferior myocardial infarction in a young man with testicular seminoma: A case report. *World J. Clin. Cases* 2021, *9*, 4040–4045. [CrossRef] [PubMed]
55. Fukuda, M.; Oka, M.; Itoh, N.; Sakamoto, T.; Mori, H.; Hayakawa, A.; Kohno, S. Vasospastic angina likely related to cisplatin-containing chemotherapy and thoracic irradiation for lung cancer. *Intern. Med.* 1999, *38*, 436–438. [CrossRef] [PubMed]
56. Rao, A.S.; Kumar, R.; Narayanan, G.S. A rare case of cisplatin-induced acute myocardial infarction in a patient receiving chemoradiation for lung cancer. *J. Cancer Res. Ther.* 2015, *11*, 983–985. [CrossRef]
57. Somov, P.; Marchak, D.; Matusov, A.; Viller, A.; Shevchenko, Y.; Miminoshvili, A. Spontaneous coronary artery dissection during cisplatin and capecitabine therapy. *Ann. Med. Surg.* 2019, *45*, 1–5. [CrossRef]
58. Brinkmann, M.; Tallone, E.M.; Wurschmidt, F.; Wulfing, C.; Dieckmann, K.P. Myocardial infarction in a young patient with seminoma during chemotherapy with cisplatinum, etoposide, and bleomycin. *Aktuelle Urol.* 2021, *52*, 54–57. [CrossRef]
59. Feldman, D.R.; Schaffer, W.L.; Steingart, R.M. Late cardiovascular toxicity following chemotherapy for germ cell tumors. *J. Natl. Compr. Cancer Netw.* 2012, *10*, 537–544. [CrossRef]
60. Bjerring, A.W.; Fossa, S.D.; Haugnes, H.S.; Nome, R.; Stokke, T.M.; Haugaa, K.H.; Kiserud, C.E.; Edvardsen, T.; Sarvari, S.I. The cardiac impact of cisplatin-based chemotherapy in survivors of testicular cancer: A 30-year follow-up. *Eur. Heart J. Cardiovasc. Imaging* 2021, *22*, 443–450. [CrossRef]
61. Cameron, A.C.; Touyz, R.M.; Lang, N.N. Vascular Complications of Cancer Chemotherapy. *Can. J. Cardiol.* 2016, *32*, 852–862. [CrossRef] [PubMed]
62. Nuver, J.; Smit, A.J.; van der Meer, J.; van den Berg, M.P.; van der Graaf, W.T.; Meinardi, M.T.; Sleijfer, D.T.; Hoekstra, H.J.; van Gessel, A.I.; van Roon, A.M.; et al. Acute chemotherapy-induced cardiovascular changes in patients with testicular cancer. *J. Clin. Oncol.* 2005, *23*, 9130–9137. [CrossRef] [PubMed]
63. Sasaki, W.; Wada, H.; Sakakura, K.; Matsuda, J.; Ibe, T.; Hayashi, T.; Ueba, H.; Momomura, S.I.; Fujita, H. Coronary vasospasm induced by cisplatin for seminoma. *Clin. Case Rep.* 2020, *8*, 190–193. [CrossRef] [PubMed]
64. Rosic, G.; Srejovic, I.; Zivkovic, V.; Selakovic, D.; Joksimovic, J.; Jakovljevic, V. The effects of N-acetylcysteine on cisplatin-induced cardiotoxicity on isolated rat hearts after short-term global ischemia. *Toxicol. Rep.* 2015, *2*, 996–1006. [CrossRef] [PubMed]
65. El-Awady, S.E.; Moustafa, Y.M.; Abo-Elmatty, D.M.; Radwan, A. Cisplatin-induced cardiotoxicity: Mechanisms and cardioprotective strategies. *Eur. J. Pharmacol.* 2011, *650*, 335–341. [CrossRef] [PubMed]
66. Knuuti, J.; Wijns, W.; Saraste, A.; Capodanno, D.; Barbato, E.; Funck-Brentano, C.; Prescott, E.; Storey, R.F.; Deaton, C.; Cuisset, T.; et al. Corrigendum to: 2019 ESC Guidelines for the diagnosis and management of chronic coronary syndromes. *Eur. Heart J.* 2020, *41*, 4242. [CrossRef]
67. Song, J.K. Coronary Artery Vasospasm. *Korean Circ. J.* 2018, *48*, 767–777. [CrossRef]
68. Willemse, P.M.; van der Meer, R.W.; Burggraaf, J.; van Elderen, S.G.; de Kam, M.L.; de Roos, A.; Lamb, H.J.; Osanto, S. Abdominal visceral and subcutaneous fat increase, insulin resistance and hyperlipidemia in testicular cancer patients treated with cisplatin-based chemotherapy. *Acta Oncol.* 2014, *53*, 351–360. [CrossRef]
69. de Haas, E.C.; Altena, R.; Boezen, H.M.; Zwart, N.; Smit, A.J.; Bakker, S.J.; van Roon, A.M.; Postma, A.; Wolffenbuttel, B.H.; Hoekstra, H.J.; et al. Early development of the metabolic syndrome after chemotherapy for testicular cancer. *Ann. Oncol.* 2013, *24*, 749–755. [CrossRef]
70. Westerink, N.L.; Nuver, J.; Lefrandt, J.D.; Vrieling, A.H.; Gietema, J.A.; Walenkamp, A.M. Cancer treatment induced metabolic syndrome: Improving outcome with lifestyle. *Crit. Rev. Oncol. Hematol.* 2016, *108*, 128–136. [CrossRef]

71. Christensen, J.F.; Bandak, M.; Campbell, A.; Jones, L.W.; Hojman, P. Treatment-related cardiovascular late effects and exercise training countermeasures in testicular germ cell cancer survivorship. *Acta Oncol.* **2015**, *54*, 592–599. [CrossRef] [PubMed]
72. Barata, P.C.; Rini, B.I. Treatment of renal cell carcinoma: Current status and future directions. *CA Cancer J. Clin.* **2017**, *67*, 507–524. [CrossRef]
73. Tian, W.; Cao, C.; Shu, L.; Wu, F. Anti-Angiogenic Therapy in the Treatment of Non-Small Cell Lung Cancer. *Onco Targets Ther.* **2020**, *13*, 12113–12129. [CrossRef] [PubMed]
74. Mossenta, M.; Busato, D.; Baboci, L.; Cintio, F.D.; Toffoli, G.; Bo, M.D. New Insight into Therapies Targeting Angiogenesis in Hepatocellular Carcinoma. *Cancers* **2019**, *11*, 1086. [CrossRef] [PubMed]
75. Capozzi, M.; von Arx, C.; de Divitiis, C.; Ottaiano, A.; Tatangelo, F.; Romano, G.M.; Tafuto, S. Antiangiogenic therapy in pancreatic neuroendocrine tumors. *Anticancer Res.* **2016**, *36*, 5025–5030. [CrossRef]
76. Fudalej, M.M.; Badowska-Kozakiewicz, A.M. Improved understanding of gastrointestinal stromal tumors biology as a step for developing new diagnostic and therapeutic schemes. *Oncol. Lett.* **2021**, *21*, 417. [CrossRef]
77. Baraniskin, A.; Buchberger, B.; Pox, C.; Graeven, U.; Holch, J.W.; Schmiegel, W.; Heinemann, V. Efficacy of bevacizumab in first-line treatment of metastatic colorectal cancer: A systematic review and meta-analysis. *Eur. J. Cancer* **2019**, *106*, 37–44. [CrossRef]
78. Ayoub, N.M.; Jaradat, S.K.; Al-Shami, K.M.; Alkhalifa, A.E. Targeting Angiogenesis in Breast Cancer: Current Evidence and Future Perspectives of Novel Anti-Angiogenic Approaches. *Front. Pharmacol.* **2022**, *13*, 838133. [CrossRef]
79. Touyz, R.M.; Herrmann, S.M.S.; Herrmann, J. Vascular toxicities with VEGF inhibitor therapies-focus on hypertension and arterial thrombotic events. *J. Am. Soc. Hypertens.* **2018**, *12*, 409–425. [CrossRef]
80. Jain, R.K.; Duda, D.G.; Clark, J.W.; Loeffler, J.S. Lessons from phase III clinical trials on anti-VEGF therapy for cancer. *Nat. Clin. Pract. Oncol.* **2006**, *3*, 24–40. [CrossRef]
81. Chen, X.L.; Lei, Y.H.; Liu, C.F.; Yang, Q.F.; Zuo, P.Y.; Liu, C.Y.; Chen, C.Z.; Liu, Y.W. Angiogenesis inhibitor bevacizumab increases the risk of ischemic heart disease associated with chemotherapy: A meta-analysis. *PLoS ONE* **2013**, *8*, e66721. [CrossRef] [PubMed]
82. Gonzalez-Pacheco, F.R.; Deudero, J.J.; Castellanos, M.C.; Castilla, M.A.; Alvarez-Arroyo, M.V.; Yague, S.; Caramelo, C. Mechanisms of endothelial response to oxidative aggression: Protective role of autologous VEGF and induction of VEGFR2 by H2O2. *Am. J. Physiol. Heart Circ. Physiol.* **2006**, *291*, H1395–H1401. [CrossRef] [PubMed]
83. Ranpura, V.; Hapani, S.; Chuang, J.; Wu, S. Risk of cardiac ischemia and arterial thromboembolic events with the angiogenesis inhibitor bevacizumab in cancer patients: A meta-analysis of randomized controlled trials. *Acta Oncol.* **2010**, *49*, 287–297. [CrossRef]
84. Scappaticci, F.A.; Skillings, J.R.; Holden, S.N.; Gerber, H.P.; Miller, K.; Kabbinavar, F.; Bergsland, E.; Ngai, J.; Holmgren, E.; Wang, J.; et al. Arterial thromboembolic events in patients with metastatic carcinoma treated with chemotherapy and bevacizumab. *J. Natl. Cancer Inst.* **2007**, *99*, 1232–1239. [CrossRef]
85. Totzeck, M.; Mincu, R.I.; Rassaf, T. Cardiovascular Adverse Events in Patients With Cancer Treated With Bevacizumab: A Meta-Analysis of More Than 20 000 Patients. *J. Am. Heart Assoc.* **2017**, *6*, e006278. [CrossRef] [PubMed]
86. Choueiri, T.K.; Schutz, F.A.; Je, Y.; Rosenberg, J.E.; Bellmunt, J. Risk of arterial thromboembolic events with sunitinib and sorafenib: A systematic review and meta-analysis of clinical trials. *J. Clin. Oncol.* **2010**, *28*, 2280–2285. [CrossRef]
87. Escudier, B.; Eisen, T.; Stadler, W.M.; Szczylik, C.; Oudard, S.; Siebels, M.; Negrier, S.; Chevreau, C.; Solska, E.; Desai, A.A.; et al. Sorafenib in advanced clear-cell renal-cell carcinoma. *N. Engl. J. Med.* **2007**, *356*, 125–134. [CrossRef]
88. Ueda, K.; Suekane, S.; Ogasawara, N.; Chikui, K.; Suyama, S.; Nakiri, M.; Nishihara, K.; Matsuo, M.; Igawa, T. Long-term response of over ten years with sorafenib monotherapy in metastatic renal cell carcinoma: A case report. *J. Med. Case Rep.* **2016**, *10*, 177. [CrossRef]
89. Zhang, D.; Zhang, X.; Zhao, C. Risk of venous and arterial thromboembolic events associated with anti-VEGF agents in advanced non-small-cell lung cancer: A meta-analysis and systematic review. *Onco Targets Ther.* **2016**, *9*, 3695–3704. [CrossRef]
90. Tebbutt, N.C.; Murphy, F.; Zannino, D.; Wilson, K.; Cummins, M.M.; Abdi, E.; Strickland, A.H.; Lowenthal, R.M.; Marx, G.; Karapetis, C.; et al. Risk of arterial thromboembolic events in patients with advanced colorectal cancer receiving bevacizumab. *Ann. Oncol.* **2011**, *22*, 1834–1838. [CrossRef]
91. Herrmann, J.; Yang, E.H.; Iliescu, C.A.; Cilingiroglu, M.; Charitakis, K.; Hakeem, A.; Toutouzas, K.; Leesar, M.A.; Grines, C.L.; Marmagkiolis, K. Vascular Toxicities of Cancer Therapies: The Old and the New–An Evolving Avenue. *Circulation* **2016**, *133*, 1272–1289. [CrossRef] [PubMed]
92. Schmidinger, M.; Zielinski, C.C.; Vogl, U.M.; Bojic, A.; Bojic, M.; Schukro, C.; Ruhsam, M.; Hejna, M.; Schmidinger, H. Cardiac toxicity of sunitinib and sorafenib in patients with metastatic renal cell carcinoma. *J. Clin. Oncol.* **2008**, *26*, 5204–5212. [CrossRef] [PubMed]
93. Zhu, X.; Wu, S.; Dahut, W.L.; Parikh, C.R. Risks of proteinuria and hypertension with bevacizumab, an antibody against vascular endothelial growth factor: Systematic review and meta-analysis. *Am. J. Kidney Dis.* **2007**, *49*, 186–193. [CrossRef]
94. Zhu, X.; Stergiopoulos, K.; Wu, S. Risk of hypertension and renal dysfunction with an angiogenesis inhibitor sunitinib: Systematic review and meta-analysis. *Acta Oncol.* **2009**, *48*, 9–17. [CrossRef] [PubMed]
95. Wu, S.; Chen, J.J.; Kudelka, A.; Lu, J.; Zhu, X. Incidence and risk of hypertension with sorafenib in patients with cancer: A systematic review and meta-analysis. *Lancet Oncol.* **2008**, *9*, 117–123. [CrossRef]

96. Pereg, D.; Lishner, M. Bevacizumab treatment for cancer patients with cardiovascular disease: A double edged sword? *Eur. Heart J.* **2008**, *29*, 2325–2326. [CrossRef]
97. Je, Y.; Schutz, F.A.B.; Choueiri, T.K. Risk of bleeding with vascular endothelial growth factor receptor tyrosine-kinase inhibitors sunitinib and sorafenib: A systematic review and meta-analysis of clinical trials. *Lancet Oncol.* **2009**, *10*, 967–974. [CrossRef]
98. Lyon, A.R.; Dent, S.; Stanway, S.; Earl, H.; Brezden-Masley, C.; Cohen-Solal, A.; Tocchetti, C.G.; Moslehi, J.J.; Groarke, J.D.; Bergler-Klein, J.; et al. Baseline cardiovascular risk assessment in cancer patients scheduled to receive cardiotoxic cancer therapies: A position statement and new risk assessment tools from the Cardio-Oncology Study Group of the Heart Failure Association of the European Society of Cardiology in collaboration with the International Cardio-Oncology Society. *Eur. J. Heart Fail.* **2020**, *22*, 1945–1960. [CrossRef]
99. Small, H.Y.; Montezano, A.C.; Rios, F.J.; Savoia, C.; Touyz, R.M. Hypertension due to antiangiogenic cancer therapy with vascular endothelial growth factor inhibitors: Understanding and managing a new syndrome. *Can. J. Cardiol.* **2014**, *30*, 534–543. [CrossRef]
100. Kruzliak, P.; Novak, J.; Novak, M. Vascular endothelial growth factor inhibitor-induced hypertension: From pathophysiology to prevention and treatment based on long-acting nitric oxide donors. *Am. J. Hypertens.* **2014**, *27*, 3–13. [CrossRef]
101. Matsuda, Y.; Akita, H.; Terashima, M.; Shiga, N.; Kanazawa, K.; Yokoyama, M. Carvedilol improves endothelium-dependent dilatation in patients with coronary artery disease. *Am. Heart J.* **2000**, *140*, 753–759. [CrossRef] [PubMed]
102. Robinson, E.S.; Khankin, E.V.; Karumanchi, S.A.; Humphreys, B.D. Hypertension induced by vascular endothelial growth factor signaling pathway inhibition: Mechanisms and potential use as a biomarker. *Semin. Nephrol.* **2010**, *30*, 591–601. [CrossRef] [PubMed]
103. Group, S.R.; Wright, J.T., Jr.; Williamson, J.D.; Whelton, P.K.; Snyder, J.K.; Sink, K.M.; Rocco, M.V.; Reboussin, D.M.; Rahman, M.; Oparil, S.; et al. A Randomized Trial of Intensive versus Standard Blood-Pressure Control. *N. Engl. J. Med.* **2015**, *373*, 2103–2116. [CrossRef] [PubMed]
104. Urbich, C.; Dernbach, E.; Zeiher, A.M.; Dimmeler, S. Double-edged role of statins in angiogenesis signaling. *Circ. Res.* **2002**, *90*, 737–744. [CrossRef]
105. Visseren, F.L.J.; Mach, F.; Smulders, Y.M.; Carballo, D.; Koskinas, K.C.; Back, M.; Benetos, A.; Biffi, A.; Boavida, J.M.; Capodanno, D.; et al. 2021 ESC Guidelines on cardiovascular disease prevention in clinical practice. *Eur. Heart J.* **2021**, *42*, 3227–3337. [CrossRef]
106. Authors/Task Force, M.; Piepoli, M.F.; Hoes, A.W.; Agewall, S.; Albus, C.; Brotons, C.; Catapano, A.L.; Cooney, M.T.; Corra, U.; Cosyns, B.; et al. 2016 European Guidelines on cardiovascular disease prevention in clinical practice: The Sixth Joint Task Force of the European Society of Cardiology and Other Societies on Cardiovascular Disease Prevention in Clinical Practice (constituted by representatives of 10 societies and by invited experts): Developed with the special contribution of the European Association for Cardiovascular Prevention & Rehabilitation (EACPR). *Eur. J. Prev. Cardiol.* **2016**, *23*, NP1–NP96. [CrossRef]
107. Lewandowski, T.; Szmit, S. Bevacizumab—cardiovascular side effects in daily practice. *Oncol. Clin. Pract.* **2016**, *12*, 136–143. [CrossRef]
108. van Nimwegen, F.A.; Schaapveld, M.; Janus, C.P.; Krol, A.D.; Petersen, E.J.; Raemaekers, J.M.; Kok, W.E.; Aleman, B.M.; van Leeuwen, F.E. Cardiovascular disease after Hodgkin lymphoma treatment: 40-year disease risk. *JAMA Intern. Med.* **2015**, *175*, 1007–1017. [CrossRef]
109. Cheng, Y.J.; Nie, X.Y.; Ji, C.C.; Lin, X.X.; Liu, L.J.; Chen, X.M.; Yao, H.; Wu, S.H. Long-Term Cardiovascular Risk After Radiotherapy in Women With Breast Cancer. *J. Am. Heart Assoc.* **2017**, *6*, e005633. [CrossRef]
110. Barthel, W.; Markwardt, F. Aggregation of blood platelets by adrenaline and its uptake. *Biochem. Pharmacol.* **1975**, *24*, 1903–1904. [CrossRef]
111. Swerdlow, A.J.; Higgins, C.D.; Smith, P.; Cunningham, D.; Hancock, B.W.; Horwich, A.; Hoskin, P.J.; Lister, A.; Radford, J.A.; Rohatiner, A.Z.; et al. Myocardial infarction mortality risk after treatment for Hodgkin disease: A collaborative British cohort study. *J. Natl. Cancer Inst.* **2007**, *99*, 206–214. [CrossRef] [PubMed]
112. Aleman, B.M.; van den Belt-Dusebout, A.W.; De Bruin, M.L.; van't Veer, M.B.; Baaijens, M.H.; de Boer, J.P.; Hart, A.A.; Klokman, W.J.; Kuenen, M.A.; Ouwens, G.M.; et al. Late cardiotoxicity after treatment for Hodgkin lymphoma. *Blood* **2007**, *109*, 1878–1886. [CrossRef] [PubMed]
113. Darby, S.C.; Ewertz, M.; McGale, P.; Bennet, A.M.; Blom-Goldman, U.; Bronnum, D.; Correa, C.; Cutter, D.; Gagliardi, G.; Gigante, B.; et al. Risk of ischemic heart disease in women after radiotherapy for breast cancer. *N. Engl. J. Med.* **2013**, *368*, 987–998. [CrossRef] [PubMed]
114. Hull, M.C.; Morris, C.G.; Pepine, C.J.; Mendenhall, N.P. Valvular dysfunction and carotid, subclavian, and coronary artery disease in survivors of hodgkin lymphoma treated with radiation therapy. *JAMA* **2003**, *290*, 2831–2837. [CrossRef]
115. Mousavi, N.; Nohria, A. Radiation-induced cardiovascular disease. *Curr. Treat Options Cardiovasc. Med.* **2013**, *15*, 507–517. [CrossRef]
116. Jaworski, C.; Mariani, J.A.; Wheeler, G.; Kaye, D.M. Cardiac complications of thoracic irradiation. *J. Am. Coll. Cardiol.* **2013**, *61*, 2319–2328. [CrossRef]
117. Taylor, C.W.; Nisbet, A.; McGale, P.; Darby, S.C. Cardiac exposures in breast cancer radiotherapy: 1950s-1990s. *Int. J. Radiat. Oncol. Biol. Phys.* **2007**, *69*, 1484–1495. [CrossRef]
118. Harris, E.E.; Correa, C.; Hwang, W.T.; Liao, J.; Litt, H.I.; Ferrari, V.A.; Solin, L.J. Late cardiac mortality and morbidity in early-stage breast cancer patients after breast-conservation treatment. *J. Clin. Oncol.* **2006**, *24*, 4100–4106. [CrossRef]

119. Bouillon, K.; Haddy, N.; Delaloge, S.; Garbay, J.R.; Garsi, J.P.; Brindel, P.; Mousannif, A.; Le, M.G.; Labbe, M.; Arriagada, R.; et al. Long-term cardiovascular mortality after radiotherapy for breast cancer. *J. Am. Coll. Cardiol.* **2011**, *57*, 445–452. [CrossRef]
120. Schubert, L.K.; Gondi, V.; Sengbusch, E.; Westerly, D.C.; Soisson, E.T.; Paliwal, B.R.; Mackie, T.R.; Mehta, M.P.; Patel, R.R.; Tome, W.A.; et al. Dosimetric comparison of left-sided whole breast irradiation with 3DCRT, forward-planned IMRT, inverse-planned IMRT, helical tomotherapy, and topotherapy. *Radiother. Oncol.* **2011**, *100*, 241–246. [CrossRef]
121. Jagsi, R.; Moran, J.; Marsh, R.; Masi, K.; Griffith, K.A.; Pierce, L.J. Evaluation of four techniques using intensity-modulated radiation therapy for comprehensive locoregional irradiation of breast cancer. *Int. J. Radiat. Oncol. Biol. Phys.* **2010**, *78*, 1594–1603. [CrossRef] [PubMed]
122. Martinou, M.; Gaya, A. Cardiac complications after radical radiotherapy. *Semin. Oncol.* **2013**, *40*, 178–185. [CrossRef] [PubMed]
123. Myrehaug, S.; Pintilie, M.; Yun, L.; Crump, M.; Tsang, R.W.; Meyer, R.M.; Sussman, J.; Yu, E.; Hodgson, D.C. A population-based study of cardiac morbidity among Hodgkin lymphoma patients with preexisting heart disease. *Blood* **2010**, *116*, 2237–2240. [CrossRef]
124. Yang, E.H.; Marmagkiolis, K.; Balanescu, D.V.; Hakeem, A.; Donisan, T.; Finch, W.; Virmani, R.; Herrman, J.; Cilingiroglu, M.; Grines, C.L.; et al. Radiation-Induced Vascular Disease-A State-of-the-Art Review. *Front. Cardiovasc. Med.* **2021**, *8*, 652761. [CrossRef] [PubMed]
125. Tukenova, M.; Guibout, C.; Oberlin, O.; Doyon, F.; Mousannif, A.; Haddy, N.; Guerin, S.; Pacquement, H.; Aouba, A.; Hawkins, M.; et al. Role of cancer treatment in long-term overall and cardiovascular mortality after childhood cancer. *J. Clin. Oncol.* **2010**, *28*, 1308–1315. [CrossRef]
126. Rademaker, J.; Schoder, H.; Ariaratnam, N.S.; Strauss, H.W.; Yahalom, J.; Steingart, R.; Oeffinger, K.C. Coronary artery disease after radiation therapy for Hodgkin's lymphoma: Coronary CT angiography findings and calcium scores in nine asymptomatic patients. *AJR Am. J. Roentgenol.* **2008**, *191*, 32–37. [CrossRef]
127. Kupeli, S.; Hazirolan, T.; Varan, A.; Akata, D.; Alehan, D.; Hayran, M.; Besim, A.; Buyukpamukcu, M. Evaluation of coronary artery disease by computed tomography angiography in patients treated for childhood Hodgkin's lymphoma. *J. Clin. Oncol.* **2010**, *28*, 1025–1030. [CrossRef]
128. Galper, S.L.; Yu, J.B.; Mauch, P.M.; Strasser, J.F.; Silver, B.; Lacasce, A.; Marcus, K.J.; Stevenson, M.A.; Chen, M.H.; Ng, A.K. Clinically significant cardiac disease in patients with Hodgkin lymphoma treated with mediastinal irradiation. *Blood* **2011**, *117*, 412–418. [CrossRef]
129. Totterman, K.J.; Pesonen, E.; Siltanen, P. Radiation-related chronic heart disease. *Chest* **1983**, *83*, 875–878. [CrossRef]
130. Stewart, F.A.; Heeneman, S.; Te Poele, J.; Kruse, J.; Russell, N.S.; Gijbels, M.; Daemen, M. Ionizing radiation accelerates the development of atherosclerotic lesions in ApoE-/- mice and predisposes to an inflammatory plaque phenotype prone to hemorrhage. *Am. J. Pathol.* **2006**, *168*, 649–658. [CrossRef]
131. Cuomo, J.R.; Javaheri, S.P.; Sharma, G.K.; Kapoor, D.; Berman, A.E.; Weintraub, N.L. How to prevent and manage radiation-induced coronary artery disease. *Heart* **2018**, *104*, 1647–1653. [CrossRef] [PubMed]
132. Orzan, F.; Brusca, A.; Conte, M.R.; Presbitero, P.; Figliomeni, M.C. Severe coronary artery disease after radiation therapy of the chest and mediastinum: Clinical presentation and treatment. *Br. Heart J.* **1993**, *69*, 496–500. [CrossRef] [PubMed]
133. Yusuf, S.W.; Sami, S.; Daher, I.N. Radiation-induced heart disease: A clinical update. *Cardiol. Res. Pract.* **2011**, *2011*, 317659. [CrossRef] [PubMed]
134. Taunk, N.K.; Haffty, B.G.; Kostis, J.B.; Goyal, S. Radiation-induced heart disease: Pathologic abnormalities and putative mechanisms. *Front. Oncol.* **2015**, *5*, 39. [CrossRef]
135. Camara Planek, M.I.; Silver, A.J.; Volgman, A.S.; Okwuosa, T.M. Exploratory Review of the Role of Statins, Colchicine, and Aspirin for the Prevention of Radiation-Associated Cardiovascular Disease and Mortality. *J. Am. Heart Assoc.* **2020**, *9*, e014668. [CrossRef]
136. Wei, T.; Cheng, Y. The cardiac toxicity of radiotherapy - a review of characteristics, mechanisms, diagnosis, and prevention. *Int. J. Radiat. Biol.* **2021**, *97*, 1333–1340. [CrossRef]
137. Darby, S.C.; Cutter, D.J.; Boerma, M.; Constine, L.S.; Fajardo, L.F.; Kodama, K.; Mabuchi, K.; Marks, L.B.; Mettler, F.A.; Pierce, L.J.; et al. Radiation-related heart disease: Current knowledge and future prospects. *Int. J. Radiat. Oncol. Biol. Phys.* **2010**, *76*, 656–665. [CrossRef]
138. Yan, Y.; Lu, Z.; Liu, Z.; Luo, W.; Shao, S.; Tan, L.; Ma, X.; Liu, J.; Drokow, E.K.; Ren, J. Dosimetric comparison between three- and four-dimensional computerised tomography radiotherapy for breast cancer. *Oncol. Lett.* **2019**, *18*, 1800–1814. [CrossRef]
139. Darapu, A.; Balakrishnan, R.; Sebastian, P.; Hussain, M.R.; Ravindran, P.; John, S. Is the Deep Inspiration Breath-Hold Technique Superior to the Free Breathing Technique in Cardiac and Lung Sparing while Treating both Left-Sided Post-Mastectomy Chest Wall and Supraclavicular Regions? *Case Rep. Oncol.* **2017**, *10*, 37–51. [CrossRef]
140. Dell'Oro, M.; Giles, E.; Sharkey, A.; Borg, M.; Connell, C.; Bezak, E. A Retrospective Dosimetric Study of Radiotherapy Patients with Left-Sided Breast Cancer; Patient Selection Criteria for Deep Inspiration Breath Hold Technique. *Cancers* **2019**, *11*, 259. [CrossRef]
141. Armenian, S.H.; Lacchetti, C.; Barac, A.; Carver, J.; Constine, L.S.; Denduluri, N.; Dent, S.; Douglas, P.S.; Durand, J.B.; Ewer, M.; et al. Prevention and Monitoring of Cardiac Dysfunction in Survivors of Adult Cancers: American Society of Clinical Oncology Clinical Practice Guideline. *J. Clin. Oncol.* **2017**, *35*, 893–911. [CrossRef] [PubMed]

142. Lai, J.; Hu, S.; Luo, Y.; Zheng, R.; Zhu, Q.; Chen, P.; Chi, B.; Zhang, Y.; Zhong, F.; Long, X. Meta-analysis of deep inspiration breath hold (DIBH) versus free breathing (FB) in postoperative radiotherapy for left-side breast cancer. *Breast Cancer* **2020**, *27*, 299–307. [CrossRef] [PubMed]
143. Hjelstuen, M.H.; Mjaaland, I.; Vikstrom, J.; Dybvik, K.I. Radiation during deep inspiration allows loco-regional treatment of left breast and axillary-, supraclavicular- and internal mammary lymph nodes without compromising target coverage or dose restrictions to organs at risk. *Acta Oncol.* **2012**, *51*, 333–344. [CrossRef] [PubMed]
144. Vikstrom, J.; Hjelstuen, M.H.; Mjaaland, I.; Dybvik, K.I. Cardiac and pulmonary dose reduction for tangentially irradiated breast cancer, utilizing deep inspiration breath-hold with audio-visual guidance, without compromising target coverage. *Acta Oncol.* **2011**, *50*, 42–50. [CrossRef]
145. Shim, J.G.; Kim, J.K.; Park, W.; Seo, J.M.; Hong, C.S.; Song, K.W.; Lim, C.H.; Jung, H.R.; Kim, C.H. Dose-Volume Analysis of Lung and Heart according to Respiration in Breast Cancer Patients Treated with Breast Conserving Surgery. *J. Breast Cancer* **2012**, *15*, 105–110. [CrossRef] [PubMed]
146. Simonetto, C.; Eidemuller, M.; Gaasch, A.; Pazos, M.; Schonecker, S.; Reitz, D.; Kaab, S.; Braun, M.; Harbeck, N.; Niyazi, M.; et al. Does deep inspiration breath-hold prolong life? Individual risk estimates of ischaemic heart disease after breast cancer radiotherapy. *Radiother. Oncol.* **2019**, *131*, 202–207. [CrossRef]
147. Mutter, R.W.; Choi, J.I.; Jimenez, R.B.; Kirova, Y.M.; Fagundes, M.; Haffty, B.G.; Amos, R.A.; Bradley, J.A.; Chen, P.Y.; Ding, X.; et al. Proton Therapy for Breast Cancer: A Consensus Statement From the Particle Therapy Cooperative Group Breast Cancer Subcommittee. *Int. J. Radiat. Oncol. Biol. Phys.* **2021**, *111*, 337–359. [CrossRef]
148. Wang, H.; Wei, J.; Zheng, Q.; Meng, L.; Xin, Y.; Yin, X.; Jiang, X. Radiation-induced heart disease: A review of classification, mechanism and prevention. *Int. J. Biol. Sci.* **2019**, *15*, 2128–2138. [CrossRef]
149. Tawakol, A.; Fayad, Z.A.; Mogg, R.; Alon, A.; Klimas, M.T.; Dansky, H.; Subramanian, S.S.; Abdelbaky, A.; Rudd, J.H.; Farkouh, M.E.; et al. Intensification of statin therapy results in a rapid reduction in atherosclerotic inflammation: Results of a multicenter fluorodeoxyglucose-positron emission tomography/computed tomography feasibility study. *J. Am. Coll. Cardiol.* **2013**, *62*, 909–917. [CrossRef]
150. Zheng, G.; Chen, J.; Lin, C.; Huang, X.; Lin, J. Effect of Statin Therapy on Fibrous Cap Thickness in Coronary Plaques Using Optical Coherence Tomography: A Systematic Review and Meta-Analysis. *J. Interv. Cardiol.* **2015**, *28*, 514–522. [CrossRef]
151. Nissen, S.E.; Nicholls, S.J.; Sipahi, I.; Libby, P.; Raichlen, J.S.; Ballantyne, C.M.; Davignon, J.; Erbel, R.; Fruchart, J.C.; Tardif, J.C.; et al. Effect of very high-intensity statin therapy on regression of coronary atherosclerosis: The ASTEROID trial. *JAMA* **2006**, *295*, 1556–1565. [CrossRef] [PubMed]
152. Marchio, P.; Guerra-Ojeda, S.; Vila, J.M.; Aldasoro, M.; Victor, V.M.; Mauricio, M.D. Targeting Early Atherosclerosis: A Focus on Oxidative Stress and Inflammation. *Oxid. Med. Cell. Longev.* **2019**, *2019*, 8563845. [CrossRef] [PubMed]
153. Ostrau, C.; Hulsenbeck, J.; Herzog, M.; Schad, A.; Torzewski, M.; Lackner, K.J.; Fritz, G. Lovastatin attenuates ionizing radiation-induced normal tissue damage in vivo. *Radiother. Oncol.* **2009**, *92*, 492–499. [CrossRef] [PubMed]
154. Doi, H.; Matsumoto, S.; Odawara, S.; Shikata, T.; Kitajima, K.; Tanooka, M.; Takada, Y.; Tsujimura, T.; Kamikonya, N.; Hirota, S. Pravastatin reduces radiation-induced damage in normal tissues. *Exp. Ther. Med.* **2017**, *13*, 1765–1772. [CrossRef]
155. Yang, H.; Huang, F.; Tao, Y.; Zhao, X.; Liao, L.; Tao, X. Simvastatin ameliorates ionizing radiation-induced apoptosis in the thymus by activating the AKT/sirtuin 1 pathway in mice. *Int. J. Mol. Med.* **2017**, *40*, 762–770. [CrossRef]
156. Ran, X.Z.; Ran, X.; Zong, Z.W.; Liu, D.Q.; Xiang, G.M.; Su, Y.P.; Zheng, H.E. Protective effect of atorvastatin on radiation-induced vascular endothelial cell injury in vitro. *J. Radiat. Res.* **2010**, *51*, 527–533. [CrossRef]
157. Zhang, K.; He, X.; Zhou, Y.; Gao, L.; Qi, Z.; Chen, J.; Gao, X. Atorvastatin Ameliorates Radiation-Induced Cardiac Fibrosis in Rats. *Radiat. Res.* **2015**, *184*, 611–620. [CrossRef]
158. Hoving, S.; Heeneman, S.; Gijbels, M.J.; te Poele, J.A.; Pol, J.F.; Gabriels, K.; Russell, N.S.; Daemen, M.J.; Stewart, F.A. Anti-inflammatory and anti-thrombotic intervention strategies using atorvastatin, clopidogrel and knock-down of CD40L do not modify radiation-induced atherosclerosis in ApoE null mice. *Radiother. Oncol.* **2011**, *101*, 100–108. [CrossRef]
159. Nubel, T.; Damrot, J.; Roos, W.P.; Kaina, B.; Fritz, G. Lovastatin protects human endothelial cells from killing by ionizing radiation without impairing induction and repair of DNA double-strand breaks. *Clin. Cancer Res.* **2006**, *12*, 933–939. [CrossRef]
160. Lenarczyk, M.; Su, J.; Haworth, S.T.; Komorowski, R.; Fish, B.L.; Migrino, R.Q.; Harmann, L.; Hopewell, J.W.; Kronenberg, A.; Patel, S.; et al. Simvastatin mitigates increases in risk factors for and the occurrence of cardiac disease following 10 Gy total body irradiation. *Pharmacol. Res. Perspect.* **2015**, *3*, e00145. [CrossRef]
161. Gaugler, M.H.; Vereycken-Holler, V.; Squiban, C.; Vandamme, M.; Vozenin-Brotons, M.C.; Benderitter, M. Pravastatin limits endothelial activation after irradiation and decreases the resulting inflammatory and thrombotic responses. *Radiat. Res.* **2005**, *163*, 479–487. [CrossRef] [PubMed]
162. Holler, V.; Buard, V.; Gaugler, M.H.; Guipaud, O.; Baudelin, C.; Sache, A.; Perez Mdel, R.; Squiban, C.; Tamarat, R.; Milliat, F.; et al. Pravastatin limits radiation-induced vascular dysfunction in the skin. *J. Invest. Dermatol.* **2009**, *129*, 1280–1291. [CrossRef] [PubMed]
163. Addison, D.; Lawler, P.R.; Emami, H.; Janjua, S.A.; Staziaki, P.V.; Hallett, T.R.; Hennessy, O.; Lee, H.; Szilveszter, B.; Lu, M.; et al. Incidental Statin Use and the Risk of Stroke or Transient Ischemic Attack after Radiotherapy for Head and Neck Cancer. *J. Stroke* **2018**, *20*, 71–79. [CrossRef] [PubMed]

164. Hoving, S.; Heeneman, S.; Gijbels, M.J.; te Poele, J.A.; Bolla, M.; Pol, J.F.; Simons, M.Y.; Russell, N.S.; Daemen, M.J.; Stewart, F.A. NO-donating aspirin and aspirin partially inhibit age-related atherosclerosis but not radiation-induced atherosclerosis in ApoE null mice. *PLoS ONE* **2010**, *5*, e12874. [CrossRef]
165. Elwood, P.C.; Morgan, G.; Delon, C.; Protty, M.; Galante, J.; Pickering, J.; Watkins, J.; Weightman, A.; Morris, D. Aspirin and cancer survival: A systematic review and meta-analyses of 118 observational studies of aspirin and 18 cancers. *Ecancermedicalscience* **2021**, *15*, 1258. [CrossRef]
166. Ferrari, R.; Fox, K. Insight into the mode of action of ACE inhibition in coronary artery disease: The ultimate 'EUROPA' story. *Drugs* **2009**, *69*, 265–277. [CrossRef] [PubMed]
167. Schmidt, B.; Drexler, H.; Schieffer, B. Therapeutic effects of angiotensin (AT1) receptor antagonists: Potential contribution of mechanisms other than AT1 receptor blockade. *Am. J. Cardiovasc. Drugs* **2004**, *4*, 361–368. [CrossRef]
168. Wu, R.; Zeng, Y. Does angiotensin II-aldosterone have a role in radiation-induced heart disease? *Med. Hypotheses* **2009**, *72*, 263–266. [CrossRef]
169. van der Veen, S.J.; Ghobadi, G.; de Boer, R.A.; Faber, H.; Cannon, M.V.; Nagle, P.W.; Brandenburg, S.; Langendijk, J.A.; van Luijk, P.; Coppes, R.P. ACE inhibition attenuates radiation-induced cardiopulmonary damage. *Radiother. Oncol.* **2015**, *114*, 96–103. [CrossRef]
170. Wei, J.; Xu, H.; Liu, Y.; Li, B.; Zhou, F. Effect of captopril on radiation-induced TGF-beta1 secretion in EA.Hy926 human umbilical vein endothelial cells. *Oncotarget* **2017**, *8*, 20842–20850. [CrossRef]
171. Charrier, S.; Michaud, A.; Badaoui, S.; Giroux, S.; Ezan, E.; Sainteny, F.; Corvol, P.; Vainchenker, W. Inhibition of angiotensin I-converting enzyme induces radioprotection by preserving murine hematopoietic short-term reconstituting cells. *Blood* **2004**, *104*, 978–985. [CrossRef] [PubMed]
172. Ghosh, S.N.; Zhang, R.; Fish, B.L.; Semenenko, V.A.; Li, X.A.; Moulder, J.E.; Jacobs, E.R.; Medhora, M. Renin-Angiotensin system suppression mitigates experimental radiation pneumonitis. *Int. J. Radiat. Oncol. Biol. Phys.* **2009**, *75*, 1528–1536. [CrossRef] [PubMed]
173. Molteni, A.; Wolfe, L.F.; Ward, W.F.; Ts'ao, C.H.; Molteni, L.B.; Veno, P.; Fish, B.L.; Taylor, J.M.; Quintanilla, N.; Herndon, B.; et al. Effect of an angiotensin II receptor blocker and two angiotensin converting enzyme inhibitors on transforming growth factor-beta (TGF-beta) and alpha-actomyosin (alpha SMA), important mediators of radiation-induced pneumopathy and lung fibrosis. *Curr. Pharm. Des.* **2007**, *13*, 1307–1316. [CrossRef]
174. Deftereos, S.; Giannopoulos, G.; Papoutsidakis, N.; Panagopoulou, V.; Kossyvakis, C.; Raisakis, K.; Cleman, M.W.; Stefanadis, C. Colchicine and the heart: Pushing the envelope. *J. Am. Coll. Cardiol.* **2013**, *62*, 1817–1825. [CrossRef]
175. Nidorf, S.M.; Eikelboom, J.W.; Budgeon, C.A.; Thompson, P.L. Low-dose colchicine for secondary prevention of cardiovascular disease. *J. Am. Coll. Cardiol.* **2013**, *61*, 404–410. [CrossRef] [PubMed]
176. Kofler, T.; Kurmann, R.; Lehnick, D.; Cioffi, G.M.; Chandran, S.; Attinger-Toller, A.; Toggweiler, S.; Kobza, R.; Moccetti, F.; Cuculi, F.; et al. Colchicine in Patients With Coronary Artery Disease: A Systematic Review and Meta-Analysis of Randomized Trials. *J. Am. Heart Assoc.* **2021**, *10*, e021198. [CrossRef]
177. O'Herron, T.; Lafferty, J. Prophylactic use of colchicine in preventing radiation induced coronary artery disease. *Med. Hypotheses* **2018**, *111*, 58–60. [CrossRef]
178. Nidorf, S.M.; Thompson, P.L. Why Colchicine Should Be Considered for Secondary Prevention of Atherosclerosis: An Overview. *Clin. Ther.* **2019**, *41*, 41–48. [CrossRef]
179. Sung, H.; Ferlay, J.; Siegel, R.L.; Laversanne, M.; Soerjomataram, I.; Jemal, A.; Bray, F. Global Cancer Statistics 2020: GLOBOCAN Estimates of Incidence and Mortality Worldwide for 36 Cancers in 185 Countries. *CA Cancer J. Clin.* **2021**, *71*, 209–249. [CrossRef]
180. Rottenberg, S.; Disler, C.; Perego, P. The rediscovery of platinum-based cancer therapy. *Nat. Rev. Cancer* **2021**, *21*, 37–50. [CrossRef]
181. Meadows, K.L.; Hurwitz, H.I. Anti-VEGF therapies in the clinic. *Cold Spring Harb. Perspect. Med.* **2012**, *2*, a006577. [CrossRef] [PubMed]
182. Ewer, M.S.; Benjamin, R.S.; Yeh, E.T.H. Cardiac complications of cancer treatment. In *Cancer Medicine*; Kufe, D.W., Pollock, R.E., Weichselbaum, R.R., Bast, J.R.C., Gansler, T.S., Holland, J.F., Frei, I.E., Eds.; BC Decker Inc.: Hamilton, ON, Canada, 2003.
183. Christensen, S.; Van der Roest, B.; Besselink, N.; Janssen, R.; Boymans, S.; Martens, J.W.M.; Yaspo, M.L.; Priestley, P.; Kuijk, E.; Cuppen, E.; et al. 5-Fluorouracil treatment induces characteristic T>G mutations in human cancer. *Nat. Commun.* **2019**, *10*, 4571. [CrossRef]
184. Lukasiewicz, S.; Czeczelewski, M.; Forma, A.; Baj, J.; Sitarz, R.; Stanislawek, A. Breast Cancer-Epidemiology, Risk Factors, Classification, Prognostic Markers, and Current Treatment Strategies-An Updated Review. *Cancers* **2021**, *13*, 4287. [CrossRef] [PubMed]
185. Cardinale, D.; Iacopo, F.; Cipolla, C.M. Cardiotoxicity of Anthracyclines. *Front. Cardiovasc. Med.* **2020**, *7*, 26. [CrossRef] [PubMed]
186. Cardinale, D.; Colombo, A.; Bacchiani, G.; Tedeschi, I.; Meroni, C.A.; Veglia, F.; Civelli, M.; Lamantia, G.; Colombo, N.; Curigliano, G.; et al. Early detection of anthracycline cardiotoxicity and improvement with heart failure therapy. *Circulation* **2015**, *131*, 1981–1988. [CrossRef]
187. Wolf, M.B.; Baynes, J.W. The anti-cancer drug, doxorubicin, causes oxidant stress-induced endothelial dysfunction. *Biochim. Biophys. Acta* **2006**, *1760*, 267–271. [CrossRef]

188. Wojcik, T.; Buczek, E.; Majzner, K.; Kolodziejczyk, A.; Miszczyk, J.; Kaczara, P.; Kwiatek, W.; Baranska, M.; Szymonski, M.; Chlopicki, S. Comparative endothelial profiling of doxorubicin and daunorubicin in cultured endothelial cells. *Toxicol. In Vitro* **2015**, *29*, 512–521. [CrossRef]
189. Murata, T.; Yamawaki, H.; Hori, M.; Sato, K.; Ozaki, H.; Karaki, H. Chronic vascular toxicity of doxorubicin in an organ-cultured artery. *Br. J. Pharmacol.* **2001**, *132*, 1365–1373. [CrossRef]
190. Eckman, D.M.; Stacey, R.B.; Rowe, R.; D'Agostino, R., Jr.; Kock, N.D.; Sane, D.C.; Torti, F.M.; Yeboah, J.; Workman, S.; Lane, K.S.; et al. Weekly doxorubicin increases coronary arteriolar wall and adventitial thickness. *PLoS ONE* **2013**, *8*, e57554. [CrossRef]
191. Galan-Arriola, C.; Vilchez-Tschischke, J.P.; Lobo, M.; Lopez, G.J.; de Molina-Iracheta, A.; Perez-Martinez, C.; Villena-Gutierrez, R.; Macias, A.; Diaz-Rengifo, I.A.; Oliver, E.; et al. Coronary microcirculation damage in anthracycline cardiotoxicity. *Cardiovasc. Res.* **2022**, *118*, 531–541. [CrossRef]
192. Laursen, A.H.; Elming, M.B.; Ripa, R.S.; Hasbak, P.; Kjaer, A.; Kober, L.; Marott, J.L.; Thune, J.J.; Hutchings, M. Rubidium-82 positron emission tomography for detection of acute doxorubicin-induced cardiac effects in lymphoma patients. *J. Nucl. Cardiol.* **2020**, *27*, 1698–1707. [CrossRef] [PubMed]
193. Kirresh, A.; White, L.; Mitchell, A.; Ahmad, S.; Obika, B.; Davis, S.; Ahmad, M.; Candilio, L. Radiation-induced coronary artery disease: A difficult clinical conundrum. *Clin. Med.* **2022**, *22*, 251–256. [CrossRef] [PubMed]
194. Herrmann, J.; Lenihan, D.; Armenian, S.; Barac, A.; Blaes, A.; Cardinale, D.; Carver, J.; Dent, S.; Ky, B.; Lyon, A.R.; et al. Defining cardiovascular toxicities of cancer therapies: An International Cardio-Oncology Society (IC-OS) consensus statement. *Eur. Heart J.* **2022**, *43*, 280–299. [CrossRef] [PubMed]

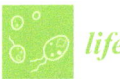

Review

The Value of Troponin as a Biomarker of Chemotherapy-Induced Cardiotoxicity

Victorita Sorodoc [1,2], Oana Sirbu [1,2,*], Catalina Lionte [1,2,*], Raluca Ecaterina Haliga [1,2], Alexandra Stoica [1,2], Alexandr Ceasovschih [1,2], Ovidiu Rusalim Petris [1,2], Mihai Constantin [1,2], Irina Iuliana Costache [2,3], Antoniu Octavian Petris [2,3], Paula Cristina Morariu [1] and Laurentiu Sorodoc [1,2]

1. Department of Internal Medicine, Clinical Emergency Hospital Sfântul Spiridon, 700111 Iasi, Romania; victorita.sorodoc@umfiasi.ro (V.S.); raluca.haliga@umfiasi.ro (R.E.H.); alexandra.rotariu@umfiasi.ro (A.S.); alexandr.ceasovschih@umfiasi.ro (A.C.); ovidiu.petris@umfiasi.ro (O.R.P.); mihai.s.constantin@umfiasi.ro (M.C.); paulacristina571@yahoo.com (P.C.M.); laurentiu.sorodoc@umfiasi.ro (L.S.)
2. Faculty of Medicine, University of Medicine and Pharmacy Grigore T. Popa, 16 Universitatii Street, 700115 Iasi, Romania; irina.costache@umfiasi.ro (I.I.C.); antoniu.petris@umfiasi.ro (A.O.P.)
3. Department of Cardiology, Clinical Emergency Hospital Sfântul Spiridon, 700111 Iasi, Romania
* Correspondence: oana.sirbu@umfiasi.ro (O.S.); catalina.lionte@umfiasi.ro (C.L.)

Abstract: In cancer survivors, cardiac dysfunction is the main cause of mortality. Cardiotoxicity represents a decline in cardiac function associated with cancer therapy, and the risk factors include smoking, dyslipidemia, an age of over 60 years, obesity, and a history of coronary artery disease, diabetes, atrial fibrillation, or heart failure. Troponin is a biomarker that is widely used in the detection of acute coronary syndromes. It has a high specificity, although it is not exclusively associated with myocardial ischemia. The aim of this paper is to summarize published studies and to establish the role of troponin assays in the diagnosis of cardiotoxicity associated with various chemotherapeutic agents. Troponin has been shown to be a significant biomarker in the diagnosis of the cardiac dysfunction associated with several types of chemotherapeutic drugs: anthracyclines, anti-human epidermal growth factor receptor 2 treatment, and anti-vascular endothelial growth factor therapy. Based on the data available at this moment, troponin is useful for baseline risk assessment, the diagnosis of cardiotoxicity, and as a guide for the initiation of cardioprotective treatment. There are currently clear regulations regarding the timing of troponin surveillance depending on the patient's risk of cardiotoxicity and the type of medication administered, but data on the cut-off values of this biomarker are still under investigation.

Keywords: cardiotoxicity; troponin; biomarkers; cancer; chemotherapy; cardiac dysfunction; heart failure

Citation: Sorodoc, V.; Sirbu, O.; Lionte, C.; Haliga, R.E.; Stoica, A.; Ceasovschih, A.; Petris, O.R.; Constantin, M.; Costache, I.I.; Petris, A.O.; et al. The Value of Troponin as a Biomarker of Chemotherapy-Induced Cardiotoxicity. *Life* 2022, *12*, 1183. https://doi.org/10.3390/life12081183

Academic Editor: Gopal J. Babu

Received: 12 June 2022
Accepted: 20 July 2022
Published: 3 August 2022

Publisher's Note: MDPI stays neutral with regard to jurisdictional claims in published maps and institutional affiliations.

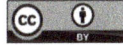

Copyright: © 2022 by the authors. Licensee MDPI, Basel, Switzerland. This article is an open access article distributed under the terms and conditions of the Creative Commons Attribution (CC BY) license (https:// creativecommons.org/licenses/by/ 4.0/).

1. Introduction

Cancer, together with heart disease, is the leading cause of death in developed countries. Advances in cancer treatment have led to significant improvements in the survival of these patients. The cardiotoxic side effects of cancer therapy have contributed to increased mortality and morbidity during and after the cancer treatment [1]. Cardiovascular mortality is up to 10-fold higher in cancer survivors than in the general population, pointing to the importance of conducting a cardiovascular toxicity risk assessment, including the early identification of the cardiac effects of cancer therapies [2].

Cardiac dysfunction associated with cancer treatment is the main cause of mortality in cancer survivors. The mortality rate is recorded to be up to 60% in the first 2 years after therapy [3]. The most commonly associated drugs with cardiotoxicity are anthracycline (AC) and monoclonal antibodies (such as trastuzumab). Other new agents, such as vascular endothelial growth factor (VEGF) inhibitors, immunotherapies, and proteasome inhibitors, can also cause cardiac dysfunction [4].

Evidence from past studies has confirmed the possibility of preventing cardiac dysfunction by promptly initiating cardio-protection with angiotensin-converting-enzyme inhibitors (ACEI) or beta blockers. Therefore, the early detection of cardiotoxicity with precise diagnostic methods and the prediction of patients that would benefit from cardioprotective treatments is essential [5].

2. Cardiotoxicity

Cancer-treatment-related cardiac dysfunction can be caused by chemotherapy, immunotherapy, and molecular targeted therapy. The cardiovascular complications associated with cancer treatments include heart failure (HF), acute and chronic coronary syndromes, arrythmias, hypertension, venous thromboembolism, and pericardial disease [3]. Cardiotoxicity represents a decline in cardiac function, with different criteria for definition over the years, and the purpose of this paper is to assess the role of troponin in the diagnosis of cardiotoxicity.

The risk factors associated with an increased risk of cardiotoxicity include an age of over 60 years old, smoking, dyslipidemia, obesity, and a history of diabetes, coronary artery disease, atrial fibrillation, or HF. Patients with any of these risk factors, together with the potential cardiotoxic effects of specific types of chemotherapy, are at a high risk of experiencing cardiac dysfunction associated with cancer treatment [6].

The diagnosis of cardiotoxicity associated with chemotherapy has evolved over the years, from endomyocardial biopsies to the imagistic detection of a decline in cardiac function, and recently, by using the association of cardiac biomarkers (NT-proBNP and troponin) that have been studied during the last years (8). The ejection fraction was proposed as the main tool for the diagnosis of cardiotoxicity by the Task Force for Cancer Treatments of the European Society of Cardiology, published in 2016. The cardiac dysfunction associated with treatments for cancer was defined as a reduction in the left ventricular ejection fraction (LVEF) to less than 50%, or a reduction in the baseline by more than 10% coupled with an LVEF of less than 55%. Global longitudinal strain, as an early sign of cardiotoxicity, may be used depending on the availability [7].

A more recent document (2022) from the International Cardio-Oncology Society divided cardiac dysfunction into asymptomatic and symptomatic groups and delivered a classification system of three grades for cardiac dysfunction in asymptomatic patients, depending on the severity of the LVEF detected by echocardiography. For all the stages, biomarkers and measurements of the GLS (global longitudinal strain) could be used in addition to assess the severity of the disfunction:

- Mild asymptomatic cardiac dysfunction consists of an LVEF > 50% with a rise in troponin (cTn) or natriuretic peptides and a reduction of >15% in the GLS from baseline;
- Moderate asymptomatic cardiac dysfunction is defined by a reduction in the LVEF of $\geq 10\%$, which would thus be in the 40–49% range, or a smaller change in the LVEF associated with a significant fall in the GLS and/or a rise in cardiac biomarkers;
- Severe asymptomatic cardiac dysfunction is defined by a reduction in the LVEF to <40% and is associated with a poor prognosis [8].

Symptomatic cardiac dysfunction associated with cancer therapy is associated with symptoms and signs of volume overload and/or inadequate perfusion caused by functional and structural changes to the heart, with a decrease in LVEF and increased biomarkers [8].

Anthracycline (AC), a class of chemotherapeutic agents, induces irreversible cardiac dysfunction, leading to severe heart failure and death in a dose-dependent manner. The changes occur predominantly in the first year following the completion of treatment, although there are cases of cardiotoxicity that appear years after the exposure. Trastuzumab toxicity is not associated with structural abnormalities, is independent of the dosage, and can be partially or completely reversed with early therapeutic interventions, such as the cessation of the causative drug or cardioprotective treatment with ACEI and beta blockers. These side effects can lead to suboptimal cancer treatment regimens and increased mortality and morbidity [9].

Different mechanisms are involved in the decline of cardiac function due to cancer therapies. The cardiomyocyte damage can be:

- Direct or endogenous (e.g., AC)—also called primary cardiomyopathy—which is a consequence of the direct toxic effects of chemotherapy on the myocardium and is caused by myocardial cell loss, necrosis, and apoptosis mediated by oxidative stress [10].
- Indirect (e.g., trastuzumab, VEGF inhibitors), which is caused by factors that do not have a direct toxic effect on cardiomyocytes, but that contribute to a decline in cardiac function. Indirect cardiomyopathy is determined by alterations in the perfusion, innervation, or hormonal background (vasoconstriction, vasospasm). Trastuzumab causes functional abnormalities, though in patients with previous AC treatment, it may exacerbate injury and myocyte death by inhibiting anti-apoptotic pathways [11].
- Caused by inflammatory cell infiltration in the myocardium, which can lead to myocarditis (immune checkpoint inhibitors—ICS) [11].

Cardiomyopathies caused by cancer therapy are rarely a consequence of a single mechanism, so this classification can be used to foster the proper selection of the care and produce the best outcomes [12]. The latest studies on the incidence and reversibility of cardiotoxicity have led to a withdrawal of the concept of type I and II cardiotoxicity, and have brought to our attention the Royal Brompton Hospital classification of myocardial toxicity [13]. This classification is more applicable to clinical practice, and includes early abnormalities that could predispose a patient to future susceptibility and identify high-risk patients that could benefit from preventive treatment. This classification includes six stages:

1. Early biochemical cardiotoxicity, which is represented by an increase in cardiac biomarkers (troponin or brain natriuretic peptide—BNP) with normal cardiac imaging.
2. Early functional cardiotoxicity, which is characterized by grade III–IV diastolic dysfunction or a reduction in the GLS and normal biomarkers.
3. Early mixed cardiotoxicity, which involves the presence of a normal LVEF with increased levels of biomarkers and a reduction in the GLS, or diastolic dysfunction.
4. Symptomatic heart failure with preserved EF.
5. Asymptomatic LV systolic dysfunction, which is indicated by a reduction in the LVEF to less than 50%, or a reduction of more than 10% resulting in a total LVEF < 55%.
6. Symptomatic LV systolic dysfunction, which is represented by a symptomatic reduction in the LVEF to <50%, or a reduction of >10% resulting in a total LVEF < 55% [14].

Echocardiographic changes used for the diagnosis of cardiotoxicity have a low diagnostic sensitivity and low predictive power for the diagnosis of subclinical myocardial injury. The lack of standardization in defining cardiac dysfunction across clinical trials and chemotherapeutic agents has led to multiple other questions regarding the role of this diagnostic tool in detecting cardiac dysfunction [15]. Echocardiographic measurements of the LVEF have several limitations, which include intra-observer or inter-observer variability and a lack of sensitivity for detecting early subclinical myocardial changes. Unfortunately, these changes appear late and are often an irreversible effect of the drugs used for chemotherapy [16]. The use of new techniques, such as three-dimensional echocardiography and contrast echocardiography, have resulted in a significant improvement to the accuracy assessment of the LVEF. The GLS can be used to detect early subclinical changes in the systolic function of the left ventricle [16].

Cardiac magnetic resonance imaging (CMR) remains the gold standard for the rigorous quantification of the LVEF, but its use is limited by the cost and the requirement for expert interpretation [4].

As a result of the complexity of the cardiovascular complications of cancer treatment and the extensions of cardiovascular toxicity beyond changes in the LVEF, there is a growing expectation for noninvasive diagnostic tools that can be used for the early detection of patients at a high risk of developing chemotherapy-induced cardiotoxicity. Finding a biomarker able to detect heart injury represents a desirable tool for the initial diagnosis of cardiotoxicity [17].

2.1. Biomarkers for Cardiotoxicity

The limitations of the mentioned imagistic method and the need to identify cardiotoxicity in early stages has led to the analysis of sensitive and specific markers of myocardial damage [18]. The most frequently used biomarkers for the diagnosis of cardiotoxicity are troponins and NT-pro BNP. A troponin assay offers a complementary diagnostic tool for patients receiving chemotherapy, and troponin assays represent a good tool for surveillance, prognosis assessment, and providing a guide for selecting and monitoring the treatment response in oncology patients [7,19].

The perfect biomarker should provide rapid and low-cost measurements, offer objectivity, be precise (the normal ranges are well-defined), be widely available, be well-studied, and offer reproducible results. The biomarker should provide better diagnostic confidence as well as information about disease progression, risk stratification, and treatment responses [20]. The detection of a specific biomarker is minimally invasive, has a significantly lower cost than echocardiography or nuclear techniques, and reflects minimal cardiomyocyte damage or small hemodynamic fluctuations. The interpretation of the results is not dependent on the expertise of the doctor, thus avoiding inter-observer variability [21]. Biomarkers have an important role in the initial evaluation and management of patients who are known to have or are at risk for cardiovascular disease. These blood tests can be good tools for identifying patients with a high risk of adverse cardiovascular effects before the initiation of therapy, and are a good addition to imaging in the detection of subclinical diseases during active therapy. For the future, an idealistic role for biomarkers would be the tailoring of oncologic regimens or the initiation of preventative cardiovascular treatments based on cardiac biomarker profiles [22].

Most of the published studies have identified the biomarkers for cardiovascular disease in patients receiving cancer treatment. However, the specificity of these biomarkers in various categories of patients is difficult to assess due to the comorbid conditions associated with cancer pathology, such as infections, hypotension, renal dysfunction, and other systemic illnesses. All these known conditions can lead to increased biomarkers in the absence of cardiac dysfunction [4].

2.2. Troponins

Troponins are biomarkers used for the diagnosis of acute coronary syndromes. Cardiac troponins (cTnI and cTnT) are largely used to detect cardiac toxicity, as they have a high specificity for cardiac injury and cardiomyocyte necrosis. The highly sensitive assays allow for the possibility of detecting small amounts of myocyte damage, enabling the application of therapeutic interventions to minimize cardiotoxicity before the development of irreversible left ventricular (LV) dysfunction. The persistent elevation of cTn I has the role of detecting a higher degree of LV dysfunction and a higher percentage of cardiac events than the transient elevation of cTn levels [11].

Troponins are a complex of regulatory proteins that are part of the skeletal and cardiac muscle, but not smooth muscle. Their function consists of regulating muscle contractions. Sarcomeres represent the fundamental units of a myofibril, and they are formed from seven actin monomers, a strand of tropomyosin, and a troponin complex [23]. There are three subunits of troponins: troponin C, cTnT, and cTnI. cTnT and cTnI have two specific isoforms that are distinct for cardiac and skeletal muscles. The two isoforms of troponin C are not different in cardiac and skeletal muscles. Each subunit of troponin has a specific function: cTnI is bound by actin and keeps the troponin–tropomyosin complex steady, cTnT anchors the components of the tropomyosin to the actin thin filament, and troponin C contains the binding sites for calcium, which help initiate contractions [24]. Diastolic relaxation occurs when cTnI binds to actin and its access to the myosin binding site is impeded, maintaining tropomyosin stability. A systolic contraction starts when a calcium influx causes the release of cTnI from actin, liberating its myosin binding site and facilitating force development [25].

High-sensitivity cardiac troponin (hs-cTn) is more specific, being able to detect levels 10- to 100-fold lower than the original technique and improving the accuracy of myocardial injury diagnoses. When hs-cTnT and hs-cTnI are compared, the latter is superior in the early detection of lesions, and its levels are not affected by the circadian rhythm [9]. There is no evidence that cTnT can be released by noncardiac tissues, but in patients with injured skeletal muscle, some proteins can be detected by cTnT assays, making the cTnT a less-specific marker of cardiac injuries [5].

The troponins cTnI and cTnT are expressed exclusively in the myocardium, and their release into circulation is an effective indicator for evaluating myocadic integrity. After cardiomyocyte necrosis, cTn is released, which has a high sensitivity and specificity for the diagnosis of myocardial infarctions. A high level of cTn can be detected before echocardiographic changes; therefore, it can become an important assessment tool for detecting subclinical cardiac dysfunction. The cTn measurement has a high specificity for the heart, but is not specific for disease [9]. Myocardial injury can be determined by reversible or irreversible impairment. If there is irreversible damage, the release of proteins from the myocardium is caused by the apoptosis or necrosis of myocardial cells [26]. If the disturbance is reversible, the release of cTn is secondary to an increased cell wall permeability or the formation and release of membrane cysts. The other mechanisms of troponin release are myocardial cell turnover and the release of cell breakdown products [5].

Changes in hs-cTn concentrations during short periods of time can discern between acute disease, when there is an acute injury of the cardiomyocyte with rapid increases and decreases in the cTn, and chronic cardiomyocyte injury, with a persistent slight elevation of hs-cTn [27].

A small concentration of cTn can be detected even in normal subjects, and the diagnosis of myocardial damage is considered pronounced if the levels of cTn are higher than the 99th percentile of the upper reference limit. High levels of cTn can be found, not only in myocardial injuries, but also in well-known inflammatory or mechanical conditions [5].

2.3. Mechanism of Troponin Release

The vast majority of cTn is stationary in the sarcomere, and a small fraction exists as a soluble pool. In patients with cardiac ischemia, the first peak of cTn release originates from the bound cTn pool. After that, the degradation of the contractile apparatus is responsible for most of the cTn release [28]. Until recently, it was believed that cardiomyocytes cannot be repaired or replenished; however, the newest evidence supports the renewal of cardiomyocytes by mitosis and cellular restoration from stem cells. The renewal of cardiomyocytes could be associated with the release of cTn into the bloodstream. cTn can be released from the myocardium in the absence of necrosis, during physiological situations (athletes after endurance exercise) or after atrial pacing or dobutamine stress test. This means that there are other mechanisms by which cTn is released from the myocardium [29]. One of the possible mechanisms is programed cellular death, which can appear in the absence of ischemia and can lead to HF. In response to myocardial injury, cTn could be released from an enhanced apoptosis rate [30]. The possibilities for the release of cTn into the bloodstream are represented in Figure 1.

Different cell wounds can lead to cardiomyocyte membrane injury. The cells have the ability to repair lesions larger than 10 μm^2 within seconds. During this period of time, some proteins could be released into the bloodstream, including cTn, which could possibly explain the high levels of cTn in the absence of myocardial necrosis. The extent of the cTn elevations explained by cell wounds that we find in clinical settings remain to be shown [30].

Another theory involves the release of cTn after bleb formation. These are buds of membrane cells that are formed after transient ischemia and contain cTn, which is released into circulation or captured into the cell after the reestablishment of the oxygen supply. Oxidative stress, reactive oxygen species, neurohormonal activation, inflammatory cytokines, acid–base disturbances, or neurohormonal activation can lead to the release of cTn into the bloodstream [23,31,32]. The understanding of different mechanisms on troponin release from a damaged myocardium could help make the distinction between high troponin levels associated with necrosis and other possible reversible causes of troponin release, which are associated with mechanisms encountered in cardiotoxicity.

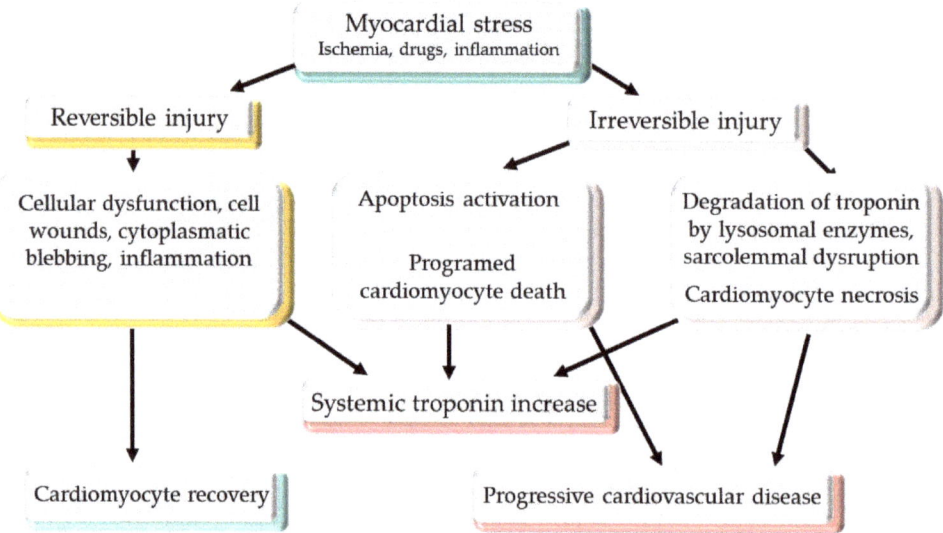

Figure 1. Potential mechanisms of troponin release from injured myocardium.

The intra-individual variability of two consecutive measurements of hs-cTn is low, so a difference in the levels of the same hs-cTn subtype in a single patient at two different moments should be considered significant if it is higher than 30% (approximately 3–5 ng/L). An increase of 3–5 ng/L in the cTn concentrations between two measurements is correlated with the necrosis of about 10–20 mg of myocardial tissue, which is undetectable even with the most sensitive cardiac imaging techniques [33]. This evidence suggests that, when using hs-cTn as a biomarker for cardiotoxicity detection, the measurement should be performed at baseline, prior to the cardiotoxic treatment, and the monitoring of the biomarker changes during the treatment should be performed using the same subtype of hs-cTn and at the same laboratory, if possible [5].

We will discuss the classes of drugs that could lead to increased levels of cTn and present the existing evidence regarding the role of cTn in the detection of cardiotoxicity and the specific indications for short- and long-term monitoring.

2.4. Anthracycline

Anthracyclines (ACs) are chemical compounds whose action is to kill tumor cells by interrupting their mitotic activity and their high metabolic demand, inhibiting DNA or RNA synthesis. Other effects of AC therapy include the inhibition of topoisomerase IIa, an enzyme involved in DNA transcription and replication, and the induction of oxidative stress, which damages DNA, lipids, and proteins by iron mediation and histone modification [12].

The incidence of cardiac dysfunction associated with AC in a study of 2625 patients followed for 5.2 years was 9%, and the majority of cases occurred within 1 year of treatment [9]. The incidence was related to the cumulative dose. If the dose of Adriamycin was 400 mg/m^2, the incidence was 5%; at a dose of 550 mg/m^2, the proportion of HF was

26%; and the incidence increased to 48% when the dosage was 700 mg/m^2 [34]. The factors associated with cardiovascular toxicity are female sex, cumulative doses, intravenous bolus administration, and a history of hypertension, cardiovascular diseases, valvular heart disease, or diabetes mellitus [1].

There are three types of cardiac dysfunction associated with AC treatment:

- Acute toxicity in less than 1% of patients, which may occur after the first cycle of treatment or the first dose and is more common in the elderly, probably owing to underlying cardiac diseases. The forms of manifestation are represented by arrythmias, pericarditis, myocarditis, and acute LV dysfunction and are usually transient [35].
- Early-onset chronic cardiotoxicity, which is more common (20–30% with asymptomatic decreases in the LVEF, or symptomatic HF in 1.6–2.1%) and can lead to irreversible cardiac dysfunction [35].
- Late or chronic cardiomyopathy related to cumulative doses of AC, with an onset after more than 1 year and which is expressed as an arrythmia or LV dysfunction [10].

It has been shown that patients receiving chemotherapy that had an elevation of cTnI levels developed LV dysfunction in the following seven months, while in patients with negative cTnI levels, the reduced LVEF was smaller and transient (less than three months). The authors concluded that cTnI is a sensitive and reliable marker for the early detection of minor cardiac dysfunction [36]. Studies that have evaluated the role of cTn in the cardiotoxicity associated with AC are summarized in Table 1. In order to assess whether high levels of hs-cTnI are associated with a long-term reduction in the LVEF, a study was conducted that evaluated 703 patients treated with high doses of chemotherapy for 3 years. In patients without increased levels of hs-cTnI, the LVEF remained at the same levels and a small number of cardiac events occurred (1%). Patients with high levels of hs-cTnI after the chemotherapy had a higher incidence of cardiac events (0.4%—sudden death; 0.3%—cardiac death; 5%—asymptomatic LV dysfunction; 7%—HF; 0.4%—acute pulmonary edema; 2%—life-threatening arrythmia; 0.3%—conduction disturbances). In these patients, careful monitoring is essential and prophylactic strategies to prevent cardiotoxicity should be implemented. The study showed that hs-cTnI has a high negative predictive value of 99% for patients with no elevation of hs-cTnI, and a positive predictive value of 84% for future cardiac events in patients with elevated hs-cTnI levels [37]. These studies suggest that measurements of hs-cTnI prior to and during therapy could identify patients at a high risk for cardiotoxicity.

A recent study that evaluated 80 patients with breast cancer treated with AC showed that the value of hs-cTnT increased gradually during AC therapy, and that it reached a maximum peak after 1 month, with similar patterns observed in patients with and without cardiotoxicity. In addition, a linear dependence of cTnT with age was observed, but it was not correlated with the level of toxicity [38].

A meta-analysis of 61 studies with 5691 patients treated with AC, AC followed by human epidermal growth factor receptor 2 (HER2) inhibitors, or HER2 inhibitors has shown that, in patients with elevated levels of cTn, the likelihood of LVEF dysfunction was higher than in patients with normal cTn levels (OR: 11.9, 95% CI: 4.4–32.1). This association was most pronounced under high-dose regimens of chemotherapy, and the specificity and sensitivity values of cTn for diagnosis were 69% and 87%, respectively. For the prediction of LV dysfunction, the negative predictive value was 93%, showing a potential benefit of cTn as a screening tool for LV dysfunction associated with cancer therapy [39].

Table 1. The role of troponin in cardiotoxicity associated with anthracycline treatment.

Study	Patients	Design	Type of Cancer	Chemotherapy	Type of cTn	Determination of cTn	Outcomes
Cardinale et al., 2000 [36]	204	PR	Breast cancer Ovarian carcinoma Small cell lung cancer Non-Hodgkin's lymphoma Hodgkin's disease	AC, radiotherapy	cTnI	Before, immediately after, and then at 12, 24, 36, and 72 h after every single cycle of high-dosage chemotherapy	LVEF decreased in cTnI group (cTnI > 0.5 ng/mL)
Auner et al., 2003 [40]	78	PR	Acute lymphoblastic leukemia Acute myeloid leukemia Non-Hodgkin's lymphoma	AC	cTnT	Baseline and after every cycle	Elevated cTnT (>0.03 ng/mL) was associated with a significantly greater decrease in LVEF
Cardinale et al., 2004 [37]	703	PR	Breast cancer Ewing's sarcoma Hodgkin's disease Myeloma Non-Hodgkin's lymphoma Ovarian carcinoma Small-cell lung cancer	AC, radiotherapy	cTnI	Baseline, after chemotherapy, at 12, 24, 36, and 72 h after every single cycle, and at 1 month after the last cycle	Patients with high levels of cTnI (>0.08 ng/mL) had a higher risk of cardiac events
Kilickap et al., 2005 [41]	41	PR	Lymphoma Breast cancer Malignant mesenchymal tumor Leukemia Nasopharyngeal carcinoma Thymic carcinoma Neuroectodermal tumor Hepatocellular carcinoma Metastasis of unknown origin Multiple myeloma	AC	cTnT	Baseline, on the 3rd and 5th days following the first dose of anthracycline, and after the last cycle of chemotherapy	High levels of cTn were associated with diastolic dysfunction (decreased E/A ratio, IRT prolongation)
Nistico et al., 2007 [42]	20	PR	Breast cancer	AC, taxanes	cTnT	Baseline, pre- and post-chemotherapy, and 12 months after the end of treatment	No cTnT serum elevations were found
Horacek et al., 2008 [43]	23	PR	Leukemia	AC	cTnT cTnI	Baseline, after the first cycle, after the last cycle, and at 6 months after completion of treatment	cTnI seemed to be superior to cTnT for the early detection of cardiac injury
Feola et al., 2011 [44]	53	PR	Breast cancer	AC	cTnI	Baseline, at 1 month, at 1 year, and at 2 years after the end of the chemotherapy	cTnI elevations were not correlated with changes in LVEF
Morris et al., 2011 [45]	95	PR	Breast cancer	AC, taxanes, trastuzumab	cTnI	Baseline, every 2 weeks during chemotherapy, and at 6, 9, and 18 months	cTnI levels did not correlate with decreased LVEF
Sawaya et al., 2012 [46]	81	PR	Breast cancer	AC, taxanes, trastuzumab	usTnI	Baseline, after AC treatment, and every 3 months until 12 months	Elevated usTnI ($\geq$30 pg/mL) at the completion of the AC treatment was predictive of cardiotoxicity
Onitilo et al., 2012 [47]	54	PR	Breast cancer	AC, trastuzumab	cTnI	Baseline and every 3 weeks until 1 year	A decrease in LVEF was not associated with the levels of cTnI

Table 1. *Cont.*

Study	Patients	Design	Type of Cancer	Chemotherapy	Type of cTn	Determination of cTn	Outcomes
Blaes et al., 2015 [48]	18	PR	Breast cancer Non-Hodgkin's lymphoma	AC	cTnT, cTnI, hs-cTnT	Baseline and at 4 weeks after completion of treatment	A decline in LVEF was associated with baseline high hscTnT levels
Malik et al., 2016 [49]	33	PR	Breast cancer	AC	cTnT	Baseline, after every cycle, and at 6 months after the end of the treatment	A decrease in the left ventricular diastolic diameter was associated with high cTnT levels
Jones et al., 2017 [19]	84	PR	Breast cancer Lymphoma Leukemia Leiomyosarcoma	AC	hs-cTnI	Baseline and after every cycle	Smaller AC doses per cycle resulted in less acute cardiomyocyte injury as indicated by hs-cTnI release
Ferreira de Souza et al., 2018 [50]	27	PR	Breast cancer	AC	cTnT	Baseline, after every cycle, and at 3 and 6 months after treatment	A reduction in LVEF and LV mass was more pronounced in patients with cTnT > 10 pg/mL
Demisei et al., 2020 [51]	323	PR	Breast cancer	AC ± trastuzumab	hs-cTnT	Baseline, at 1 month, and after the end of AC treatment at 2 and 4 months	Elevated hs-cTnT (>14 ng/L) was associated with a double risk of cardiotoxicity
Michel et al., 2020 [39]	61 research articles and 5691 patients	Meta-analysis	Various	AC, various high doses of chemotherapy	cTnI, cTnT	Various	In patients with elevated levels of cTn, the likelihood of LVEF dysfunction was higher than in patients with normal cTn
Diaz-Anton et al., 2022 [38]	72	PR	Breast cancer	AC ± trastuzumab	hs-cTnT	Before and after each cycle and at 1, 3, 6, and 12 months after completion of treatment	hs-cTnT increased gradually, reaching a maximum peak at 1 month after the completion of anthracycline treatment

AC—anthracycline, cTn—troponin, hs-cTn—high-sensitivity troponin, LV—left ventricle, LVEF—left ventricular ejection fraction, PR—prospective, us-cTnI—ultrasensitive troponin I.

A study on 323 patients treated with doxorubicin showed that an increased level of hs-cTnT over 14 ng/L after AC treatment increased the risk of cardiac dysfunction by 2-fold (hazard ratio: 2.01; 95% CI: 1.00–4.06, $p = 0.052$). The sensitivity and specificity of hs-cTnT were 60.3% and 62.5%, respectively, for the prediction of cardiac dysfunction within 1 year after the finalization of the doxorubicin treatment. In contrast, patients with levels of hs-cTnT < 5 ng/L at the end of AC treatment had a sensitivity of 100% for cardiac dysfunction at 1 year [51].

Another study of 41 patients receiving AC therapy suggested an association between the levels of cTn and the diastolic dysfunction assessed by the E/A ratio and isovolemic relaxation time (IRT) [41].

A small study on 23 patients treated with AC for leukemia suggested that an assessment of cTnI could be superior to cTnT for the early detection of cardiac dysfunction because of the molecular weight and the release kinetics of the two forms of troponin [43].

The goal of a study including 81 patients treated with AC, followed by taxanes and trastuzumab, was to assess the role of blood biomarkers and myocardial strain in cardiotoxicity prediction. Cardiotoxicity was developed by 32% of the patients, and the study showed that us-cTnI (ultra-sensitive cTnI) and the peak systolic longitudinal myocardial strain at the finalization of treatment predicted cardiotoxicity. Concentration levels of us-cTnI $\geq$ 30 pg/mL after AC treatment were predictive of cardiotoxicity ($p = 0.04$). A combination of us-cTnI and longitudinal strain increased the sensitivity of the cardiotoxicity diagnosis from 74% to 87%, with a negative value of 91% [46].

Not all the studies performed have shown an association between high levels of cTn and cardiac outcomes [44,45,47]. A study on 53 patients with breast cancer treated with AC failed to demonstrate that an elevation of cTn measured 1 month post-treatment could predict cardiac outcomes. The cTn levels were not different between the patients with and without cardiac events [47].

As presented, there are some studies that have highlighted the beneficial role of measuring cTn levels during AC therapy, and others that could not find an association between the levels of cTn and cardiovascular toxicity. Potential explanations for the discrepancies between these studies include a difference in the timing of biomarker measurement, the cutoff values used, and the type of chemotherapy administered [4].

Regardless of the predictive role of cTn in detecting the clinical manifestation of cardiac dysfunction, its increase is an index of subclinical cardiac damage. In this context, some authors have suggested that the administration of ACEI and beta blockers in patients with elevated cTn levels is effective in preventing the development of LV dysfunction [52,53]. Cardinale et al. established that the response to HF treatment (increased LVEF) is determined by the time between the end of chemotherapy and the initiation of HF treatment (beta blockers and ACEI) [54].

The presented studies show that, in patients treated with anthracycline, a positive value of cTn is acceptable, but possibly the best benefit of monitoring cTn in these patients is the ability to exclude subjects that will not develop cardiac dysfunction. Although we do not have specific data about the cut-off values of cTn after chemotherapy, a recent study has evaluated the increase in cTn after radiation treatment and concluded that the cut-off levels for cardiac events were 10 ng/L for hs-cTnT before the initiation of radiation, 16 ng/L for hs-cTnT during treatment, and 12 ng/L for hs-cTnT after radiation [55].

In 2020, the Cardio-Oncology Study Group of the Heart Failure Association and the Cardio-Oncology Council of the European Society of Cardiology published a position statement regarding the type and duration of biomarker monitoring, depending on the cardiotoxicity risk of the patient. Cardiotoxicity risk is evaluated according to the patient's cardiovascular profile and risk factors relating to preexisting cardiovascular disease and the type or dose of cancer treatment [13].

Patients at low risk are adults treated with low dose of AC, liposomal products or trastuzumab without AC. Patients with moderate risk are more than 50 and less than 64 years old, present 1–2 cardiovascular risk factors (smoking, dyslipidemia, insulin resistance, obesity), are treated with modest dose of AC (doxorubicin 200–400 mg/m^2, epirubicin 300–600 mg/m^2), with AC before trastuzumab, or are treated with one of the following classes of drugs: vascular endothelial growth factor (VEGF), tyrosine kinase inhibitors (TKI), Second- and third-generation Bcr-Abl TKI, Proteasome inhibitors, Combination immune checkpoint inhibitors. Patients with high risk of cardiotoxicity are more than 65 years old and presents more than 2 cardiovascular risk factors, cardiovascular disease (severe valvular heart disease, cardiomyopathy, coronary artery disease, heart failure, peripheral artery disease) presented prior cancer therapy and the LVEF is reduced before the initiation of treatment (50–54% or less) and the cTn levels are increased after AC treatment. The patients with high risk are treated with a combination of AC with trastuzumab or VEGF-TKI after AC therapy, high doses of AC (doxorubicin > 400 mg/m^2, epirubicin > 600 mg/m^2) and radiation therapy with a modest dose of AC or with a high dose (heart in the radiation field with >30 Gr) [13].

The position statement of the ESC suggests that, in patients with a low or medium cardiotoxicity risk treated with anthracycline, an assessment of cTn should be performed at the baseline, before the fifth cycle, and at 12 months after the end of treatment. For patients with a high cardiovascular risk, the measurement should be made before cycles two, four, and six or before every cycle and at three, six, and twelve months after the final cycle of treatment [13].

2.5. Trastuzumab

Almost 20% of breast cancers express human epidermal growth factor receptor 2 (HER2). An anti-HER2 agent—trastuzumab—was developed and was demonstrated to reduce the disease progression by 40%. HER2 isoforms are also expressed in cardiomyocytes; therefore, trastuzumab treatment is associated with LV dysfunction and HF [56]. This review focused on trastuzumab because is the most studied in the class of HER2 direct therapies. Five approved trastuzumab biosimilars demonstrate similar rates of cardiotoxicity [57].

The studies available on the role of cTn in cardiac dysfunction associated with trastuzumab are presented in Table 2. The exact mechanism of trastuzumab-induced cardiotoxicity is still unknown, but some studies have suggested the following possibilities: the inhibition of cardiomyocyte repair by blocking the HER2 downstream pathway and neuregulin 1, and/or the inhibition of topoisomerase IIb, leading to the increased formation of reactive oxygen species and apoptosis [58].

Table 2. The role of troponin in cardiotoxicity associated with trastuzumab treatment.

Study	Patients	Design	Type of Cancer	Chemotherapy	Type of cTn	Determination of cTn	Outcomes
Cardinale et al., 2010 [59]	251	PR	Breast cancer	TRA	cTnI	Baseline and before and after each trastuzumab cycle	cTnI > 0.08 ng/mL was the strongest independent predictor of cardiotoxicity
Fallah-Rad et al., 2011 [60]	42	-	Breast cancer	AC, TRA	cTnT	Before AC, before trastuzumab therapy, and 3, 6, 9, and 12 months after the initiation of trastuzumab	cTnT did not show any significant changes over 1 year of follow-up
Ky et al., 2014 [61]	78	PR	Breast cancer	AC, taxanes, TRA	us-cTnI	Baseline and every 3 months (maximum 15 months)	cTnI was associated with the risk of cardiotoxicity
Zardavas et al., 2016 [62]	533	PR	Breast cancer	TRA	us-cTnI hs-cTnT	Baseline; weeks 13, 25, and 52; and months 18, 24, 30, and 36	High-baseline cTnT and cTnI was associated with a 4-fold increased risk of cardiac dysfunction
Yu et al., 2016 [63]	69	Phase 2 sub-study	Breast cancer	Paclitaxel, TRA, pertuzumab	cTnI	Baseline and before every cycle	cTnI (>0.06 ng/mL) was not associated with a decline in LVEF
de Vries Schultink et al., 2017 [64]	206	Secondary analysis of randomized placebo-controlled clinical trial	Breast cancer	AC, TRA	cTnT	Before AC treatment, before starting trastuzumab treatment, and 3, 12, 24, 36, 52, 64, 78, and 92 weeks afterwards	Maximum concentration of cTnT after AC treatment was an important determinant of reduced LVEF
Ponde et al., 2018 [65]	280	Phase III trial sub-study	Breast cancer	Lapatinib, TRA, paclitaxel	cTnT	Baseline and on weeks 2 and 18	No correlation between high cTnT levels and cardiac events
Ben Kridis et al., 2020 [66]	50	PR	Breast cancer	AC, taxanes, TRA	us-cTnI	Baseline and at 3, 6, 9, 12, and 15 months	Levels of us-cTnI at the completion of AC treatment were predictive of the occurrence of cardiotoxicity
Kirkman et al., 2022 [56]	94	Secondary analysis of randomized controlled trial	Breast cancer	TRA	cTnI	Before trastuzumab treatment, post-cycle 4, and post-cycle 17	No significant changes in cTnI were detected

AC—anthracycline, cTn—troponin, hs-cTn—high-sensitivity troponin, LV—left ventricle, LVEF—left ventricular ejection fraction, PR—prospective, TRA—trastuzumab, us-cTnI—ultrasensitive troponin I.

One of the major side effects of trastuzumab treatment is cardiotoxicity expressed as an asymptomatic decrease in the LVEF and HF. After treatment with trastuzumab alone, the incidence of cardiac dysfunction ranged from 3 to 7% and reached 27% when the treatment was performed in combination with AC [67]. A meta-analysis including 9117 patients across five studies showed that the likelihood of cardiotoxicity after trastuzumab use was 2.45-fold higher than the likelihood without trastuzumab use (95% CI: 1.89–3.16) [68].

The clinical outcome of cardiotoxicity associated with trastuzumab treatment is more favorable than that associated with AC, because it is not dependent on the dosage and can be reversed by discontinuing the treatment or by using standard cardiac therapy. Other data have shown that, in patients treated with AC and trastuzumab, the cardiac function does not recover, so it is difficult to separate the cardiotoxicity induced by AC or trastuzumab in patients receiving both chemotherapies [21].

The risk increased in patients that received a combination of chemotherapy, especially including AC; when there was a short duration between the two types of treatment; with increasing age of the patient (>65 years); with chest wall irradiation; for patients with other comorbidities (hypertension, obesity, or diabetes); and for patients with previous cardiac dysfunction [44]. Based on these risk factors, a Canadian study evaluated a score model that predicts the possibility of cardiotoxicity, and established that a low score was associated with a negative predictive probability of 94% for permanent toxicity, and a high score was associated with a positive predictive value of 0.17 [68].

Despite all these data, an elevation of cTn in patients with trastuzumab therapy is usually seen at the shift between the AC and trastuzumab treatments, leading to cardiac injury and dysfunction [12].

One of the largest studies evaluating the role of cTnT and cTnI in predicting the cardiac dysfunction of patients [69] with trastuzumab treatment established that an increased baseline of cTnT and cTnI was associated with a 4-fold increased risk of cardiac dysfunction [62]. A study that included 251 patients with breast cancer receiving trastuzumab treatment, with or without AC in combination, revealed that cardiotoxicity occurred in 17% of the patients and affected mostly the patients with elevated cTnI (62% vs. 5%, $p < 0.001$). The recovery of the LVEF was present in 60% of these patients, and an improvement in the LVEF was less likely in patients with positive cTnI levels during treatment (35% vs. 100%; $p < 0.001$). In a multivariate analysis, the cTnI levels were the only independent predictor for cardiotoxicity related to trastuzumab treatment (HR: 22.9; 95% CI: 11.6–45.5; $p < 0.001$) and of the absence of LV function recovery (HR: 2.88; 95% CI: 1.78–4.65; $p < 0.001$). The patients who received a combination of drugs with AC prior to trastuzumab were more likely to present with positive levels of cTnI, suggesting that the high levels of cTn were determined by the preexisting myocardial damage secondary to the AC treatment [21]. Similar results, confirming that the levels of us-cTnI at the end of AC treatment were a predictor of cardiotoxicity in patients treated with trastuzumab, were demonstrated by a study performed in Tunisia [66].

These studies raise some questions regarding the elevation of cTn levels. The most important is related to the relationship between the increased levels of cTn after AC treatment and patients that continue on to receive trastuzumab. If increased levels of cTn occur mostly in patients treated previously with AC and drop over time, regardless of trastuzumab treatment, this could be explained by two mechanisms. First, the mechanism suggests that the increased levels of cTn appear as a consequence of the AC treatment, and are not related to trastuzumab. This possibility is supported by the high levels of cTn detected before trastuzumab treatment and the high levels of cTn that can persist for months after AC treatment. Another possibility is that the increased levels of cTn occur by the direct trastuzumab damage of the already-vulnerable heart after AC administration. Considering the fact that myocardial HER2 expression increases early after AC treatment and disperses in time, this mechanism is also plausible [70]. The studies to come should shed light on this dilemma.

Despite the results presented above, a study on 54 patients receiving adjuvant therapy with trastuzumab did not find an association between the levels of cTn and the risk of cardiac dysfunction [44]. Another study evaluated 95 patients with breast cancer receiving trastuzumab after chemotherapy with AC, and showed that an increase in cTnI at 14 weeks after the beginning of chemotherapy preceded the maximum deterioration of the LVEF, but did not predict or relate to the maximum decline in the LVEF [45]. However, a study aimed at finding a pharmacokinetic–pharmacodynamic (biomarker) model for the prediction of LVEF decreases showed that the maximum concentration of cTnT after AC treatment was an important determinant for reduced LVEF levels resulting from trastuzumab treatment [63].

The studies performed until now have shown conflicting results for the association between cTn and cardiac dysfunction. The most likely explanation for these results is the timing of cTn detection and the previous AC treatment [58]. In this context, major studies to detect a association between the levels of troponin and cardiotoxicity from trastuzumab (with or without AC association) are needed in order to specify the exact timing of cTn detection and its relationship with the presentation of cardiac dysfunction.

An interesting study showed that cTnI could predict the reversibility of cardiotoxicity induced by trastuzumab. All patients with cardiac dysfunction with cTnI levels < 0.08 ng/mL recovered their normal cardiac function, while only 35% patients with cTnI levels over this threshold recovered [53].

The available recommendations for cTn measurements in patients receiving trastuzumab treatment depend on the cardiotoxicity risk of the patients. For all patients, cTn should be measured before the beginning of the treatment and at 12 months after the completion of therapy. In patients with a low risk, cTn should be measured every four cycles; in medium-risk patients, it should be measured before alternate cycles for 3–6 months and every three cycles for the remaining treatment until 1 year. At 3–6 months after the final cycle, a cTn assay should be performed. Patients with a high risk should have an assessment of cTn before and after every cycle for the first 3–6 months, then every three cycles until 1 year. After the end of the treatment, another measurement should be performed at every 3 months [13].

2.6. Immunotherapy

Immune checkpoint inhibitors (ICSs) belong to a class of anticancer treatment that magnifies T cell-mediated immune feedback against cancer cells. The cardiotoxic effects of ICS include myocarditis, cardiomyopathy, arrhythmias, and vasculitis, but myocarditis is the side effect associated with major morbidity and high mortality [71].

The incidence of myocarditis associated with ICS treatment was 0.27% in patients receiving a combination of therapies and 0.09% in patients receiving a single ICS. A multi-center registry noted a prevalence of 1.14% for a single treatment, which increased to 2.4% for a combination of therapies [71]. Although myocarditis can appear at any time during ICS treatment, it usually appears early, in most cases occurring in the first 3 months of therapy, and it is associated with a very high mortality rate (38–46%) and a high number of nonfatal major cardiovascular events, such as HF, complete heart block, ventricular arrhythmias, cardiac arrest, or cardiogenic shock [72].

According to the recommendations for the diagnosis of myocarditis associated with chemotherapy, the gold standard is a myocardial biopsy. Cardiac magnetic resonance (CMR) is the preferred imagistic modality for diagnosis because of its tissue characterization techniques. Positron emission tomography can be used in certain conditions, especially when CMR is not suitable or when the results are equivocal. Biomarkers of cardiac necrosis, especially cTn (the most specific marker for myocardial injury), are used as a minor criterion for the diagnosis of myocarditis associated with chemotherapy [73].

Patients treated with ICS and diagnosed with myocarditis (associated with chemotherapy) by endomyocardial biopsy on autopsy had elevated levels of cTn (94%), and 46% of these patients developed major cardiac events: cardiovascular death, cardiogenic shock, cardiac arrest, or complete heart block with hemodynamic instability. A cTn level > 1.5 ng/mL was associated with a 4-fold increased risk of major cardiac events (HR: 4.0; 95% CI: 1.5–10.9; p = 0.003) [58]. Although elevated levels of cTn are not a specific indicator of cardiotoxicity induced by ICS, they predict a poor prognosis and should be interpreted as an indication of adverse cardiac events [74].

A study on 252 patients with lung cancer treated with ICS showed that the incidence of major cardiovascular events was similar in patients treated with ICS and patients treated with other therapies. Nevertheless, ICS-associated cardiotoxicity occurred early during therapy, was dose-independent, and was associated with elevated levels of cTnI [75].

The prompt recognition and risk stratification of myocarditis in patients receiving ICS treatment, especially for those with diabetes, autoimmune diseases, or cardiovascular conditions, can be helpful for reducing mortality and cardiovascular complications. The highest sensitivity for the early diagnosis of myocarditis is obtained by using ECG and hs-cTn; therefore, cTn measurements according to the latest recommendations could be important [71].

The available guidelines of the ESC suggest measurements of cTn before the initiation of treatment and at any moment of the treatment if new cardiovascular symptoms appear during the treatment (e.g., dyspnea, chest pain, palpitations, syncope, or presyncope). In high-risk patients, assessments of cTn should be performed before the second, third, and fourth doses. If the measurements are normal, the measurements can be reduced to alternating doses until the 12th dose, and then every three doses until the completion of treatment [13].

2.7. Anti-Vascular Endothelial Growth Factor-Targeted Therapy

Anti-vascular endothelial growth factor (VEGF) therapy includes agents that block the binding of VEGF to receptors, antibodies that arrest the communication through receptors, and tyrosine kinase inhibitors (TKI) that impede the kinase activity on VEGF receptors. These drugs have been associated with hypertension and LV dysfunction, and the possible mechanisms for the development of the latter could be increased ventricular overload, direct toxicity to cardiomyocytes, or microvascular dysfunction [27].

Tyrosine kinase inhibitors (TKI) belong to a class of drugs that target the VEGF receptor, which suppresses the angiogenic response in cancerous tissue. The incidence of asymptomatic LV dysfunction is 30%, and symptomatic heart failure appears in 3–15% of patients receiving TKI treatment [15].

Data on the role of cTn in these patients are scarce, and the largest study in this area, which evaluated 90 patients treated with TKI inhibitors, could not find a connection between the elevation of cTn levels and cardiac dysfunction as evaluated by magnetic resonance imaging, echocardiography, and coronary angiograms [76]. At this moment, we do not have an official recommendation for assessing the levels of cTn during treatment with VEGF [27].

3. Conclusions

During risk assessment for the cardiotoxicity of different chemotherapy drugs, cTn is an important tool for the early detection of cardiac injury and could predict subsequent changes in the LVEF and the development of HF. The assessment of cTn can be a very useful tool for identifying patients that would benefit from cardiotoxicity prevention treatments, and for monitoring the responses of the patient to treatment. Although much progress has been made so far, and cTn is an important assay in the evaluation of cancer patients, we have little data about the cut-off values of cTn over which patients are certain to develop cardiotoxicity and the levels that suggest a discontinuation of treatment. In this context, an estimation of other confounding factors that could be associated with cTn increases should be assessed and the confirmation of cardiotoxicity should be made by imagistic methods.

An increase in the cTn isolated from other identifiable changes in the cardiac structure and function should not be used as a justifiable reason for chemotherapy cessation. An elevated cTn level should be assessed by the medical team of the patient (oncologist and cardiologist), the risks and benefits should be discussed, and the best decision regarding patient's treatment and well-being should be taken according to the available information. Elevated cTn levels could lead to increased monitoring frequency, provoke further cardiovascular investigation, or initiate cardioprotective treatment [13]. According to the recommendations of the ESC, patients should be monitored depending on their cardiotoxicity risk, not by their cTn level. If their baseline value of cTn is high, the monitoring frequency should increase and other imagistic methods should be used in order to establish the diagnosis of cardiotoxicity, considering the fact that cTn is not a tool for diagnosis, but a marker of increased risk [8].

Author Contributions: Conceptualization, V.S., O.S. and L.S.; methodology, R.E.H.; investigation, P.C.M. and M.C.; data curation, A.S., A.C. and O.R.P.; writing—original draft preparation, O.S. and M.C.; writing—review and editing, C.L., I.I.C. and A.O.P.; visualization, V.S.; supervision, L.S. All authors have read and agreed to the published version of the manuscript.

Funding: This research received no external funding.

Data Availability Statement: Not applicable.

Acknowledgments: We would like to thank the Critical Patient Medicine Association for the donations received.

Conflicts of Interest: The authors declare no conflict of interest.

References

1. Michel, L.; Rassaf, T.; Totzeck, M. Biomarkers for the detection of apparent and subclinical cancer therapy-related cardiotoxicity. *J. Thorac. Dis.* **2018**, *10* (Suppl. 35), S4282–S4295. [CrossRef] [PubMed]
2. Gong, F.F.; Cascino, G.J.; Murtagh, G.; Akhter, N. Circulating Biomarkers for Cardiotoxicity Risk Prediction. *Curr. Treat. Options Oncol.* **2021**, *22*, 46. [CrossRef] [PubMed]
3. Berliner, D.; Beutel, G.; Bauersachs, J. Echocardiography and biomarkers for the diagnosis of cardiotoxicity. *Herz* **2020**, *45*, 637–644. [CrossRef] [PubMed]
4. Vohra, A.; Asnani, A. Biomarker Discovery in Cardio-Oncology. *Curr. Cardiol. Rep.* **2018**, *20*, 52. [CrossRef] [PubMed]
5. Semeraro, G.C.; Cipolla, C.M.; Cardinale, D.M. Role of Cardiac Biomarkers in Cancer Patients. *Cancers* **2021**, *13*, 5426. [CrossRef]
6. Rao, V.U.; Reeves, D.J.; Chugh, A.R.; O'Quinn, R.; Fradley, M.G.; Raghavendra, M.; Dent, S.; Barac, A.; Lenihan, D. Clinical Approach to Cardiovascular Toxicity of Oral Antineoplastic Agents: JACC State-of-the-Art Review. *J. Am. Coll. Cardiol.* **2021**, *77*, 2693–2716. [CrossRef]
7. Zamorano, J.L.; Lancellotti, P.; Rodriguez Muñoz, D.; Aboyans, V.; Asteggiano, R.; Galderisi, M.; Habib, G.; Lenihan, D.J.; Lip, G.Y.H.; Lyon, A.R.; et al. 2016 ESC Position Paper on cancer treatments and cardiovascular toxicity developed under the auspices of the ESC Committee for Practice Guidelines: The Task Force for cancer treatments and cardiovascular toxicity of the European Society of Cardiology (ESC). *Eur. Heart J.* **2016**, *37*, 2768–2801. [CrossRef] [PubMed]
8. Herrmann, J.; Lenihan, D.; Armenian, S.; Barac, A.; Blaes, A.; Cardinale, D.; Carver, J.; Dent, S.; Ky, B.; Lyon, A.R.; et al. Defining cardiovascular toxicities of cancer therapies: An International Cardio-Oncology Society (IC-OS) consensus statement. *Eur. Heart J.* **2022**, *43*, 280–299. [CrossRef]
9. Xiao, H.; Wang, X.; Li, S.; Liu, Y.; Cui, Y.; Deng, X. Advances in Biomarkers for Detecting Early Cancer Treatment-Related Cardiac Dysfunction. *Front. Cardiovasc. Med.* **2021**, *8*, 753313. [CrossRef]
10. Bojan, A.; Torok-Vistai, T.; Parvu, A. Assessment and Management of Cardiotoxicity in Hematologic Malignancies. *Dis. Markers.* **2021**, *2021*, 6616265. [CrossRef] [PubMed]
11. Ananthan, K.; Lyon, A.R. The Role of Biomarkers in Cardio-Oncology. *J. Cardiovasc. Transl. Res.* **2020**, *13*, 431–450. [CrossRef] [PubMed]
12. Herrmann, J. Adverse cardiac effects of cancer therapies: Cardiotoxicity and arrhythmia. *Nat. Rev. Cardiol.* **2020**, *17*, 474–502. [CrossRef] [PubMed]
13. Čelutkienė, J.; Pudil, R.; López-Fernández, T.; Grapsa, J.; Nihoyannopoulos, P.; Bergler-Klein, J.; Cohen-Solal, A.; Farmakis, D.; Tocchetti, C.G.; von Haehling, S.; et al. Role of cardiovascular imaging in cancer patients receiving cardiotoxic therapies: A position statement on behalf of the Heart Failure Association (HFA), the European Association of Cardiovascular Imaging (EACVI) and the Cardio-Oncology Council of the European Society of Cardiology (ESC). *Eur. J. Heart Fail.* **2020**, *22*, 1504–1524. [PubMed]
14. Pareek, N.; Cevallos, J.; Moliner, P.; Shah, M.; Tan, L.L.; Chambers, V.; Baksi, A.J.; Khattar, R.S.; Sharma, R.; Rosen, S.D.; et al. Activity and outcomes of a cardio-oncology service in the United Kingdom-a five-year experience. *Eur. J. Heart Fail.* **2018**, *20*, 1721–1731. [CrossRef] [PubMed]
15. Stevens, P.L.; Lenihan, D.J. Cardiotoxicity due to Chemotherapy: The Role of Biomarkers. *Curr. Cardiol. Rep.* **2015**, *17*, 603. [CrossRef] [PubMed]
16. Yu, A.F.; Ky, B. Roadmap for biomarkers of cancer therapy cardiotoxicity. *Heart* **2016**, *102*, 425–430. [CrossRef] [PubMed]

17. Horacek, J.M.; Vasatova, M.; Pudil, R.; Tichy, M.; Zak, P.; Jakl, M.; Jebavy, L.; Maly, J. Biomarkers for the early detection of anthracycline-induced cardiotoxicity: Current status. *Biomed. Pap. Med. Fac. Univ. Palacky Olomouc Czech Repub.* **2014**, *158*, 511–517. [CrossRef] [PubMed]
18. Semeraro, G.C.; Lamantia, G.; Cipolla, C.M.; Cardinale, D. How to identify anthracycline-induced cardiotoxicity early and reduce its clinical impact in everyday practice. *Kardiol. Pol.* **2021**, *79*, 114–122. [CrossRef]
19. Jones, M.; O'Gorman, P.; Kelly, C.; Mahon, N.; Fitzgibbon, M.C. High-sensitive cardiac troponin-I facilitates timely detection of subclinical anthracycline-mediated cardiac injury. *Ann. Clin. Biochem.* **2017**, *54*, 149–157. [CrossRef]
20. Tan, L.L.; Lyon, A.R. Role of Biomarkers in Prediction of Cardiotoxicity During Cancer Treatment. *Curr Treat. Options Cardiovasc. Med.* **2018**, *20*, 55. [CrossRef]
21. Cardinale, D.; Sandri, M.T. Role of biomarkers in chemotherapy-induced cardiotoxicity. *Prog. Cardiovasc. Dis.* **2010**, *53*, 121–129. [CrossRef]
22. Shah, K.S.; Yang, E.H.; Maisel, A.S.; Fonarow, G.C. The Role of Biomarkers in Detection of Cardio-toxicity. *Curr. Oncol. Rep.* **2017**, *19*, 42. [CrossRef]
23. Muthu, V.; Kozman, H.; Liu, K.; Smulyan, H.; Villarreal, D. Cardiac troponins: Bench to bedside interpretation in cardiac disease. *Am. J. Med. Sci.* **2014**, *347*, 331–337. [CrossRef] [PubMed]
24. O'Brien, P.J. Cardiac troponin is the most effective translational safety biomarker for myocardial injury in cardiotoxicity. *Toxicology* **2008**, *245*, 206–218. [CrossRef] [PubMed]
25. Soetkamp, D.; Raedschelders, K.; Mastali, M.; Sobhani, K.; Bairey Merz, C.N.; Van Eyk, J. The continuing evolution of cardiac troponin I biomarker analysis: From protein to proteoform. *Expert. Rev. Proteom.* **2017**, *14*, 973–986. [CrossRef] [PubMed]
26. Sorodoc, V.; Sorodoc, L.; Ungureanu, D.; Sava, A.; Jaba, I.M. Cardiac troponin T and NT-proBNP as biomarkers of early myocardial damage in amitriptyline-induced cardiovascular toxicity in rats. *Int. J. Toxicol.* **2013**, *32*, 351–357. [CrossRef] [PubMed]
27. Pudil, R.; Mueller, C.; Čelutkienė, J.; Henriksen, P.A.; Lenihan, D.; Dent, S.; Barac, A.; Stanway, S.; Moslehi, J.; Suter, T.M.; et al. Role of serum biomarkers in cancer patients receiving cardiotoxic cancer therapies: A position statement from the Cardio-Oncology Study Group of the Heart Failure Association and the Cardio-Oncology Council of the European Society of Cardiology. *Eur. J. Heart Fail.* **2020**, *22*, 1966–1983. [CrossRef] [PubMed]
28. Agewall, S.; Giannitsis, E. Troponin elevation in coronary ischemia and necrosis. *Curr. Atheroscler. Rep.* **2014**, *16*, 396. [CrossRef] [PubMed]
29. Mair, J.; Lindahl, B.; Hammarsten, O.; Müller, C.; Giannitsis, E.; Huber, K.; Möckel, M.; Plebani, M.; Thygesen, K.; Jaffe, A.S. How is cardiac troponin released from injured myocardium? *Eur. Heart J. Acute Cardiovasc. Care* **2018**, *7*, 553–560. [CrossRef] [PubMed]
30. Hammarsten, O.; Mair, J.; Möckel, M.; Lindahl, B.; Jaffe, A.S. Possible mechanisms behind cardiac troponin elevations. *Biomarkers* **2018**, *23*, 725–734. [CrossRef]
31. Gresslien, T.; Agewall, S. Troponin and exercise. *Int. J. Cardiol.* **2016**, *221*, 609–621. [CrossRef] [PubMed]
32. Hickman, P.E.; Potter, J.M.; Aroney, C.; Koerbin, G.; Southcott, E.; Wu, A.H.; Roberts, M.S. Cardiac troponin may be released by ischemia alone, without necrosis. *Clin. Chim. Acta* **2010**, *411*, 318–323. [CrossRef] [PubMed]
33. Clerico, A.; Zaninotto, M.; Passino, C.; Aspromonte, N.; Piepoli, M.F.; Migliardi, M.; Perrone, M.; Fortunato, A.; Padoan, A.; Testa, A.; et al. Evidence on clinical relevance of cardiovascular risk evaluation in the general population using cardio-specific biomarkers. *Clin. Chem. Lab. Med.* **2020**, *59*, 79–90. [CrossRef] [PubMed]
34. Swain, S.M.; Whaley, F.S.; Ewer, M.S. Congestive heart failure in patients treated with doxorubicin: A retrospective analysis of three trials. *Cancer* **2003**, *97*, 2869–2879. [CrossRef] [PubMed]
35. Fornaro, A.; Olivotto, I.; Rigacci, L.; Ciaccheri, M.; Tomberli, B.; Ferrantini, C.; Coppini, R.; Girolami, F.; Mazzarotto, F.; Chiostri, M.; et al. Comparison of long-term outcome in anthracycline-related versus idiopathic dilated cardiomyopathy: A single centre experience. *Eur. J. Heart Fail.* **2018**, *20*, 898–906. [CrossRef] [PubMed]
36. Cardinale, D.; Sandri, M.T.; Martinoni, A.; Tricca, A.; Civelli, M.; Lamantia, G.; Cinieri, S.; Martinelli, G.; Cipolla, C.M.; Fiorentini, C. Left ventricular dysfunction predicted by early troponin I release after high-dose chemotherapy. *J. Am. Coll. Cardiol.* **2000**, *36*, 517–522. [CrossRef]
37. Cardinale, D.; Sandri, M.T.; Colombo, A.; Colombo, N.; Boeri, M.; Lamantia, G.; Civelli, M.; Peccatori, F.; Martinelli, G.; Fiorentini, C.; et al. Prognostic value of troponin I in cardiac risk stratification of cancer patients undergoing high-dose chemotherapy. *Circulation* **2004**, *109*, 2749–2754. [CrossRef]
38. Díaz-Antón, B.; Madurga, R.; Zorita, B.; Wasniewski, S.; Moreno-Arciniegas, A.; López-Melgar, B.; Ramírez Merino, N.; Martín-Asenjo, R.; Barrio, P.; Amado Escañuela, M.G.; et al. Early detection of anthracycline- and trastuzumab-induced cardiotoxicity: Value and optimal timing of serum biomarkers and echocardiographic parameters. *ESC Heart Fail.* **2022**, *9*, 1127–1137. [CrossRef] [PubMed]
39. Michel, L.; Mincu, R.I.; Mahabadi, A.A.; Settelmeier, S.; Al-Rashid, F.; Rassaf, T.; Totzeck, M. Troponins and brain natriuretic peptides for the prediction of cardiotoxicity in cancer patients: A meta-analysis. *Eur. J. Heart Fail.* **2020**, *22*, 350–361. [CrossRef] [PubMed]
40. Auner, H.W.; Tinchon, C.; Linkesch, W.; Tiran, A.; Quehenberger, F.; Link, H.; Sill, H. Prolonged monitoring of troponin T for the detection of anthracycline cardiotoxicity in adults with hematological malignancies. *Ann. Hematol.* **2003**, *82*, 218–222. [CrossRef] [PubMed]

41. Kilickap, S.; Barista, I.; Akgul, E.; Aytemir, K.; Aksoyek, S.; Aksoy, S.; Celik, I.; Kes, S.; Tekuzman, G. cTnT can be a useful marker for early detection of anthracycline cardiotoxicity. *Ann. Oncol.* **2005**, *16*, 798–804. [CrossRef] [PubMed]
42. Nisticò, C.; Bria, E.; Cuppone, F.; Carpino, A.; Ferretti, G.; Vitelli, G.; Sperduti, I.; Calabretta, F.; Toglia, G.; Tomao, S.; et al. Troponin-T and myoglobin plus echocardiographic evaluation for monitoring early cardiotoxicity of weekly epirubicin-paclitaxel in metastatic breast cancer patients. *Anticancer Drugs.* **2007**, *18*, 227–232. [CrossRef] [PubMed]
43. Horacek, J.M.; Pudil, R.; Tichy, M.; Jebavy, L.; Strasova, A.; Ulrychova, M.; Zak, P.; Maly, J. Cardiac troponin I seems to be superior to cardiac troponin T in the early detection of cardiac injury associated with anthracycline treatment. *Onkologie* **2008**, *31*, 559–560. [CrossRef] [PubMed]
44. Feola, M.; Garrone, O.; Occelli, M.; Francini, A.; Biggi, A.; Visconti, G.; Albrile, F.; Bobbio, M.; Merlano, M. Cardiotoxicity after anthracycline chemotherapy in breast carcinoma: Effects on left ventricular ejection fraction, troponin I and brain natriuretic peptide. *Int. J. Cardiol.* **2011**, *148*, 194–198. [CrossRef] [PubMed]
45. Morris, P.G.; Chen, C.; Steingart, R.; Fleisher, M.; Lin, N.; Moy, B.; Come, S.; Sugarman, S.; Abbruzzi, A.; Lehman, R.; et al. Troponin I and C-reactive protein are commonly detected in patients with breast cancer treated with dose-dense chemotherapy incorporating trastuzumab and lapatinib. *Clin. Cancer Res.* **2011**, *17*, 3490–3499. [CrossRef]
46. Sawaya, H.; Sebag, I.A.; Plana, J.C.; Januzzi, J.L.; Ky, B.; Tan, T.C.; Cohen, V.; Banchs, J.; Carver, J.R.; Wiegers, S.E.; et al. Assessment of echocardiography and biomarkers for the extended prediction of cardiotoxicity in patients treated with anthracyclines, taxanes, and trastuzumab. *Circ. Cardiovasc. Imaging* **2012**, *5*, 596–603. [CrossRef] [PubMed]
47. Onitilo, A.A.; Engel, J.M.; Stankowski, R.V.; Liang, H.; Berg, R.L.; Doi, S.A. High-sensitivity C-reactive protein (hs-CRP) as a biomarker for trastuzumab-induced cardiotoxicity in HER2-positive early-stage breast cancer: A pilot study. *Breast Cancer Res. Treat.* **2012**, *134*, 291–298. [CrossRef]
48. Blaes, A.H.; Rehman, A.; Vock, D.M.; Luo, X.; Menge, M.; Yee, D.; Missov, E.; Duprez, D. Utility of high-sensitivity cardiac troponin T in patients receiving anthracycline chemotherapy. *Vasc. Health Risk Manag.* **2015**, *11*, 591–594. [CrossRef]
49. Malik, A.; Jeyaraj, P.A.; Calton, R.; Uppal, B.; Negi, P.; Shankar, A.; Patil, J.; Mahajan, M.K. Are Biomarkers Predictive of Anthracycline-Induced Cardiac Dysfunction? *Asian Pac. J. Cancer Prev.* **2016**, *17*, 2301–2305. [CrossRef] [PubMed]
50. Ferreira de Souza, T.; Quinaglia AC Silva, T.; Osorio Costa, F.; Shah, R.; Neilan, T.G.; Velloso, L.; Nadruz, W.; Brenelli, F.; Sposito, A.C.; Matos-Souza, J.R.; et al. Anthracycline Therapy Is Associated with Cardiomyocyte Atrophy and Preclinical Manifestations of Heart Disease. *JACC Cardiovasc. Imaging* **2018**, *11*, 1045–1055. [CrossRef]
51. Demissei, B.G.; Hubbard, R.A.; Zhang, L.; Smith, A.M.; Sheline, K.; McDonald, C.; Narayan, V.; Domchek, S.M.; DeMichele, A.; Shah, P.; et al. Changes in Cardiovascular Biomarkers with Breast Cancer Therapy and Associations with Cardiac Dysfunction. *J. Am. Heart Assoc.* **2020**, *9*, e014708. [CrossRef]
52. Cardinale, D.; Colombo, A.; Sandri, M.T.; Lamantia, G.; Colombo, N.; Civelli, M.; Martinelli, G.; Veglia, F.; Fiorentini, C.; Cipolla, C.M. Prevention of high-dose chemotherapy-induced cardiotoxicity in high-risk patients by angiotensin-converting enzyme inhibition. *Circulation* **2006**, *114*, 2474–2481. [CrossRef]
53. Cardinale, D.; Ciceri, F.; Latini, R.; Franzosi, M.G.; Sandri, M.T.; Civelli, M.; Cucchi, G.; Menatti, E.; Mangiavacchi, M.; Cavina, R.; et al. ICOS-ONE Study Investigators. Anthracycline-induced cardiotoxicity: A multicenter randomised trial comparing two strategies for guiding prevention with enalapril: The International CardioOncology Society-one trial. *Eur. J. Cancer.* **2018**, *94*, 126–137. [CrossRef] [PubMed]
54. Cardinale, D.; Colombo, A.; Lamantia, G.; Colombo, N.; Civelli, M.; De Giacomi, G.; Rubino, M.; Veglia, F.; Fiorentini, C.; Cipolla, C.M. Anthracycline-induced cardiomyopathy: Clinical relevance and response to pharmacologic therapy. *J. Am. Coll. Cardiol.* **2010**, *55*, 213–220. [CrossRef]
55. Xu, T.; Meng, Q.H.; Gilchrist, S.C.; Lin, S.H.; Lin, R.; Xu, T.; Milgrom, S.A.; Gandhi, S.J.; Wu, H.; Zhao, Y.; et al. Assessment of Prognostic Value of High-Sensitivity Cardiac Troponin T for Early Prediction of Chemoradiation Therapy-Induced Cardiotoxicity in Patients with Non-Small Cell Lung Cancer: A Secondary Analysis of a Prospective Randomized Trial. *Int. J. Radiat. Oncol. Biol. Phys.* **2021**, *111*, 907–916. [CrossRef]
56. Kirkham, A.A.; Pituskin, E.; Thompson, R.B.; Mackey, J.R.; Koshman, S.L.; Jassal, D.; Pitz, M.; Haykowsky, M.J.; Pagano, J.J.; Chow, K.; et al. Cardiac and cardiometabolic phenotyping of trastuzumab-mediated cardiotoxicity: A secondary analysis of the MANTICORE trial. *Eur. Heart J. Cardiovasc. Pharmacother.* **2022**, *8*, 130–139. [CrossRef]
57. Dempsey, N.; Rosenthal, A.; Dabas, N.; Kropotova, Y.; Lippman, M.; Bishopric, N.H. Trastuzumab-induced cardiotoxicity: A review of clinical risk factors, pharmacologic prevention, and cardiotoxicity of other HER2-directed therapies. *Breast Cancer Res. Treat.* **2021**, *188*, 21–36. [CrossRef] [PubMed]
58. Bouwer, N.I.; Jager, A.; Liesting, C.; Kofflard, M.J.M.; Brugts, J.J.; Kitzen, J.J.E.M.; Boersma, E.; Levin, M.D. Cardiac monitoring in HER2-positive patients on trastuzumab treatment: A review and implications for clinical practice. *Breast* **2020**, *52*, 33–44. [CrossRef] [PubMed]
59. Cardinale, D.; Colombo, A.; Torrisi, R.; Sandri, M.T.; Civelli, M.; Salvatici, M.; Lamantia, G.; Colombo, N.; Cortinovis, S.; Dessanai, M.A.; et al. Trastuzumab-induced cardiotoxicity: Clinical and prognostic implications of troponin I evaluation. *J. Clin. Oncol.* **2010**, *28*, 3910–3916. [CrossRef] [PubMed]

60. Fallah-Rad, N.; Walker, J.R.; Wassef, A.; Lytwyn, M.; Bohonis, S.; Fang, T.; Tian, G.; Kirkpatrick, I.D.; Singal, P.K.; Krahn, M.; et al. The utility of cardiac biomarkers, tissue velocity and strain imaging, and cardiac magnetic resonance imaging in predicting early left ventricular dysfunction in patients with human epidermal growth factor receptor II-positive breast cancer treated with adjuvant trastuzumab therapy. *J. Am. Coll. Cardiol.* **2011**, *57*, 2263–2270. [PubMed]
61. Ky, B.; Putt, M.; Sawaya, H.; French, B.; Januzzi JLJr Sebag, I.A.; Plana, J.C.; Cohen, V.; Banchs, J.; Carver, J.R.; Wiegers, S.E.; et al. Early increases in multiple biomarkers predict subsequent cardiotoxicity in patients with breast cancer treated with doxorubicin, taxanes, and trastuzumab. *J. Am. Coll. Cardiol.* **2014**, *63*, 809–816. [CrossRef] [PubMed]
62. Zardavas, D.; Suter, T.M.; Van Veldhuisen, D.J.; Steinseifer, J.; Noe, J.; Lauer, S.; Al-Sakaff, N.; Piccart-Gebhart, M.J.; de Azambuja, E. Role of Troponins I and T and N-Terminal Prohormone of Brain Natriuretic Peptide in Monitoring Cardiac Safety of Patients with Early-Stage Human Epidermal Growth Factor Receptor 2-Positive Breast Cancer Receiving Trastuzumab: A Herceptin Adjuvant Study Cardiac Marker Substudy. *J. Clin. Oncol.* **2017**, *35*, 878–884. [PubMed]
63. Yu, A.F.; Manrique, C.; Pun, S.; Liu, J.E.; Mara, R.; Fleisher, M.; Patil, S.; Jones, L.W.; Steingart, R.M.; Hudis, C.A.; et al. Cardiac Safety of Paclitaxel Plus Trastuzumab and Pertuzumab in Patients with HER2-Positive Metastatic Breast Cancer. *Oncologist* **2016**, *21*, 418–424. [CrossRef] [PubMed]
64. de Vries Schultink, A.H.M.; Boekhout, A.H.; Gietema, J.A.; Burylo, A.M.; Dorlo, T.P.C.; van Hasselt, J.G.C.; Schellens, J.H.M. Huitema, A.D.R. Pharmacodynamic modeling of cardiac biomarkers in breast cancer patients treated with anthracycline and trastuzumab regimens. *J. Pharmacokinet. Pharmacodyn.* **2018**, *45*, 431–442. [CrossRef] [PubMed]
65. Ponde, N.; Bradbury, I.; Lambertini, M.; Ewer, M.; Campbell, C.; Ameels, H.; Zardavas, D.; Di Cosimo, S.; Baselga, J.; Huober, J.; et al. Cardiac biomarkers for early detection and prediction of trastuzumab and/or lapatinib-induced cardiotoxicity in patients with HER2-positive early-stage breast cancer: A NeoALTTO sub-study (BIG 1-06). *Breast Cancer Res. Treat.* **2018**, *168*, 631–638. [CrossRef]
66. Ben Kridis, W.; Sghaier, S.; Charfeddine, S.; Toumi, N.; Daoud, J.; Kammoun, S.; Khanfir, A. A Prospective Study About Trastuzumab-induced Cardiotoxicity in HER2-positive Breast Cancer. *Am. J. Clin. Oncol.* **2020**, *43*, 510–516. [CrossRef] [PubMed]
67. Seidman, A.; Hudis, C.; Pierri, M.K.; Shak, S.; Paton, V.; Ashby, M.; Murphy, M.; Stewart, S.J.; Keefe, D. Cardiac dysfunction in the trastuzumab clinical trials experience. *J. Clin. Oncol.* **2002**, *20*, 1215–1221. [CrossRef]
68. Rushton, M.; Johnson, C.; Dent, S. Trastuzumab-induced cardiotoxicity: Testing a clinical risk score in a real-world cardio-oncology population. *Curr. Oncol.* **2017**, *24*, 176–180. [CrossRef]
69. Viani, G.A.; Afonso, S.L.; Stefano, E.J.; De Fendi, L.I.; Soares, F.V. Adjuvant trastuzumab in the treatment of her-2-positive early breast cancer: A meta-analysis of published randomized trials. *BMC Cancer* **2007**, *7*, 153. [CrossRef]
70. Witteles, R.M. Biomarkers as Predictors of Cardiac Toxicity from Targeted Cancer Therapies. *J. Card Fail.* **2016**, *22*, 459–464. [CrossRef] [PubMed]
71. Ganatra, S.; Parikh, R.; Neilan, T.G. Cardiotoxicity of Immune Therapy. *Cardiol Clin.* **2019**, *37*, 385–397. [CrossRef] [PubMed]
72. Mahmood, S.S.; Fradley, M.G.; Cohen, J.V.; Nohria, A.; Reynolds, K.L.; Heinzerling, L.M.; Sullivan, R.J.; Damrongwatanasuk, R.; Chen, C.L.; Gupta, D.; et al. Myocarditis in Patients Treated with Immune Checkpoint Inhibitors. *J. Am. Coll. Cardiol.* **2018**, *71*, 1755–1764. [CrossRef] [PubMed]
73. Bonaca, M.P.; Olenchock, B.A.; Salem, J.E.; Wiviott, S.D.; Ederhy, S.; Cohen, A.; Stewart, G.C.; Choueiri, T.K.; Di Carli, M.; Allenbach, Y.; et al. Myocarditis in the Setting of Cancer Therapeutics: Proposed Case Definitions for Emerging Clinical Syndromes in Cardio-Oncology. *Circulation* **2019**, *140*, 80–91. [CrossRef] [PubMed]
74. Spallarossa, P.; Tini, G.; Sarocchi, M.; Arboscello, E.; Grossi, F.; Queirolo, P.; Zoppoli, G.; Ameri, P. Identification and Management of Immune Checkpoint Inhibitor-Related Myocarditis: Use Troponin Wisely. *J. Clin. Oncol.* **2019**, *37*, 2201–2205. [CrossRef] [PubMed]
75. Chitturi, K.R.; Xu, J.; Araujo-Gutierrez, R.; Bhimaraj, A.; Guha, A.; Hussain, I.; Kassi, M.; Bernicker, E.H.; Trachtenberg, B.H. Immune Checkpoint Inhibitor-Related Adverse Cardiovascular Events in Patients with Lung Cancer. *JACC Cardio Oncol.* **2019**, *1*, 182–192. [CrossRef] [PubMed]
76. Ederhy, S.; Massard, C.; Dufaitre, G.; Balheda, R.; Meuleman, C.; Rocca, C.G.; Izzedine, H.; Cohen, A.; Soria, J.C. Frequency and management of troponin I elevation in patients treated with molecular targeted therapies in phase I trials. *Investig. New Drugs* **2012**, *30*, 611–615. [CrossRef] [PubMed]

life

Review

New Insights into Non-Alcoholic Fatty Liver Disease and Coronary Artery Disease: The Liver-Heart Axis

Georgiana-Diana Cazac [1,2,†], Cristina-Mihaela Lăcătușu [1,2,*,†], Cătălina Mihai [3,4,†], Elena-Daniela Grigorescu [1,*,†], Alina Onofriescu [1,2,†] and Bogdan-Mircea Mihai [1,2,†]

1 Unit of Diabetes, Nutrition and Metabolic Diseases, "Grigore T. Popa" University of Medicine and Pharmacy, 700115 Iași, Romania
2 Clinical Center of Diabetes, Nutrition and Metabolic Diseases, "St. Spiridon" County Clinical Emergency Hospital, 700111 Iași, Romania
3 Institute of Gastroenterology and Hepatology, "Sf. Spiridon" Emergency Hospital, 700111 Iași, Romania
4 Unit of Medical Semiology and Gastroenterology, "Grigore T. Popa" University of Medicine and Pharmacy, 700115 Iasi, Romania
* Correspondence: cristina.lacatusu@umfiasi.ro (C.-M.L.); elena-daniela-gh-grigorescu@umfiasi.ro (E.-D.G.); Tel.: +40-72-321-1116 (C.-M.L.); +40-74-209-3749 (E.-D.G.)
† These authors contributed equally to this work.

Abstract: Non-alcoholic fatty liver disease (NAFLD) represents the hepatic expression of the metabolic syndrome and is the most prevalent liver disease. NAFLD is associated with liver-related and extrahepatic morbi-mortality. Among extrahepatic complications, cardiovascular disease (CVD) is the primary cause of mortality in patients with NAFLD. The most frequent clinical expression of CVD is the coronary artery disease (CAD). Epidemiological data support a link between CAD and NAFLD, underlain by pathogenic factors, such as the exacerbation of insulin resistance, genetic phenotype, oxidative stress, atherogenic dyslipidemia, pro-inflammatory mediators, and gut microbiota. A thorough assessment of cardiovascular risk and identification of all forms of CVD, especially CAD, are needed in all patients with NAFLD regardless of their metabolic status. Therefore, this narrative review aims to examine the available data on CAD seen in patients with NAFLD, to outline the main directions undertaken by the CVD risk assessment and the multiple putative underlying mechanisms implicated in the relationship between CAD and NAFLD, and to raise awareness about this underestimated association between two major, frequent and severe diseases.

Keywords: non-alcoholic fatty liver disease; coronary artery disease; cardiovascular risk; liver-heart axis

1. Introduction

Non-alcoholic fatty liver disease (NAFLD) is a chronic liver disease constantly on the rise among patients with metabolic syndrome (MS), leading to an emerging worldwide epidemic. Therefore, a growing volume of research tries to describe its pathogenesis, to determine the most appropriate therapy, and to identify the most accurate predictors for its evolution and prognosis [1].

Already recognized as the most widespread cause of chronic liver disease around the world, NAFLD is a growing public health problem extending to a prevalence of about 25% in the general population. Well-developed countries display the highest prevalences, due to the current unhealthy, sedentary lifestyle [2,3]. Reports of NAFLD involve more than 50% of persons with type 2 diabetes mellitus (T2DM) and 90% of people with severe obesity [3]. Advanced fibrosis is present in approximately 10–15% of patients with NAFLD in the United States and Europe [3]. Moreover, patients with histologically proven non-alcoholic steatohepatitis (NASH) have an increased risk of liver-related death [3,4]. The global prevalence of NAFLD is expected to increase in line with the rates of obesity and T2DM.

NAFLD is characterized by excessive hepatic accumulation of lipids caused by abdominal obesity and insulin resistance [5]. NAFLD is classically defined by the presence of steatosis affecting more than 5% of all hepatocytes (documented histologically by liver biopsy), in the absence of excessive alcohol consumption and after excluding other causes of steatosis such as drugs, or viral hepatitis, autoimmune diseases, hereditary liver disease or hypothyroidism [5,6]. In a recent move to redefine NAFLD as metabolic dysfunction associated fatty liver disease (MAFLD), criteria in a recent consensus include detection of hepatic steatosis in addition to one of three criteria represented by overweight/obesity, T2DM, or at least two metabolic risk factors [7]. NAFLD encompasses a spectrum of progressive pathological conditions ranging from simple steatosis to NASH, advanced fibrosis, liver cirrhosis, or even hepatocellular carcinoma (HCC) [5,6]. As mentioned above, advanced liver disease due to NAFLD is associated with a worsened prognosis. Therefore, the progression of NAFLD to these late stages of liver histology needs to be prevented.

Since the most important trigger of hepatic insulin resistance is the accumulation of lipids within the liver, NAFLD is perceived today as the hepatic manifestation of the MS [8]. Besides focusing on insulin resistance as the main target of the therapeutic strategy, ongoing studies provide new evidence on additional mechanisms that need to be dealt with in order to intervene on all MS components and to ameliorate all risk factors not only for advanced liver disease, but also for cardiovascular disease (CVD). This constellation of metabolic conditions also includes abdominal obesity, hyperlipidemia, hyperuricemia, chronic kidney disease, and T2DM [9].

Recent epidemiological research has identified a close relationship between these two global health problems, NAFLD and CVD. The progression of NAFLD displays the closest correlation with CVD, followed by extra-hepatic cancers and other liver-associated complications [10]. CVD represents a leading cause of death in the general population, with a prevalence of at least 40% among patients with NAFLD [2,11]. NAFLD is a predictor and a risk factor for the development of CVD, as it increases the risk of morbidity and mortality and impacts the progress to other extrahepatic manifestations [9]. Therefore, the highest mortality in NAFLD seems to be due to the aggravation of the CVD risk driven by metabolic comorbidities, and not to the evolution towards HCC or end-stage liver disease [12,13].

However, a minority of studies have not succeeded to demonstrate this significant association of NAFLD with the risk of CVD. Olubamwo et al. showed that incident CVD can be predicted in patients with NAFLD using a non-invasive test (NIT), but the results were not significant after adjustments based on metabolic factors [14]. Shah and colleagues reported no correlation between hepatic fat and atherosclerotic CVD (ASCVD), demonstrating instead a correlation between the rising incidence of ASCVD and a higher pericardial fat content [15].

In contrast with the few studies that failed to prove that hepatic steatosis significantly contributes to an increased cardiovascular risk, a greater number of researchers demonstrated a link existing between fatty liver and subclinical CVD, independently of traditional cardiovascular risk factors or other MS elements [16–18]. Differences in the inclusion criteria and the high variability of tools used for NAFLD and CVD diagnosis may be the explanation of this discrepancy between results [19].

Therefore, there is a high probability that NAFLD is an independent risk factor for CVD, regardless of other associated metabolic risk factors. The multiple conventional risk factors like dyslipidemia, hypertension, obesity, tobacco smoking, and T2DM are also strongly correlated with the incidence and severity of atherosclerosis. A well represented body of evidence supports the hypothesis that atherosclerosis and NAFLD share a handful of common cardiometabolic risk factors [20,21]. NAFLD not only promotes atherosclerosis, but also predisposes to the evolution towards coronary artery disease (CAD), valvular heart disease, left ventricular dysfunction, heart failure, arrhythmia, and stroke [22,23]. A longer duration and the progression to advanced stages of NAFLD are associated with an increased cardiovascular risk, including coronary lesions [24,25], high arterial stiffness [26], impaired endothelial function, or a greater risk for carotid intima-media thickening [27].

Further pathogenesis-related research is needed to identify all mechanisms and then develop targeted therapies able to decrease the additional CVD risk related to NAFLD. The evolution towards cardiovascular events and mortality could be prevented by a sustained screening for cardiovascular risk and an early intervention to reduce it. Since CAD is one of the most frequent forms of ASCVD, such an approach would surely serve to lower, in particular, the prevalence of coronary events and to reduce CAD-related morbidity and death.

In this review, we summarize the current knowledge on the pathogenesis linking together NAFLD and CAD and revise the available evidence validating the hypothesis that these two conditions share key pathological features. We also highlight the results of CAD risk assessment in patients with NAFLD, independently of their metabolic status, and the need for approaches to improve their outcome.

2. Epidemiology of the Relationship between NAFLD and CAD

Compared to non-NAFLD individuals, it appears that patients with NAFLD are associated with an important risk of fatal and non-fatal cardiovascular events such as angina, myocardial infarction, coronary revascularization, or stroke [28]. An extensive meta-analysis of six studies carried out on 25,837 adults, including nearly 6000 cases of NAFLD showed that patients with NAFLD had an increased risk of clinical cardiovascular events compared to those without NAFLD (14.9% vs. 6.3%) [29].

Narrowing the hypothesis that NAFLD is a risk factor for CVD, the fatty liver also appears to be a risk factor for CAD, independently of common risk factors, such as age, sex, family history of CVD, dyslipidemia, obesity, arterial hypertension, and diabetes [23].

Multiple publications indicate that patients at high risk for both diseases, such as those with diabetes, dyslipidemia, high level of low-density lipoprotein cholesterol, smoking, or family history of CAD, also have a high risk for non-calcified plaques (NCPs) [30–32].

A cohort study of 3756 North American individuals evaluated for NAFLD using computed tomography (CT) and for CAD using coronary computed angiography (CCTA) demonstrated that hepatic steatosis is associated with major adverse cardiovascular events (MACE) irrespective of other cardiovascular risk factors or of CAD extent, assessed by measurements of coronary stenosis or plaques [33]. According to Choi et al., the intensity of NAFLD was closely related to the severity of angiography-proven coronary artery stenosis in an Asian population. NAFLD kept its value of CAD predictor independently of common risk factors like age, gender, body mass index (BMI), or glycemic control [34].

In a recent meta-analysis, the prevalence of subclinical CAD in 67,070 patients with NAFLD reached 38.7% (95% confidence interval [CI]: 29.8%–48.5%) of asymptomatic patients (odds ratio [OR]: 1.22; CI: 1.13–1.31, $p < 0.001$), and clinical CAD was present in 55.4% (CI: 39.6%–70.1%) of symptomatic patients (OR: 2.18, CI: 1.69–2.81, $p < 0.0001$); both forms significantly correlated with NAFLD. Non-obstructive CAD had a 43.5% prevalence (CI: 30.3%–57.8%), higher than obstructive CAD, with a 33.5% prevalence (CI: 19.6%–51.1%) [35].

The research conducted by Lee et al. pointed out that only NCPs are independently associated with NAFLD, while the incidence of calcified or mixed plaques did not vary between people with or without NAFLD [36]. NCPs are suggestive of instability and predisposition to acute coronary events, whilst calcified plaques (CPs) add a less vulnerable feature [37]. Considering these findings, the mechanism leading to sudden, unexpected cardiac events in asymptomatic patients with NAFLD may be related to the NCPs instability and the elevated risk of plaque rupture [36].

During NAFLD progression, some data suggests that advanced fibrosis worsens the CAD state. Moreover, NASH has a lower risk for the liver fibrosis stage than for CAD lesions and cardiovascular events [38,39].

Furthermore, research adjusting for cardiometabolic risk factors found NAFLD severity to be independently associated with coronary atherosclerosis, especially with mixed type plaques. Moreover, even the population without associated metabolic risk factors had a higher risk for CAD and mixed atherosclerotic plaques when hepatic steatosis was more severe [40]. A study comparing NASH patients to controls with hepatic steatosis found the former to have a higher risk of coronary lesions (stenosis, NCPs and calcium score) [38].

Another example proving the existence of advanced, high-risk coronary plaques in patients with NAFLD is represented by a cohort study derived from The ROMICAT II trial (Rule Out Myocardial Infarction using Computer Assisted Tomography). Assessment by CCTA and hepatic CT demonstrated an increased prevalence of high-risk plaques compared to patients without NAFLD, irrespective of cardiovascular risk factors and CAD severity. Moreover, NAFLD added an approximately 6-fold higher risk for the development of acute coronary syndromes [41]. The risk of progression from subclinical coronary and carotid atherosclerosis also correlates with NAFLD [42].

Asymptomatic patients with NAFLD submitted to coronary angiography have a higher risk for needing percutaneous coronary interventions or bypass grafting surgery, with an increased risk for fatal and non-fatal outcomes. Among patients with NAFLD meeting the criteria for coronary artery bypass grafting surgery, levels of inflammatory markers were elevated in comparison to patients without NAFLD [43,44].

The prospective and retrospective studies focused on the relationship between NAFLD and clinical and subclinical forms of CAD, are listed in Tables 1 and 2 (all references are detailed within the tables).

Table 1. Summary of studies that evaluated the association between NAFLD and clinical CAD.

Author, Year, Ref.	Country	Study Type	NAFLD Diagnosis	CAD Diagnosis	Patients Characteristics	Impact of NAFLD on CAD/ Results
Thévenot et al., 2022 [45]	France	Prospective (CORONASH)	NIT FibroScan	Coronary angiography	189	5.3% advanced liver fibrosis (LSM ≥ 8 kPa) eLIFT, NFS—good sensitivity and specificity as first-line screening test for liver fibrosis
Hsu et al., 2021 [40]	Taiwan	Retrospective	US APRI	CCTA	1502 893 NAFLD 581 CAD	Steatosis severity associated with mixed plaque pattern ($p = 0.043$)
Fiorentino et al., 2020 [46]	Italy	Retrospective	US	Coronary angiography	1254 601 NAFLD 130 CAD	prediabetes and NAFLD—increased risk of CVD or CAD by 2.3 and 2 fold T2DM with NAFLD—2.3 and 2 fold higher risk of CVD or CAD
Niikura et al., 2020 [38]	Japan	Prospective	Liver biopsy	CCTA CACS (CT)	101 NAFLD 51 CACS	NASH and fibrosis—independent RF for CAS NASH—not significantly associated with presence of CACS NASH independent RF for high-risk plaque
Seba et al., 2020 [47]	India	Prospective	US FibroScan	Coronary angiography SINTAX Score	300 CAD 165 NAFLD	NAFLD associated with CAD No correlation between NAFLD grades and CAD
Liu HH et al., 2019 [48]	China	Prospective	US	Coronary angiography	162 CAD 40 NAFLD	NAFLD—independent predictor of CVD outcomes in patients with stable, new-onset CAD (OR: 2.72, 95% CI: 1.16–6.39, $p = 0.022$)
Langroudi TF et al., 2018 [49]	Iran	Retrospective	US	Coronary angiography	264 191 NAFLD 127 CHD	NAFLD presence and grade not correlated with coronary arteries ATS and its severity in non-diabetic patients
Pulimaddi et al., 2016 [50]	India	Cross-sectional	US	ECG/ coronary angiogram/angioplasty	150 T2DM >30 years	59.3% prevalence of CAD in the NAFLD group (significant statistically)
Sinn et al., 2017 [51]	South Korea	Retrospective	US	CACS	4731 2088 NAFLD	NAFLD significantly associated with the development of CAC independent of CV and metabolic RF
Idilman et al., 2015 [52]	Turkey	Retrospective	CT	CCTA	273 T2DM 59 NAFLD 44 CAD	NAFLD—associated with CAD in T2DM $p = 0.04$
Osawa K et al., 2015 [53]	Japan	Retrospective	CT	CT	414 64 NAFLD 22 CHD	NAFLD—independent predictor of high-risk plaques (OR: 4.60; 95% CI: 1.94–9.07, $p < 0.01$
Puchner SB et al., 2014 [41]	USA	Prospective	CT	CCTA	445 205 CP 190 NCP	NAFLD—significantly associated with the presence of high-risk plaque (adjusted OR: 2.13; 95% CI: 1.18, 3.85), adjusted for CV RF and the extent and severity of CAD

Table 1. Cont.

Author, Year, Ref.	Country	Study Type	NAFLD Diagnosis	CAD Diagnosis	Patients Characteristics	Impact of NAFLD on CAD/ Results
Agaç et al., 2013 [54]	Turkey	Prospective	US	Coronary angiography	80, acute coronary syndrome	81.2% patients with NAFLD and acute coronary syndrome; NAFLD associated with higher SYNTAX score (OR: 13.20; 95% CI: 2.52–69.15)
Ballestri S et al., 2014 [55]	Italy	Retrospective	US Fetuin-A	Coronary angiography	29 NAFLD 20 CAD	High Fetuin-A associated with NAFLD and lower risk of CAD
Choi DH et al., 2013 [34]	South Korea	Prospective	US	Coronary angiography	134	NAFLD—independent predictor for CAD ($p = 0.03$, OR: 1.685; 95% CI: 1.051–2.702); Increased proportion of severe fatty liver in higher grade CAD; Adiponectin level decreased once the CAD progressed
Josef et al., 2013 [56]	Israel	Retrospective	CT	CCTA	29 NAFLD 9 CHD	Smaller retinal AVR (<0.7)—increased risk for CAD and carotid atherosclerosis in NAFLD even without hypertension or diabetes
Wong VW-S et al., 2011 [57]	Hong Kong	Prospective	US	Coronary angiography	612 356 NAFLD 301 CAD	Steatosis (adjusted OR: 2.31; 95% CI: 1.46–3.64) and alanine aminotransferase level (adjusted OR: 1.01; 95% CI: 1.00–1.02) independently associated with CAD
Assy et al., 2010 [58]	Israel	Prospective	CT	CT	29 NAFLD 11 CHD	NAFLD—associated with high prevalence of CP and NCP, independently of the MS and CRP
Açikel M et al., 2009 [59]	Turkey	Retrospective	US	Coronary angiography	355 215 NAFLD 153 CHD	NAFLD—independent predictor of CHD (>50% stenosis of ≥1 major coronary artery) after adjustment for CVD risk factors
Arslan U et al., 2007 [60]	Turkey	Retrospective	US	Coronary angiography	65 NAFLD 39 CHD	NAFLD—independent predictor of CHD (>50% stenosis of ≥1 major coronary artery) after adjustment for CVD risk factors and MS

Table 2. Summary of studies that evaluated the association between NAFLD and subclinical CAD.

Author, Year, Ref.	Country	Study Type	NAFLD Diagnosis	CAD Diagnosis	Patients Characteristics	Impact of NAFLD on CAD/Results
Carter et al., 2022 [61]	Scotland	Post-hoc analysis of Prospective Scottish Computed Tomography of HEART trial	CT	CT (CACS)	1726 155 hepatic steatosis	Hepatic steatosis associated with increased prevalence of CAD. No difference in MI in those with and without steatosis (1.9% vs. 2.4%, $p = 0.92$)
Ichikawa et al., 2022 [62]	Japan	Prospective	CT	CCTA	1148 247 hepatic steatosis 977 suspected CAD	High association between hepatic steatosis and increased risk of MACE in suspected stable CAD
Wang X et al., 2022 [63]	China	Retrospective	FIB-4 score	Coronary angiography Gensini score	342 105 NAFLD	NAFLD severity—associated with CAS. High FIB-4 score—high CAC
Chen et al., 2021 [25]	Taiwan	Prospective	US	CACS (CT)	545 437 NAFLD 242 CAC	1.36-fold greater risk of developing CAC in patients with different severity of NAFLD vs. those without NAFLD (OR: 1.36, 95% CI: 1.07–1.77, $p = 0.016$)
Ichikawa et al., 2021 [64]	Japan	Prospective	CT	CACS FRS	529 T2DM	NAFLD, CACS, and FRS-associated with CVE (HR and 95% CI: 5.43, 2.82–10.44, $p < 0.001$; 1.56, 1.32–1.86, $p < 0.001$; 1.23, 1.08–1.39, $p = 0.001$, respectively)
Meyersohn NM et al., 2021 [33]	North America	Nested cohort study	CT	CCTA	3756	Hepatic steatosis associated with MACE (4.4% vs. 2.6% in those without steatosis) indepently of other CV RF/extent of CAD
Saraya et al., 2021 [65]	Egypt	Prospective	CT	CCTA	800 440 CAD	NAFLD and high-risk plaque features: Napkin ring sign, Positive remodeling, Low HU, and Spotty calcium (OR: 7.88, 95% CI (4.39–14.12), $p < 0.001$, OR: 5.84, 95% CI (3.85–8.85), $p < 0.001$, OR: 7.25, 95% CI (3.31–15.90), $p < 0.001$ and OR: 6.66, 95% CI (3.75–11.82), $p < 0.001$)
Bae YS et al., 2020 [66]	South Korea	Retrospective	US NFS, FIB-4 index	CCTA	3693 244 CAS 1588 NAFLD	NAFLD associated with CAS (≥50% stenosis) stronger in women, but absolute risk higher in men
Ismael H et al., 2020 [19]	Egypt	Prospective	FibroScan	Coronary angiography Gensini score	100 42 NAFLD	S2-S3 NAFLD and CVD (OR: 24, 95% CI: 17–31)
Koo BK et al., 2020 [67]	USA	Retrospective	CT	CCTA	719 NAFLD 443 CHD	NAFLD significantly associated with coronary calcification (OR: 1.28; 95% CI: 1.07–1.53)
Chang Y et al., 2019 [68]	South Korea	Retrospective	US FIB-4 score, APRI	CACS	105328 34382 NAFLD 5249 CAD	NAFLD, AFLD associated with CAC

Table 2. Cont.

Author, Year, Ref.	Country	Study Type	NAFLD Diagnosis	CAD Diagnosis	Patients Characteristics	Impact of NAFLD on CAD/Results
Oni E et al., 2019 [69]	USA	Retrospective	CT	CACS CIMT	4123 729 NAFLD 386 CHD	NAFLD—independently associated with CAC> 0 and CIMT > 1 mm
Pais et al., 2019 [70]	France	Retrospective	FLI	FRS CACS (CT)	2617 930 NAFLD	High prevalence of CAC (183 ± 425 vs. 117 ± 288, $p < 0.001$) in those with hepatic steatosis vs. without
Park HE et al., 2019 [71]	South Korea	Retrospective	CAP	CCTA Coronary plaque >1.5 mm^2	330 NAFLD 186 CAD 147 NCP	CAP-defined NAFLD significantly associated with NCP, independent from cardiometabolic RF (adjusted OR: 3.528, 95% CI: 1.463–8.511, $p = 0.005$), no significant correlation with CP ($p = 0.171$)
Sinn DH et al., 2019 [51]	South Korea	Retrospective	US NFS	Hospitalization for MI	111492 37263 NAFLD 183 MI	NAFLD associated with increased incidence of MI independent of RF
Gummesson et al., 2018 [72]	Sweden	Retrospective	CT	CACS (CT)	106 NAFLD 73 CHD	NAFLD and CACS association in subjects with few other metabolic risk factors (60% subjects of the total cohort) with 0 or 1 of the 7 predefined RF; OR: 5.94, 95% CI: 2.13 ± 16.6
Lee SB et al., 2018 [36]	South Korea	Retrospective	US, FLI, NFS	CCTA	5121 38.6% NAFLD	NAFLD associated with NCP; significant association of FLI ≥30 with NCP (1.37, 95% CI: 1.14–1.65, $p = 0.001$) and NFS ≥ −1.455 with NCP (1.20, 95% CI: 1.08–1.42, $p = 0.030$)
Wu R et al., 2017 [73]	China	Retrospective	US	CACS (CT)	2345 1272 NAFLD 237 CHD	NAFLD—significantly associated with the development of coronary artery calcifications (adjusted OR: 1.348, 95% CI: 1.030–1.765)
Jacobs K et al., 2016 [74]	USA	Retrospective	US	CACS (CT) (VAT)	250 71 NAFLD 52 CHD	NAFLD and CAC—no clear association Increased CAC, VAT with age, but no increased NAFLD
Kim JB et al., 2016 [75]	South Korea	Retrospective	US	CT EFV	1472 677 NAFLD 147 CHD	Higher EFV levels and NAFLD prevalence in individuals with MS than those without MS (81.0 cm^3 vs. 57.3 cm^3, $p < 0.001$; 75.6% vs. 36.5%, $p < 0.001$)
Park HE et al., 2016 [76]	South Korea	Retrospective	US	CCTA (CAC)	1732 846 NAFLD 413 CAC	NAFLD associated with CAC development independent of other metabolic RF in those without CAC at baseline, but not with CAC progression in those with CAC at baseline DM risk factor for CAC progression

Table 2. Cont.

Author, Year, Ref.	Country	Study Type	NAFLD Diagnosis	CAD Diagnosis	Patients Characteristics	Impact of NAFLD on CAD/Results
Al Rifai M et al., 2015 [18]	USA	Retrospective	CT	CACS (CT)	3976 670 NAFLD 362 CAC	NAFLD—associated with inflammation and CAC
Kim MK et al., 2015 [77]	South Korea	Retrospective	US	CACS (CT)	919 Postmenopausal women 294 NAFLD 81 CAC	OR for prevalence of CAC: no NAFLD, 1.0; mild NAFLD, 1.34 (95% CI: 0.92–2.16); moderate to severe NAFLD, 1.83 (95% CI: 1.06–3.16) NAFLD—not independent factor for CAD in postmenopausal women
Kang MK et al., 2015 [78]	South Korea	Retrospective	US	CT	346 NAFLD 173 CHD	NAFLD—associated with coronary plaques OR: 1.48; 95% CI: 1.05–2.08, $p = 0.025$
Lee M-K et al., 2015 [79]	South Korea	Retrospective	US	CACS (CT)	10063 NAFLD 1843 CAD 340 CACS>100	NAFLD relatively increased risk for CAC vs. non-NAFLD; higher OR than that in subjects with abdominal obesity [1.360; 95% CI: 1.253–1.476) vs. (1.220; 95% CI: 1.122–1.326)]
Efe D et al., 2014 [80]	Turkey	Retrospective	CT	CT	372 204 NAFLD 107 CAD	Higher prevalence of CAD in NAFLD than non-NAFLD
VanWagner et al., 2014 [81]	USA	Retrospective	CT	CACS (CT)	2424 232 NAFLD 88 CAD	Increased CAC (37.9% vs. 26.0%, $p < 0.001$) in NAFLD cases Obesity attenuates NAFLD-ATS relation
Chhabra et al., 2013 [82]	USA	Retrospective	CT	CACS (CT)	400 43 NAFLD 15 CAD	Hepatic steatosis—independent predictor of CACS
Juarez-Rojas et al., 2013 [83]	Mexico	Retrospective	CT	CACS (CT)	765 163 NAFLD 64 CHD	Fatty liver associated with T2DM and MS
Khashper et al., 2013 [84]	Israel	Retrospective	CT	CACS (CT)	318 93 NAFLD 70 CAD	Increased VAT in patients with coronary artery plaques, $p < 0.001$
Sung KC et al., 2013 [85]	South Korea	Retrospective	US	CACS (CT)	7371 39.5% NAFLD 4.5% CACS > 0	Steatosis and baPWV are independently associated with the presence of CAC
Arslan et al., 2012 [86]	Turkey	Prospective	US	Coronary angiography	151 98 NAFLD	64.9% patients with NAFLD NAFLD associated with poor coronary collateral development

Table 2. Cont.

Author, Year, Ref.	Country	Study Type	NAFLD Diagnosis	CAD Diagnosis	Patients Characteristics	Impact of NAFLD on CAD/Results
Kim D et al., 2012 [26]	South Korea	Prospective	US	CACS (CT)	4023 1617 NAFLD 649 CAD	High CACS significantly associated with the presence of NAFLD (OR: 1.28, 95% CI: 1.04–1.59, $p = 0.023$) independent of visceral adiposity
Sung KC et al., 2012 [87]	South Korea	Retrospective	US	CACS (CT)	3784 NAFLD 510 CAD	Steatosis (OR: 1.21, 95% CI: 1.01–1.45, $p = 0.04$) and HOMA-IR (1.10; 1.02–1.18, $p = 0.02$) associated with CACS > 0
Agarwal et al., 2011 [88]	India	Prospective	US	CIMT	124 T2DM 71 NAFLD 43 CAD	60.5% CAD of the patients with NAFLD; 45.2% of the ones without NAFLD NAFLD—risk marker for CAD in T2DM

Abbreviations: NAFLD, non-alcoholic fatty liver disease; NASH, non-alcoholic steatohepatitis; CAD, coronary artery disease; CHD, coronary heart disease; CCTA, coronary computed tomography angiography; CAC, coronary artery calcification; CACS, coronary artery calcium score; CT, computed tomography; FLI, Fatty Liver Index; NFS, NAFLD Fibrosis Score; US, ultrasonography; ECG, electrocardiogram; T2DM, type 2 diabetes; MS, metabolic syndrome; CP, calcified plaques; NCP, non-calcified plaques; ATS, atherosclerosis; CAS, coronary artery stenosis; CV, cardiovascular; CVE, cardiovascular events; CVD, cardiovascular disease; MI, myocardial infarction; RF, risk factor; LSM, liver stiffness measurement; APRI, AST to platelet ratio index; baPWV, brachial-ankle pulse wave velocity; CIMT, carotid intima-media tissue; VAT, visceral abdominal adipose tissue; EFV, epicardial fat volume; FRS, Framingham score; VAI, visceral adipose tissue; CRP, C-reactive protein; HOMA-IR, homeostatic model assessment for insulin resistance; HR, hazard ratio; OR, odd ratio; CI, confidence interval.

3. Screening and Diagnosis

3.1. CAD in Patients Assessed for NAFLD

The "gold standard" tool for NAFLD diagnosis and quantification is the liver biopsy, which identifies macrovesicular steatosis. Since it is an invasive method, with many potential complications, biopsy indications are limited to patients with NAFLD at high risk of NASH and/or advanced fibrosis and patients with suspected NAFLD in whom other etiologies of steatosis cannot be ruled out without a liver biopsy [6,89].

The early findings correlating NAFLD and CVD focused on the elevation of liver enzymes. Increased values of serum alanine aminotransferase (ALT) [90], gamma-glutamyl transferase [91], or alkaline phosphatase [92] were associated with other forms of CVD like arterial hypertension and peripheral vascular disease [93].

Non-invasive tests such as clinical scores, serum biomarkers and liver elastographic evaluation provide a good alternative to the diagnosis and staging of NAFLD [89]. According to European guidelines, clinical scores should be used in all patients with NAFLD [5]. A retrospective cross-sectional study involving 34,890 asymptomatic subjects evaluated by ultrasonography (US) analyzed 665 subjects undergoing CCTA imaging. Multiple non-invasive scores, including fatty liver index (FLI), hepatic steatosis index (HSI), Fibrosis-4 score (FIB-4), NAFLD fibrosis score (NFS), Forn's index, and AST to platelet ratio index (APRI), were applied. Values of NFS, FIB-4, and Forn's index were higher when coronary artery calcium scoring (CACS) increased. The authors concluded that fibrosis markers incorporating risk factors for CAD demonstrated a good discriminatory power in the prediction of CACS levels over 100 [94].

Another non-invasive test of NAFLD is represented by the liver fat score (LFS), used in a study, including 17,244 participants of the United States National Health and Nutrition Survey (US NHANES) database. LFS showed associations with CAD (adjusted OR: 1.09 per standard deviation [SD], 95% CI: 1.03–1.15, $p = 0.003$), angina (1.08, 1.02–1.13, $p = 0.005$) and congestive heart failure (1.11, 1.04–1.18, $p = 0.003$), but not with myocardial infarction or stroke [95].

Currently available imaging methods for hepatic steatosis and fibrosis are represented by US, liver stiffness measurement (LSM) and controlled attenuation parameter (CAP) by transient elastography (VCTE or FibroScan®), CT, magnetic resonance imaging, magnetic resonance spectroscopy (MRS), and magnetic resonance elastography (MRE) [89,96].

Transient elastography is a non-invasive imagistic method that remarked as a clinical tool for staging both liver fibrosis indicated by LSM and hepatic steatosis assessed by CAP, allowing an early detection of NAFLD even in asymptomatic individuals without overt liver disease [97,98]. Use of VCTE measurements in patients from the Framingham Heart Study showed that hepatic fibrosis is significantly correlated with cardiometabolic risk factors represented by high values of BMI and waist circumference, elevated serum transaminases, poor glycemic control, higher systolic and diastolic blood pressure, modified lipid profile [99]. Some studies using FibroScan for the assessment of NAFLD showed an independent link between liver stiffness and CACS [71,100]. A retrospective cohort study highlighted the association between NAFLD and CVD using CAP by transient elastography and found an independent correlation between the degree of steatosis and the incidence of CVD. The results suggest an optimal cut-off CAP value set at 295 dB/m for stratifying the associated CVD risk [101].

The Multi-Ethnic Study of Atherosclerosis (MESA) [102] assessed NAFLD by CT and the cardiovascular risk by CACS in selected patients [15]. Interestingly, these findings identified only pericardial fat, but not fatty liver, to be associated with cardiovascular outcomes, including CAD, calling into question the role of inflammation and insulin resistance.

3.2. NAFLD in Patients Assessed for CAD

Current guidelines recommend the assessment of CVD risk in asymptomatic adults using the Framingham Risk Score (FRS), the European SCORE-2 and SCORE-2 OP, and the ASCVD algorithm, each based on the identification of several risk factors [103]. All these models fail to correctly identify NAFLD-related CVD, because features like insulin resistance are not included in the evaluation [95]. The Framingham Risk Score underestimate CVD risk in patients with MS; hence, this category could be subject to a late mitigation of cardiovascular risk. It is therefore reasonable to hypothesize that NAFLD evaluation could help in accurately assessing cardiovascular risk in the general population [95,104].

The CACS is an accurate assessment tool for the presence and development of coronary atherosclerosis, and can be used for monitoring the disease progression, detecting cardiac outcomes, and oversee therapeutic effectiveness [76]. The association between NAFLD and coronary artery calcification has been most frequently demonstrated by calculating the Agatston CACS by CT [26]. Ichikawa et al. propose in their prospective study on patients with T2DM the stratification of NAFLD-associated risk for cardiovascular events using CACS and FRS [64]. Another study including an Austrian screening cohort and using the FRS to assess the CVD risk showed an independent association of NAFLD with CV risk [105].

CCTA is another non-invasive assessment method of coronary arteries that allows their measurement and identification of plaque composition [71]. The lipid-rich coronary plaques are more vulnerable to sudden rupture and predict an increased risk of CV morbi-mortality [53,106]. Increased CACS measured by cardiac multiple detector CT is followed by a negative impact on patients' outcome, reflecting the total burden of atherosclerosis. NAFLD is related to CACS progression and high-risk plaques, irrespective of traditional CV risk factors [51]. As mentioned in the previous pages, Meyersohn and colleagues showed, using CCTA scan, that the addition of NAFLD to every grade of CAD (no significant CAD, non-obstructive CAD, obstructive CAD) was associated with a higher risk for cardiovascular events than in patients without fatty liver [33].

4. Potential Pathogenic Links between NAFLD and CAD

The pathogenic mechanisms associating NAFLD and CAD are still poorly understood. Several mechanisms have been proposed as promoters of both conditions (Figure 1), among which systemic inflammation, gut microbiota, endothelial dysfunction (ED), oxidative stress, or cardiometabolic comorbidities like glucose dysregulation, insulin resistance, dyslipidemia, obesity, and hypertension; all of these usually display a genetic predisposition; a growing line of evidence suggests that the NAFLD–CAD association is tightly linked to dysfunctional secretion of fatty acids, enzymes, cytokine-related anomalies, and pro-atherogenic microRNAs [22,107,108].

Following recent research, MAFLD may be a more appropriate acronym that highlights better the relevant risk factors and NAFLD pathogenesis [109]. The heterogeneity of MAFLD emphasizes the need for individualization, an absolute requisite for the development of new effective treatments for each patient, depending on the dominant subphenotype [110].

Pathogenic features such as insulin resistance, lipid disturbances, oxidative stress, and inflammation can induce NASH and aggravate CVD progression. It is therefore reasonable to suppose that NASH modifications significantly associated with worse coronary artery lesions than hepatic steatosis [40].

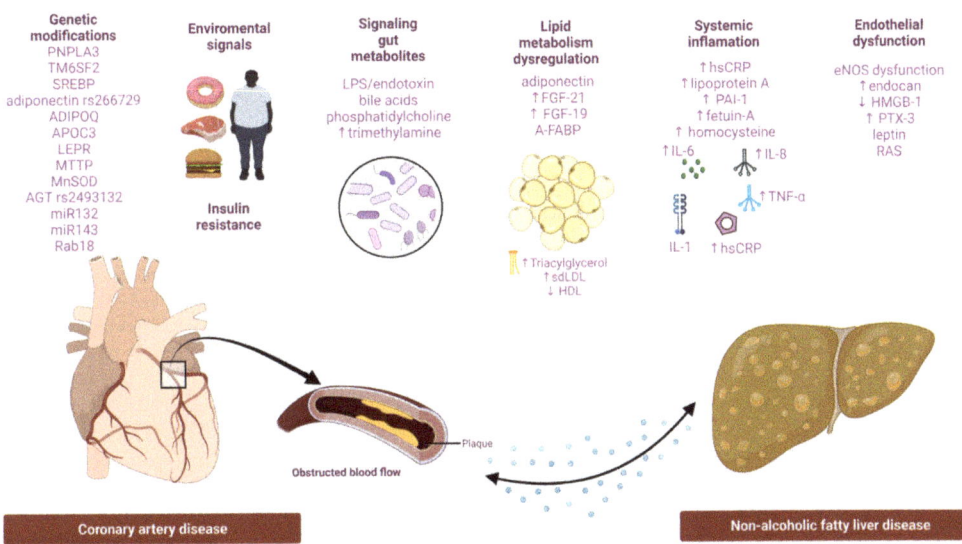

Figure 1. Summary of suggested pathophysiological mechanisms underlying the NAFLD–CAD interconnection. *Abbreviations:* PNPLA3, patatin-like phospholipase domain-containing protein-3; TM6SF2, transmembrane 6 superfamily member 2; SREBP, sterol regulatory element-binding proteins; ADIPOQ, adiponectin-encoding gene, APOC3, apolipoprotein C3; LEPR, leptin receptor; MTTP, microsomal triglyceride transfer protein; MnSOD, manganese superoxide dismutase; AGT, angiotensin; LPS, lipopolysaccharides; FGF-21, fibroblast growth factor-21; FGF-19, fibroblast growth factor-19; A-FABP, adipocyte fatty acid-binding protein; hsCRP, high-sensitive C-protein reaction; PAI-1, plasminogen activator inhibitor-1; IL-1, interleukin-1; IL-6, interleukin-6; IL-8, interleukin-8; TNF-α, tumor necrosis factor-alpha; HMGB-1, high mobility group box 1; PTX-3. petraxin-3; RAS, renin-angiotensin system.

4.1. Common Risk Factors

The well-established risk factors for CAD are represented by age, gender, family history of premature CVD, hypertension, hyperlipidemia, overweight, T2DM, chronic smoking, or other comorbidities increasing CVD risk [103]. It seems that some residual risk factors remain even after the classical risk factors are mitigated. For example, a study including individuals without classical cardiovascular risk factors showed that even normal levels of low-density lipoprotein (LDL)-cholesterol are associated with subclinical atherosclerosis [111].

The decisive factors leading to NAFLD progression are related to unhealthy lifestyle and eating behavior (excessive intake of saturated fatty acids or fructose, de novo lipogenesis caused by excessive carbohydrate intake), microbiome-related metabolites, and metabolic comorbidities (insulin resistance, dyslipidemia, obesity, T2DM, MS, hypothyroidism) [5,112].

It is therefore obvious that NAFLD and CVD share several common risk factors, e.g., obesity, T2DM, dyslipidemia, and physical inactivity, supporting the idea of a shared pathogenesis [113]. At its turn, insulin resistance is associated both with NAFLD and with endothelial dysfunction and ASCVD [41].

4.2. Genetics, Epigenetics Modifications

Also correlating with NAFLD stages, three genetic forms represented by patatin-like phospholipase domain-containing protein-3 (PNPLA3), transmembrane 6 superfamily member 2 (TM6SF2), and sterol regulatory element-binding proteins (SREBP) were found to have a protective effect against CAD [5,95]. The possible negative correlation between

PNPLA3 and CAD seems to be influenced by the triglyceride metabolism and NAFLD severity related to PNPLA3 rs738409 mutation [114,115].

CARDIoGRAMplusC4D (Coronary Artery Disease Genomewide Replication and Meta-analysis (CARDIoGRAM) plus the Coronary Artery Disease (C4D)) included a cohort of cases with and without CAD [116]. In this study, TM6SF2 had a protective role for CAD, while the new NAFLD susceptibility gene of the membrane-bound O-acyltransferase domain-containing protein 7 (MBOAT7) had a neutral effect on CAD risk [117].

Other newly identified gene polymorphisms apparently involved in the NAFLD–CAD relationship are represented by: adiponectin rs266729 [118], adiponectin-encoding gene (ADIPOQ), apolipoprotein C3 (APOC3), leptin receptor (LEPR), peroxisome proliferator activated receptors (PPAR), tumor necrosis factor-alpha (TNF-α), microsomal triglyceride transfer protein (MTTP), and manganese superoxide dismutase (MnSOD) [105,119]. The angiotensin (AGT) rs2493132 genotype displayed a significantly increased risk of developing CAD in a Chinese Han population with NAFLD [120]. Rab18 gene expression seems to be linked to increased adiposity and lipotoxicity [121].

Circulating microRNAs are secreted and released in biological fluids and maintain intracellular balance. Metha et al. investigated the expression of microRNAs related to NAFLD and CAD. The researchers found that miR132 circulatory level was reduced in patients with both diseases (0.24 ± 0.16 vs. 0.30 ± 0.11, $p = 0.03$) and miR-143 circulatory level was increased compared to controls with NAFLD, but without CAD (0.96 ± 0.90 vs. 0.64 ± 0.77, $p = 0.02$). Hence, miRNAs could be utilized as biomarkers to identify and monitor the disease progression [122].

4.3. Lipid and Cholesterol Metabolism

Lipid profiles with a pro-atherogenic feature appear to be influenced by the hepatic lipid concentration and the peripheral, adipose insulin resistance; such profiles include an increased proportion of small dense LDL and very low-density lipoproteins (VLDL), high apolipoprotein B to apolipoprotein A-1 ratio, and low high-density lipoprotein (HDL)-cholesterol concentration [6]. Some authors argue that patients with NASH have reduced levels of VLDL due to the decrease of microsomal triglyceride transfer protein and reduced VLDL synthesis. This precursor of the small dense LDL particles that transports an abundance of triglyceride thus becomes a pivotal atherosclerosis risk factor [38]. Prolonged hypertriglyceridemia can determine postprandial hyperlipidemia in patients with NAFLD, which further progresses to an accelerated postprandial atherogenesis and a higher CVD risk [22].

High levels of triglyceride-rich lipoprotein-related elements are related to either calcified or non-calcified coronary lesions in patients with NAFLD [123,124]. Studies such as GREACE (The Greek Atorvastatin and Coronary-heart-disease Evaluation) support the need to prevent major coronary events in patients with elevated plasma liver enzymes caused by NAFLD [125].

Another suggested driver of metabolic and cardiovascular complications seems to be the exhaustion of adipose tissue expansion and ectopic lipid accumulation in non-adipose cells, which in turn causes lipotoxicity [126].

The NAFLD–CVD link is also influenced by lipid profile modifications determined by adipokines like adiponectin, fibroblast growth factor 21 (FGF-21), and adipocyte fatty acid-binding protein (A-FABP) [127,128]. FGF-21 concentrations are elevated in obesity and T2DM, which involves it in NAFLD development. Therefore, the administration of FGF-21 analog can reduce lipogenesis and fatty acid oxidation and can also protect against atherosclerosis progression [129,130]. The association of A-FABP with NAFLD-related CVD is amplified by insulin resistance and arterial inflammation [95]. Fibroblast growth factor 19 (FGF-19) hormone levels were negatively correlated with CAD (defined by coronary angiography), independently of BMI, hypertension, dyslipidemia, and diabetes [131]. Levels of FGF-19 are decreased in patients with obesity, regardless of the degree of insulin resistance. FGF-19 analogs currently under research can suppress *de novo* bile acid synthesis and *de novo* lipogenesis [129,132].

4.4. Systemic Inflammation and Cytokines

NAFLD-associated pro-inflammatory status changes the structure of the coronary wall, leading to CAD and increased CVD mortality [133].

The inflammatory syndrome and the increased oxidative stress play a crucial role in CAD associated with NAFLD. Plaque vulnerability is influenced by the inflammatory status of NAFLD. Underlying mechanisms include increased levels of high-sensitive C-reactive protein (hsCRP) and lipoprotein A reported in these patients [40]. Other markers associated both with NAFLD and a high risk for CAD include homeostatic and fibrinolytic function markers, such as fibrinogen, tissue plasminogen activator, and plasminogen activator inhibitor 1 (PAI-1), fetuin-A [55], or homocysteine [50].

The heart-liver axis is related to the MS and acts as a direct connection between the white adipose tissue, the liver and the heart by a systemic signaling led by organic cytokines such as adipokines, hepatokines, and cardiomyokines, predicting the NAFLD-related CVD risk [134]. The adipose tissue produces cytokines with complex outcomes, including a pro-inflammatory effect, such as interleukin 6 (IL-6), interleukin 8 (IL-8), and tumor necrosis factor α (TNF-α). The cumulative pathogenic effects of the disturbed cytokine secretion, the oxidative stress, and the lipotoxicity lead both to NAFLD development and to coronary atherosclerosis, irrespective of conventional cardiovascular risk factors [41,135,136].

Contrary to other studies, Choi et al. did not find insulin, hsCRP, IL-6, and TNF-α levels to be related to CAD; however, the authors found reduced levels serum of adiponectin once the CAD progressed, which indicates a possible dual role that also extends to NAFLD pathogenesis [34]. Adiponectin inhibits hepatic gluconeogenesis and lipogenesis. Therefore, hypoadiponectinemia can determine impaired glucose tolerance, but also CAD in patients without diabetes [137]. In patients with NAFLD, hypoadiponectinemia associates with increased inflammation and oxidative stress. It seems that the early onset of atherosclerosis and CAD is also related to lower serum adiponectin levels, which suggests that hypoadiponectinemia may predict atherosclerosis [138]. The CANTOS (Canakinumab Anti-inflammatory Thrombosis Outcome Study) trial highlighted the key role of interleukin 1 (IL-1), a cytokine related to the evolution of NAFLD, as a therapeutic strategy for atherosclerosis. The results showed a positive outcome on CVD events and morbi-mortality [139].

4.5. Endothelial Dysfunction and Oxidative Stress

Endothelial dysfunction developed during NAFLD progression is considered an independent risk factor for CAD occurrence [140]. An impaired coronary flow reserve was described in patients with NAFLD compared to controls without fatty liver after adjustment for cardiometabolic risk factors [141]. An impaired flow-mediated vasodilatation (FMD) can also influence the emergence of vulnerable coronary plaques and the high risk for ischemic heart syndromes in patients with NAFLD [133]. Moreover, NAFLD was associated with a higher short-term mortality and a worsened long-term prognosis in patients with ST-segment elevation myocardial infarction [142].

It was shown that patients with NAFLD may have an impaired endothelial nitric oxide synthase (eNOS) function due to insulin resistance, leading to a reduction in the nitric oxide (NO) substrate production and an imbalance in the induction of platelet-mediated vasorelaxation. Hence, eNOS dysfunction plays a key role in modifying the endothelial function in patients with NAFLD and may determine an increased cardiovascular risk [143].

The role of adipocyte-derived hormone leptin and angiotensin are also investigated for their role in endothelial function as vasoactive factors [144]. Hyperleptinemia in obesity and NAFLD is significantly correlated with the development of atherosclerosis and cardiovascular diseases [145,146]. Stimulation of the renin-angiotensin system and leptin resistance appears to be correlated with arterial hypertension associated with obesity. Moreover, angiotensin II can also participate to the NAFLD pathophysiology by stimulation of lipogenesis, insulin resistance or pro-inflammatory cytokine production [145,147].

Several endothelial biomarkers were studied as possible determinants of the pathophysiological relationship between NAFLD and CAD. Increased endocan levels and decreased levels of high mobility group box 1 (HMGB-1) were correlated with the severity of CAD in NAFLD, while anti-endothelial cell antibodies (AECA) has not yet proven any significance [148,149]. The levels of circulating petraxin-3 (PTX-3), an acute-phase protein, were found to be elevated and strongly correlated with endothelial dysfunction in patients with NAFLD [150].

4.6. Gut Microbiota

Compared to healthy individuals, patients with NAFLD, obesity and diabetes display an increased intestinal permeability and increased bacterial growth in the small intestine (endotoxemia) [108]. Metabolic endotoxemia can occur in the form of lipopolysaccharides (LPS) entering portal circulation and impairing the immune response by binding to toll-like receptor 4 (TLR) and activating the inflammatory cascade [108,151]. This process acts on the insulin signaling, favors hepatic steatosis and progression to NASH; on the other hand, it promotes endothelial dysfunction, LDL oxidation, and thrombogenesis, destabilizing the atherosclerotic plaques [152].

Gut dysbiosis was discovered in patients with both CAD and NAFLD. The intestinal microbiota might be different in patients with NAFLD and CAD than in those with just CAD. Studies focused on gut microbiota composition in patients with NAFLD and CAD [152] showed increased levels of *Coprococcus* and *Veillonella*, and decreased levels of Bacteroides fragilis, *Parabacterioides, Bifidobacterium longum* subsp. *infantis, Ruminococcus gnavus, Bacteroides dorei*, which could underlie the intestinal alterations that cause a higher risk for adverse CVD outcomes less witnessed in NAFLD-free CAD. The abundance of *Coprococcus* could favor MS in patients with CAD and NAFLD due to its positive correlation with BMI [153]. Another potential cause of the progression of NAFLD and CAD could be the abundance of *Collinsella* and *Proteobacteria* [154].

Circulating bile acids (BA) are also implicated in metabolic liver diseases associated with CVD. Glycochenodeoxycholic acid (GCDCA), a marker for reduced serum concentrations of BA, predicts CAD. Interestingly, this defect is reversible under statin therapy [155].

Gut microbiome-related metabolites, such as phosphatidylcholine (PC) and trimethylamine N-oxide (TMAO), are also studied for their association with an increased cardiovascular risk [152]. TMAO is a metabolite linked with the PC metabolism and modulates glucose and lipid homeostasis, thus influencing the liver, precipitating intra-adipose inflammation and impairing platelet function. High levels of TMAO seem to be involved in the progression of NAFLD-related CAD, probably due to intestinal dysbiosis influenced by dietary factors [105]. TMAO was found able to predict cardiovascular events in a cohort of patients submitted to coronary angiography, independently of other risk factors [156]. Among current attempts for therapeutic strategies aiming at gut microbiota in CAD, an inhibitor targeting a pair of microbial TMA-generating enzymes was developed, which was able to reduce the risk of atherothrombotic events and prevent coronary complications [157].

5. The Challenge of Lean NAFLD and Cardiovascular Risk

Patients with NAFLD usually are overweight or obese and associate insulin resistance, T2DM, dyslipidemia, hypertriglyceridemia, or hypertension, all of these being MS components and CVD risk factors [105]. However, it appears that CVD risk is increased even in individuals with NAFLD but normal BMI, who became categorized as lean patients with NAFLD (BMI <25 kg/m^2 in Caucasians and <23 kg/m^2 in Asians) [158]. The prevalence of lean NAFLD ranges from 10% to 20%, and despite the absence of obesity these individuals have a similar cardiovascular risk to patients with obese NAFLD [159].

In lean NAFLD, the risk of cardiometabolic conditions is elevated compared to NAFLD-free subjects of all BMI categories [160]. When lean NAFLD was compared with a healthy control group, an increased prevalence of metabolic impairment and cardiovascular risk was noticed [161]. An analysis on 5375 lean participants selected from the NHANES III survey showed that NAFLD presence was associated with a major increase in all-cause and cardiovascular mortality compared to controls [162].

While most opinions support an important role for obesity in patients with both NAFLD and CVD, some recent studies suggest a new theory of a particular lean NAFLD phenotype displaying a higher CVD risk than overweight people [163]. This hypothesis suggests that visceral adiposity has a higher contribution to the waist circumference value in lean NAFLD persons; this ectopic adipose accumulation leads to endothelial dysfunction and a pro-inflammatory effect [164]. Visceral fat accumulation in lean Asian people was correlated with the severity of NAFLD [95].

Despite the seemingly favorable metabolic risk profile, lean NAFLD is associated with a higher rate of cardiovascular events compared to the obese NAFLD group, as shown in a recent subgroup analysis study [165]. Likewise, another retrospective *post hoc* analysis showed the risk for incident CVD of various types (CAD, ischemic stroke, and cerebral hemorrhage) in lean patients with NAFLD to be higher than in overweight patients with NAFLD (8.8% vs. 3.3%) [166]. Therefore, NAFLD also needs an increased attention in lean individuals to prevent cardiovascular events.

The differences between lean and obese NAFLD include genetic predisposition, body composition, environmental risk factors, and gut microbiota, all related to the incidence of cardiovascular disease [167,168]. The metabolic dysfunction in NAFLD is weight-dependent. A recent meta-analysis showed lean people with NAFLD have significantly lower values of systolic and diastolic blood pressure and fasting glycemia than patients with NAFLD and obesity [169]. According to a study by Kim and colleagues, lean patients with NAFLD had a significantly higher ASCVD score (defined as an ASCVD risk of >10%) compared to patients with NAFLD and obesity (51.6% vs. 39.8%) and NAFLD-free controls (25.5%) [170]. NAFLD influences the incidence of CVD more than the presence of any degree excess weight, indicating that NAFLD-triggered mechanisms favor ASCVD independently of overweight or obesity [166].

The impact of lean NAFLD on the long-term prognosis of such patients is not completely understood, but it could be labeled as not being a benign condition [171]. The fact that NAFLD is also found in normal weight patients is usually overlooked, delaying the diagnosis and risking the progression of hepatic steatosis to NASH or fibrosis, with an increased associated CVD risk [172]. The conundrum of lean NAFLD being linked to CVD risk needs clarification in future studies.

At this moment, no data are available on the incidence and progression of coronary artery disease in lean NAFLD.

6. Conclusions

The available findings strongly support the fact that NAFLD and CAD are two conditions closely related to the MS. Similar to NAFLD being named the hepatic MS manifestation, we could say that CAD is its cardiac manifestation, closely related to the former. Consistent data showed that CAD has a high prevalence among patients with NAFLD, leading to an increased mortality. NAFLD is significantly associated with clinical and subclinical CAD, independently of the conventional cardiometabolic risk factors.

Many putative mechanisms are considered relevant in NALFD-related CAD, including genetics, inflammation, oxidative stress, lipotoxicity, atherogenic dyslipidemia, or gut microbiota. Key questions for future research refer to the complex mechanisms linking NAFLD to CAD, to the nature of optimal personalized lifestyle modification and appropriate pharmacologic approaches for both conditions, and to whether NAFLD-directed therapeutic strategies can also reduce CVD risk.

Author Contributions: Conceptualization, G.-D.C., C.-M.L. and B.-M.M.; methodology, G.-D.C., C.-M.L. and E.-D.G.; validation, G.-D.C., C.-M.L. and B.-M.M.; formal analysis, C.M., E.-D.G. and A.O.; investigation, C.M., E.-D.G. and A.O.; resources, G.-D.C., C.-M.L. and E.-D.G.; writing—original draft preparation, G.-D.C., C.-M.L. and E.-D.G.; writing—review and editing, C.M., A.O. and B.-M.M.; visualization, G.-D.C. and C.-M.L.; supervision, B.-M.M.; project administration, C.-M.L. and E.-D.G. All authors have read and agreed to the published version of the manuscript.

Funding: This research received no external funding.

Institutional Review Board Statement: Not applicable.

Informed Consent Statement: Not applicable.

Data Availability Statement: Not applicable.

Conflicts of Interest: The authors declare no conflict of interest.

References

1. Younossi, Z.; Anstee, Q.M.; Marietti, M.; Hardy, T.; Henry, L.; Eslam, M.; George, J.; Bugianesi, E. Global burden of NAFLD and NASH: Trends, predictions, risk factors and prevention. *Nat. Rev. Gastroenterol. Hepatol.* **2017**, *15*, 11–20. [CrossRef] [PubMed]
2. Younossi, Z.M.; Koenig, A.B.; Abdelatif, D.; Fazel, Y.; Henry, L.; Wymer, M. Global Epidemiology of Nonalcoholic Fatty Liver Disease—Meta-analytic Assessment of Prevalence, Incidence, and Outcomes. *Hepatology* **2016**, *64*, 73–84. [CrossRef] [PubMed]
3. Younossi, Z.M.; Henry, L. Epidemiology of non-alcoholic fatty liver disease and hepatocellular carcinoma. *JHEP Rep.* **2021**, *3*, 100305. [CrossRef]
4. Younossi, Z.M.; Golabi, P.; de Avila, L.; Paik, J.M.; Srishord, M.; Fukui, N.; Qiu, Y.; Burns, L.; Afendy, A.; Nader, F. The global epidemiology of NAFLD and NASH in patients with type 2 diabetes: A systematic review and meta-analysis. *J. Hepatol.* **2019**, *71*, 793–801. [CrossRef]
5. European Association for the Study of the Liver (EASL); European Association for the Study of Diabetes (EASD); European Association for the Study of Obesity (EASO). EASL-EASD-EASO Clinical Practice Guidelines for the management of non-alcoholic fatty liver disease. *J. Hepatol.* **2016**, *64*, 1388–1402. [CrossRef]
6. Chalasani, N.; Younossi, Z.; LaVine, J.E.; Charlton, M.; Cusi, K.; Rinella, M.; Harrison, S.A.; Brunt, E.M.; Sanyal, A.J. The diagnosis and management of nonalcoholic fatty liver disease: Practice guidance from the American Association for the Study of Liver Diseases. *Hepatology* **2018**, *67*, 328–357. [CrossRef]
7. Eslam, M.; Newsome, P.N.; Sarin, S.K.; Anstee, Q.M.; Targher, G.; Romero-Gomez, M.; Zelber-Sagi, S.; Wong, V.W.-S.; Dufour, J.-F.; Schattenberg, J.M.; et al. A new definition for metabolic dysfunction-associated fatty liver disease: An international expert consensus statement. *J. Hepatol.* **2020**, *73*, 202–209. [CrossRef]
8. Kotronen, A.; Yki-Järvinen, H. Fatty Liver. *Arter. Thromb. Vasc. Biol.* **2008**, *28*, 27–38. [CrossRef]
9. Targher, G.; Tilg, H.; Byrne, C.D. Non-alcoholic fatty liver disease: A multisystem disease requiring a multidisciplinary and holistic approach. *Lancet Gastroenterol. Hepatol.* **2021**, *6*, 578–588. [CrossRef]
10. Wijarnpreecha, K.; Aby, E.S.; Ahmed, A.; Kim, D. Evaluation and management of extrahepatic manifestations of nonalcoholic fatty liver disease. *Clin. Mol. Hepatol.* **2021**, *27*, 221–235. [CrossRef] [PubMed]
11. Duell, P.B.; Welty, F.K.; Miller, M.; Chait, A.; Hammond, G.; Ahmad, Z.; Cohen, D.E.; Horton, J.D.; Pressman, G.S.; Toth, P.P. Nonalcoholic Fatty Liver Disease and Cardiovascular Risk: A Scientific Statement from the American Heart Association. *Arter. Thromb. Vasc. Biol.* **2022**, *42*. [CrossRef]
12. Luo, J.; Xu, L.; Li, J.; Zhao, S. Nonalcoholic fatty liver disease as a potential risk factor of cardiovascular disease. *Eur. J. Gastroenterol. Hepatol.* **2015**, *27*, 193–199. [CrossRef]
13. Alexander, M.; Loomis, A.K.; Van Der Lei, J.; Duarte-Salles, T.; Prieto-Alhambra, D.; Ansell, D.; Pasqua, A.; Lapi, F.; Rijnbeek, P.; Mosseveld, M.; et al. Non-alcoholic fatty liver disease and risk of incident acute myocardial infarction and stroke: Findings from matched cohort study of 18 million European adults. *BMJ* **2019**, *367*, l5367. [CrossRef]
14. Olubamwo, O.O.; Virtanen, J.K.; Voutilainen, A.; Kauhanen, J.; Pihlajamäki, J.; Tuomainen, T.-P. Association of fatty liver index with the risk of incident cardiovascular disease and acute myocardial infarction. *Eur. J. Gastroenterol. Hepatol.* **2018**, *30*, 1047–1054. [CrossRef]
15. Shah, R.V.; Anderson, A.; Ding, J.; Budoff, M.; Rider, O.; Petersen, S.; Jensen, M.K.; Koch, M.; Allison, M.; Kawel-Boehm, N.; et al. Pericardial, But Not Hepatic, Fat by CT Is Associated with CV Outcomes and Structure. *JACC Cardiovasc. Imaging* **2017**, *10*, 1016–1027. [CrossRef]
16. Liu, C.-J. Prevalence and risk factors for non-alcoholic fatty liver disease in Asian people who are not obese. *J. Gastroenterol. Hepatol.* **2012**, *27*, 1555–1560. [CrossRef]
17. Oni, E.T.; Agatston, A.S.; Blaha, M.J.; Fialkow, J.; Cury, R.; Sposito, A.; Erbel, R.; Blankstein, R.; Feldman, T.; Al-Mallah, M.H.; et al. A systematic review: Burden and severity of subclinical cardiovascular disease among those with nonalcoholic fatty liver; Should we care? *Atherosclerosis* **2013**, *230*, 258–267. [CrossRef]
18. Al Rifai, M.; Silverman, M.G.; Nasir, K.; Budoff, M.J.; Blankstein, R.; Szklo, M.; Katz, R.; Blumenthal, R.S.; Blaha, M.J. The association of nonalcoholic fatty liver disease, obesity, and metabolic syndrome, with systemic inflammation and subclinical atherosclerosis: The Multi-Ethnic Study of Atherosclerosis (MESA). *Atherosclerosis* **2015**, *239*, 629–633. [CrossRef]
19. Ismael, H.; Tag-Adeen, M.; Abdel-Rady, A.; Shazly, M.; Hussein, A. Non-Alcoholic Fatty Liver Disease as a Coronary Heart Disease Severity Predictor. *Int. J. Clin. Med.* **2020**, *11*, 182–192. [CrossRef]

20. Gaudio, E.; Nobili, V.; Franchitto, A.; Onori, P.; Carpino, G. Nonalcoholic fatty liver disease and atherosclerosis. *Intern. Emerg. Med.* **2012**, *7*, 297–305. [CrossRef]
21. Baharvand-Ahmadi, B.; Sharifi, K.; Namdari, M. Prevalence of non-alcoholic fatty liver disease in patients with coronary artery disease. *ARYA Atheroscler.* **2016**, *12*, 201–205.
22. Ismaiel, A.; Dumitraşcu, D.L. Cardiovascular Risk in Fatty Liver Disease: The Liver-Heart Axis—Literature Review. *Front. Med.* **2019**, *6*, 202. [CrossRef]
23. Przybyszewski, E.M.; Targher, G.; Roden, M.; Corey, K.E. Nonalcoholic Fatty Liver Disease and Cardiovascular Disease. *Clin. Liver Dis.* **2021**, *17*, 19–22. [CrossRef]
24. Akabame, S.; Hamaguchi, M.; Tomiyasu, K.-I.; Tanaka, M.; Kobayashi-Takenaka, Y.; Nakano, K.; Oda, Y.; Yoshikawa, T. Evaluation of Vulnerable Coronary Plaques and Non-Alcoholic Fatty Liver Disease (NAFLD) by 64-Detector Multislice Computed Tomography (MSCT). *Circ. J.* **2007**, *72*, 618–625. [CrossRef] [PubMed]
25. Chen, C.-C.; Hsu, W.-C.; Wu, H.-M.; Wang, J.-Y.; Yang, P.-Y.; Lin, I.-C. Association between the Severity of Nonalcoholic Fatty Liver Disease and the Risk of Coronary Artery Calcification. *Medicina* **2021**, *57*, 807. [CrossRef] [PubMed]
26. Kim, D.; Choi, S.-Y.; Park, E.H.; Lee, W.; Kang, J.H.; Kim, W.R.; Kim, Y.J.; Yoon, J.-H.; Jeong, S.H.; Lee, D.H.; et al. Nonalcoholic fatty liver disease is associated with coronary artery calcification. *Hepatology* **2012**, *56*, 605–613. [CrossRef] [PubMed]
27. Li, X.; Xia, M.; Ma, H.; Hofman, A.; Hu, Y.; Yan, H.; He, W.; Lin, H.; Jeekel, J.; Zhao, N.; et al. Liver fat content is associated with increased carotid atherosclerosis in a Chinese middle-aged and elderly population: The Shanghai Changfeng study. *Atherosclerosis* **2012**, *224*, 480–485. [CrossRef]
28. Arab, J.P.; Dirchwolf, M.; Álvares-Da-Silva, M.R.; Barrera, F.; Benítez, C.; Castellanos-Fernandez, M.; Castro-Narro, G.; Chavez-Tapia, N.; Chiodi, D.; Cotrim, H.; et al. Latin American Association for the study of the liver (ALEH) practice guidance for the diagnosis and treatment of non-alcoholic fatty liver disease. *Ann. Hepatol.* **2020**, *19*, 674–690. [CrossRef]
29. Mahfood Haddad, T.; Hamdeh, S.; Kanmanthareddy, A.; Alla, V.M. Nonalcoholic fatty liver disease and the risk of clinical cardiovascular events: A systematic review and meta-analysis. *Diabetes Metab. Syndr.* **2017**, *11* (Suppl. S1), S209–S216. [CrossRef]
30. Park, G.-M.; Yun, S.-C.; Cho, Y.-R.; Gil, E.-H.; Her, S.H.; Kim, S.H.; Joon-Won, K.; Lee, M.S.; Lee, S.-W.; Kim, Y.-H.; et al. Prevalence of coronary atherosclerosis in an Asian population: Findings from coronary computed tomographic angiography. *Int. J. Cardiovasc. Imaging* **2015**, *31*, 659–668. [CrossRef]
31. Virmani, R.; Burke, A.P.; Farb, A.; Kolodgie, F.D. Pathology of the Vulnerable Plaque. *J. Am. Coll. Cardiol.* **2006**, *47*, C13–C18. [CrossRef]
32. Lim, S.; Shin, H.; Lee, Y.; Yoon, J.W.; Kang, S.M.; Choi, S.H.; Park, K.S.; Jang, H.C.; Choi, S.I.; Chun, E.J. Effect of Metabolic Syndrome on Coronary Artery Stenosis and Plaque Characteristics as Assessed with 64–Detector Row Cardiac CT. *Radiology* **2011**, *261*, 437–445. [CrossRef]
33. Meyersohn, N.M.; Mayrhofer, T.; Corey, K.E.; Bittner, D.O.; Staziaki, P.V.; Szilveszter, B.; Hallett, T.; Lu, M.T.; Puchner, S.B.; Simon, T.G.; et al. Association of Hepatic Steatosis with Major Adverse Cardiovascular Events, Independent of Coronary Artery Disease. *Clin. Gastroenterol. Hepatol.* **2020**, *19*, 1480–1488.e14. [CrossRef]
34. Choi, D.H.; Lee, S.J.; Kang, C.D.; Park, M.O.; Choi, N.W.; Kim, T.S.; Lee, W.; Cho, B.R.; Kim, Y.H.; Lee, B.-K.; et al. Nonalcoholic fatty liver disease is associated with coronary artery disease in Koreans. *World J. Gastroenterol.* **2013**, *19*, 6453–6457. [CrossRef]
35. Toh, J.Z.K.; Pan, X.-H.; Tay, P.W.L.; Ng, C.H.; Yong, J.N.; Xiao, J.; Koh, J.H.; Tan, E.Y.; Tan, E.X.X.; Dan, Y.Y.; et al. A Meta-Analysis on the Global Prevalence, Risk factors and Screening of Coronary Heart Disease in Nonalcoholic Fatty Liver Disease. *Clin. Gastroenterol. Hepatol.* **2021**; in press. [CrossRef]
36. Lee, S.B.; Park, G.-M.; Lee, J.-Y.; Lee, B.U.; Park, J.H.; Kim, B.G.; Jung, S.W.; Du Jeong, I.; Bang, S.-J.; Shin, J.W.; et al. Association between non-alcoholic fatty liver disease and subclinical coronary atherosclerosis: An observational cohort study. *J. Hepatol.* **2018**, *68*, 1018–1024. [CrossRef]
37. Thomsen, C.; Abdulla, J. Characteristics of high-risk coronary plaques identified by computed tomographic angiography and associated prognosis: A systematic review and meta-analysis. *Eur. Heart J. Cardiovasc. Imaging* **2015**, *17*, 120–129. [CrossRef]
38. Niikura, T.; Imajo, K.; Ozaki, A.; Kobayashi, T.; Iwaki, M.; Honda, Y.; Kessoku, T.; Ogawa, Y.; Yoneda, M.; Kirikoshi, H.; et al. Coronary Artery Disease is More Severe in Patients with Non-Alcoholic Steatohepatitis than Fatty Liver. *Diagnostics* **2020**, *10*, 129. [CrossRef]
39. Baratta, F.; Pastori, D.; Angelico, F.; Balla, A.; Paganini, A.M.; Cocomello, N.; Ferro, D.; Violi, F.; Sanyal, A.J.; Del Ben, M. Nonalcoholic Fatty Liver Disease and Fibrosis Associated with Increased Risk of Cardiovascular Events in a Prospective Study. *Clin. Gastroenterol. Hepatol.* **2020**, *18*, 2324–2331.e4. [CrossRef]
40. Hsu, P.; Wang, Y.; Lin, C.; Wang, Y.; Ding, Y.; Liou, T.; Huang, S.; Lu, T.; Chan, W.; Lin, S.; et al. The association of the steatosis severity in fatty liver disease with coronary plaque pattern in general population. *Liver Int.* **2020**, *41*, 81–90. [CrossRef]
41. Puchner, S.B.; Lu, M.T.; Mayrhofer, T.; Liu, T.; Pursnani, A.; Ghoshhajra, B.; Truong, Q.A.; Wiviott, S.D.; Fleg, J.L.; Hoffmann, U.; et al. High-Risk Coronary Plaque at Coronary CT Angiography Is Associated with Nonalcoholic Fatty Liver Disease, Independent of Coronary Plaque and Stenosis Burden: Results from the ROMICAT II Trial. *Radiology* **2015**, *274*, 693–701. [CrossRef]
42. Targher, G.; Corey, K.E.; Byrne, C.D. NAFLD, and cardiovascular and cardiac diseases: Factors influencing risk, prediction and treatment. *Diabetes Metab.* **2020**, *47*, 101215. [CrossRef]
43. Wong, V.W.-S.; Wong, G.L.-H.; Yeung, J.C.-L.; Fung, C.Y.-K.; Chan, J.K.-L.; Chang, Z.H.-Y.; Kwan, C.T.-Y.; Lam, H.-W.; Limquiaco, J.; Chim, A.M.-L.; et al. Long-term clinical outcomes after fatty liver screening in patients undergoing coronary angiogram: A prospective cohort study. *Hepatology* **2015**, *63*, 754–763. [CrossRef]

44. Wang, L.; Li, Y.; Gong, X. Changes in inflammatory factors and prognosis of patients complicated with non-alcoholic fatty liver disease undergoing coronary artery bypass grafting. *Exp. Ther. Med.* **2017**, *15*, 949–953. [CrossRef] [PubMed]
45. Thévenot, T.; Vendeville, S.; Weil, D.; Akkouche, L.; Calame, P.; Canivet, C.M.; Vanlemmens, C.; Richou, C.; Cervoni, J.-P.; Seronde, M.-F.; et al. Systematic screening for advanced liver fibrosis in patients with coronary artery disease: The CORONASH study. *PLoS ONE* **2022**, *17*, e0266965. [CrossRef]
46. Fiorentino, T.V.; Succurro, E.; Sciacqua, A.; Andreozzi, F.; Perticone, F.; Sesti, G. Non-alcoholic fatty liver disease is associated with cardiovascular disease in subjects with different glucose tolerance. *Diabetes/Metabolism Res. Rev.* **2020**, *36*, e3333. [CrossRef] [PubMed]
47. Jana, S.B.; Paul, K.; Roy, B.; Mandal, S.C. A Correlation Study between Non-Alcoholic Fatty Liver Disease and Severity of Coronary Artery Disease. *J. Med Sci. Clin. Res.* **2020**, *8*, 4688–4699. [CrossRef]
48. Liu, H.-H.; Cao, Y.-X.; Sun, D.; Jin, J.-L.; Guo, Y.-L.; Wu, N.-Q.; Zhu, C.-G.; Gao, Y.; Dong, Q.-T.; Zhao, X.; et al. Impact of Non-Alcoholic Fatty Liver Disease on Cardiovascular Outcomes in Patients with Stable Coronary Artery Disease: A Matched Case–Control Study. *Clin. Transl. Gastroenterol.* **2019**, *10*, e00011. [CrossRef]
49. Langroudi, T.F.; Haybar, H.; Parsa, S.A.; Mahjoorian, M.; Khaheshi, I.; Naderian, M. The severity of coronary artery disease was not associated with non-alcoholic fatty liver disease in a series of 264 non-diabetic patients who underwent coronary angiography. *Romanian J. Intern. Med.* **2018**, *56*, 167–172. [CrossRef]
50. Pulimaddi, R.; Parveda, A.R.; Dasari, D. Prevalence of Non-Alcoholic Fatty Liver Disease (NAFLD) in Type 2 Diabetic Patients in Correlation with Coronary Artery Disease. *Int. Arch. Integr. Med.* **2016**, *3*, 118–128.
51. Sinn, D.H.; Kang, D.; Chang, Y.; Ryu, S.; Gu, S.; Kim, H.; Seong, D.; Cho, S.J.; Yi, B.-K.; Park, H.-D.; et al. Non-alcoholic fatty liver disease and progression of coronary artery calcium score: A retrospective cohort study. *Gut* **2016**, *66*, 323–329. [CrossRef]
52. Idilman, I.S.; Akata, D.; Hazirolan, T.; Erdogan, B.D.; Aytemir, K.; Karcaaltincaba, M. Nonalcoholic fatty liver disease is associated with significant coronary artery disease in type 2 diabetic patients: A computed tomography angiography study. *J. Diabetes* **2014**, *7*, 279–286. [CrossRef]
53. Osawa, K.; Miyoshi, T.; Yamauchi, K.; Koyama, Y.; Nakamura, K.; Sato, S.; Kanazawa, S.; Ito, H. Nonalcoholic Hepatic Steatosis Is a Strong Predictor of High-Risk Coronary-Artery Plaques as Determined by Multidetector CT. *PLoS ONE* **2015**, *10*, e0131138. [CrossRef]
54. Ağaç, M.T.; Korkmaz, L.; Çavuşoğlu, G.; Karadeniz, A.G.; Ağaç, S.; Bektas, H.; Erkan, H.; Varol, M.O.; Vatan, M.B.; Acar, Z.; et al. Association Between Nonalcoholic Fatty Liver Disease and Coronary Artery Disease Complexity in Patients with Acute Coronary Syndrome. *Angiology* **2013**, *64*, 604–608. [CrossRef]
55. Ballestri, S.; Meschiari, E.; Baldelli, E.; Musumeci, F.E.; Romagnoli, D.; Trenti, T.; Zennaro, R.G.; Lonardo, A.; Loria, P. Relationship of Serum Fetuin-A Levels with Coronary Atherosclerotic Burden and NAFLD in Patients Undergoing Elective Coronary Angiography. *Metab. Syndr. Relat. Disord.* **2013**, *11*, 289–295. [CrossRef]
56. Josef, P.; Ali, I.; Ariel, P.; Alon, M.; Nimer, A. Relationship between Retinal Vascular Caliber and Coronary Artery Disease in Patients with Non-Alcoholic Fatty Liver Disease (NAFLD). *Int. J. Environ. Res. Public Health* **2013**, *10*, 3409–3423. [CrossRef]
57. Wong, V.W.-S.; Wong, G.L.-H.; Yip, G.W.K.; Lo, A.O.S.; Limquiaco, J.; Chu, W.C.W.; Chim, A.M.-L.; Yu, C.-M.; Yu, J.; Chan, H.L.Y.; et al. Coronary artery disease and cardiovascular outcomes in patients with non-alcoholic fatty liver disease. *Gut* **2011**, *60*, 1721–1727. [CrossRef]
58. Assy, N.; Djibre, A.; Farah, R.; Grosovski, M.; Marmor, A. Presence of Coronary Plaques in Patients with Nonalcoholic Fatty Liver Disease. *Radiology* **2010**, *254*, 393–400. [CrossRef]
59. Açikel, M.; Sunay, S.; Koplay, M.; Gündoğdu, F.; Karakelleoğlu, S. Evaluation of ultrasonographic fatty liver and severity of coronary atherosclerosis, and obesity in patients undergoing coronary angiography. *Anadolu Kardiyol. Derg. AKD Anatol. J. Cardiol.* **2009**, *9*, 273–279.
60. Arslan, U.; Türkoğlu, S.; Balcioğlu, S.; Tavil, Y.; Karakan, T.; Çengel, A. Association between nonalcoholic fatty liver disease and coronary artery disease. *Coron. Artery Dis.* **2007**, *18*, 433–436. [CrossRef]
61. Carter, J.; Heseltine, T.D.; Meah, M.N.; Tzolos, E.; Kwiecinski, J.; Doris, M.; McElhinney, P.; Moss, A.J.; Adamson, P.D.; Hunter, A.; et al. Hepatosteatosis and Atherosclerotic Plaque at Coronary CT Angiography. *Radiol. Cardiothorac. Imaging* **2022**, *4*, e210260. [CrossRef]
62. Ichikawa, K.; Miyoshi, T.; Osawa, K.; Miki, T.; Toda, H.; Ejiri, K.; Yoshida, M.; Nakamura, K.; Morita, H.; Ito, H. Incremental prognostic value of non-alcoholic fatty liver disease over coronary computed tomography angiography findings in patients with suspected coronary artery disease. *Eur. J. Prev. Cardiol.* **2021**, *28*, 2059–2066. [CrossRef]
63. Wang, X.; Shen, L.; Shen, Y.; Han, F.; Ji, Z. Association between Non-alcoholic Fatty Liver Disease and the Severity of Coronary Artery Stenosis in Eastern Chinese Population. *Zahedan J. Res. Med Sci.* **2022**, *21*, 1–7. [CrossRef]
64. Ichikawa, K.; Miyoshi, T.; Osawa, K.; Miki, T.; Toda, H.; Ejiri, K.; Yoshida, M.; Nanba, Y.; Yoshida, M.; Nakamura, K.; et al. Prognostic value of non-alcoholic fatty liver disease for predicting cardiovascular events in patients with diabetes mellitus with suspected coronary artery disease: A prospective cohort study. *Cardiovasc. Diabetol.* **2021**, *20*, 8. [CrossRef]
65. Saraya, S.; Saraya, M.; Mahmoud, M.; Galal, M.; Soliman, H.H.; Raafat, M. The associations between coronary artery disease, and non-alcoholic fatty liver disease by computed tomography. *Egypt. Hear. J.* **2021**, *73*, 96. [CrossRef]
66. Bae, Y.S.; Ko, Y.S.; Yun, J.M.; Eo, A.Y.; Kim, H. Association and Prediction of Subclinical Atherosclerosis by Nonalcoholic Fatty Liver Disease in Asymptomatic Patients. *Can. J. Gastroenterol. Hepatol.* **2020**, *2020*, 8820445. [CrossRef]
67. Koo, B.K.; Allison, M.A.; Criqui, M.H.; Denenberg, J.O.; Wright, C.M. The association between liver fat and systemic calcified atherosclerosis. *J. Vasc. Surg.* **2019**, *71*, 204–211.e4. [CrossRef] [PubMed]

68. Chang, Y.; Cho, Y.K.; Cho, J.; Jung, H.-S.; Yun, K.E.; Ahn, J.; Sohn, C.I.; Shin, H.; Ryu, S. Alcoholic and Nonalcoholic Fatty Liver Disease and Liver-Related Mortality: A Cohort Study. *Am. J. Gastroenterol.* **2019**, *114*, 620–629. [CrossRef] [PubMed]
69. Oni, E.; Budoff, M.J.; Zeb, I.; Li, D.; Veledar, E.; Polak, J.F.; Blankstein, R.; Wong, N.D.; Blaha, M.J.; Agatston, A.; et al. Nonalcoholic Fatty Liver Disease Is Associated with Arterial Distensibility and Carotid Intima-Media Thickness: (from the Multi-Ethnic Study of Atherosclerosis). *Am. J. Cardiol.* **2019**, *124*, 534–538. [CrossRef]
70. Pais, R.; Redheuil, A.; Cluzel, P.; Ratziu, V.; Giral, P. Relationship Among Fatty Liver, Specific and Multiple-Site Atherosclerosis, and 10-Year Framingham Score. *Hepatology* **2019**, *69*, 1453–1463. [CrossRef] [PubMed]
71. Park, H.E.; Lee, H.; Choi, S.-Y.; Kwak, M.-S.; Yang, J.I.; Yim, J.Y.; Chung, G.E. Clinical significance of hepatic steatosis according to coronary plaque morphology: Assessment using controlled attenuation parameter. *J. Gastroenterol.* **2018**, *54*, 271–280. [CrossRef]
72. Gummesson, A.; Strömberg, U.; Schmidt, C.; Kullberg, J.; Angerås, O.; Lindgren, S.; Hjelmgren, O.; Torén, K.; Rosengren, A.; Fagerberg, B.; et al. Non-alcoholic fatty liver disease is a strong predictor of coronary artery calcification in metabolically healthy subjects: A cross-sectional, population-based study in middle-aged subjects. *PLoS ONE* **2018**, *13*, e0202666. [CrossRef]
73. Wu, R.; Hou, F.; Wang, X.; Zhou, Y.; Sun, K.; Wang, Y.; Liu, H.; Wu, J.; Zhao, R.; Hu, J. Nonalcoholic Fatty Liver Disease and Coronary Artery Calcification in a Northern Chinese Population: A Cross Sectional Study. *Sci. Rep.* **2017**, *7*, 9933. [CrossRef]
74. Jacobs, K.; Brouha, S.; Bettencourt, R.; Barrett-Connor, E.; Sirlin, C.; Loomba, R. Association of Nonalcoholic Fatty Liver Disease With Visceral Adiposity but Not Coronary Artery Calcification in the Elderly. *Clin. Gastroenterol. Hepatol.* **2016**, *14*, 1337–1344.e3. [CrossRef]
75. Kim, B.J.; Kim, H.S.; Kang, J.G.; Kim, B.S.; Kang, J.H. Association of epicardial fat volume and nonalcoholic fatty liver disease with metabolic syndrome: From the CAESAR study. *J. Clin. Lipidol.* **2016**, *10*, 1423–1430.e1. [CrossRef]
76. Park, H.E.; Kwak, M.-S.; Kim, D.; Kim, M.-K.; Cha, M.-J.; Choi, S.-Y. Nonalcoholic Fatty Liver Disease is Associated with Coronary Artery Calcification Development: A longitudinal study. *J. Clin. Endocrinol. Metab.* **2016**, *101*, 3134–3143. [CrossRef]
77. Kim, M.K.; Ahn, C.W.; Nam, J.S.; Kang, S.; Park, J.S.; Kim, K.R. Association between nonalcoholic fatty liver disease and coronary artery calcification in postmenopausal women. *Menopause* **2015**, *22*, 1323–1327. [CrossRef]
78. Kang, M.K.; Kang, B.H.; Kim, J.H. Nonalcoholic Fatty Liver Disease Is Associated with the Presence and Morphology of Subclinical Coronary Atherosclerosis. *Yonsei Med. J.* **2015**, *56*, 1288–1295. [CrossRef]
79. Lee, M.-K.; Park, H.-J.; Jeon, W.S.; Park, S.E.; Park, C.-Y.; Lee, W.-Y.; Oh, K.-W.; Park, S.-W.; Rhee, E.-J. Higher association of coronary artery calcification with non-alcoholic fatty liver disease than with abdominal obesity in middle-aged Korean men: The Kangbuk Samsung Health Study. *Cardiovasc. Diabetol.* **2015**, *14*, 88. [CrossRef]
80. Efe, D.; Aygün, F. Assessment of the Relationship between Non-Alcoholic Fatty Liver Disease and CAD using MSCT. *Arq. Bras. Cardiol.* **2013**, *102*, 10–18. [CrossRef]
81. Van Wagner, L.B.; Ning, H.; Lewis, C.E.; Shay, C.M.; Wilkins, J.; Carr, J.J.; Terry, J.G.; Lloyd-Jones, D.M.; Jacobs, D.R.; Carnethon, M.R. Associations between nonalcoholic fatty liver disease and subclinical atherosclerosis in middle-aged adults: The Coronary Artery Risk Development in Young Adults Study. *Atherosclerosis* **2014**, *235*, 599–605. [CrossRef]
82. Chhabra, R.; O'Keefe, J.H.; Patil, H.; O'Keefe, E.; Thompson, R.C.; Ansari, S.; Kennedy, K.F.; Lee, L.W.; Helzberg, J.H. Association of Coronary Artery Calcification with Hepatic Steatosis in Asymptomatic Individuals. *Mayo Clin. Proc.* **2013**, *88*, 1259–1265. [CrossRef]
83. Juárez-Rojas, J.G.; Medina-Urrutia, A.X.; Jorge-Galarza, E.; González-Salazar, C.; Kimura-Hayama, E.; Cardoso-Saldaña, G.; Posadas-Sánchez, R.; Martínez-Alvarado, R.; Posadas-Romero, C. Fatty Liver Increases the Association of Metabolic Syndrome with Diabetes and Atherosclerosis. *Diabetes Care* **2013**, *36*, 1726–1728. [CrossRef]
84. Khashper, A.; Gaspar, T.; Azencot, M.; Dobrecky-Mery, I.; Peled, N.; Lewis, B.S.; Halon, D.A. Visceral abdominal adipose tissue and coronary atherosclerosis in asymptomatic diabetics. *Int. J. Cardiol.* **2013**, *162*, 184–188. [CrossRef]
85. Sung, K.-C.; Lim, Y.-H.; Park, S.; Kang, S.-M.; Park, J.B.; Kim, B.-J.; Shin, J.-H. Arterial stiffness, fatty liver and the presence of coronary artery calcium in a large population cohort. *Cardiovasc. Diabetol.* **2013**, *12*, 162. [CrossRef]
86. Arslan, U.; Kocaoğlu, I.; Balcı, M.; Duyuler, S.; Korkmaz, A. The association between impaired collateral circulation and non-alcoholic fatty liver in patients with severe coronary artery disease. *J. Cardiol.* **2012**, *60*, 210–214. [CrossRef] [PubMed]
87. Sung, K.-C.; Wild, S.H.; Kwag, H.J.; Byrne, C.D. Fatty Liver, Insulin Resistance, and Features of Metabolic Syndrome. *Diabetes Care* **2012**, *35*, 2359–2364. [CrossRef]
88. Agarwal, A.K.; Jain, V.; Singla, S.; Baruah, B.P.; Arya, V.; Yadav, R.; Singh, V.P. Prevalence of non-alcoholic fatty liver disease and its correlation with coronary risk factors in patients with type 2 diabetes. *J. Assoc. Physicians India* **2011**, *59*, 351–354. [PubMed]
89. Cotter, T.G.; Rinella, M. Nonalcoholic Fatty Liver Disease 2020: The State of the Disease. *Gastroenterology* **2020**, *158*, 1851–1864. [CrossRef] [PubMed]
90. Schindhelm, R.K.; Dekker, J.M.; Nijpels, G.; Bouter, L.M.; Stehouwer, C.D.; Heine, R.J.; Diamant, M. Alanine aminotransferase predicts coronary heart disease events: A 10-year follow-up of the Hoorn Study. *Atherosclerosis* **2007**, *191*, 391–396. [CrossRef] [PubMed]
91. Kunutsor, S.; Apekey, T.A.; Cheung, B.M. Gamma-glutamyltransferase and risk of hypertension. *J. Hypertens.* **2015**, *33*, 2373–2381. [CrossRef]
92. Webber, M.; Krishnan, A.; Thomas, N.G.; Cheung, B.M. Association between serum alkaline phosphatase and C-reactive protein in the United States National Health and Nutrition Examination Survey 2005–2006. *Clin. Chem. Lab. Med. (CCLM)* **2009**, *48*, 167–173. [CrossRef]
93. Cheung, B.M.; Ong, K.L.; Wong, L.Y. Elevated serum alkaline phosphatase and peripheral arterial disease in the United States National Health and Nutrition Examination Survey 1999–2004. *Int. J. Cardiol.* **2009**, *135*, 156–161. [CrossRef]

94. Song, D.S.; Chang, U.I.; Kang, S.-G.; Song, S.-W.; Yang, J.M. Noninvasive Serum Fibrosis Markers are Associated with Coronary Artery Calcification in Patients with Nonalcoholic Fatty Liver Disease. *Gut Liver* **2019**, *13*, 658–668. [CrossRef]
95. Lee, C.-O.; Li, H.-L.; Tsoi, M.-F.; Cheung, C.-L.; Cheung, B.M.Y. Association between the liver fat score (LFS) and cardiovascular diseases in the national health and nutrition examination survey 1999–2016. *Ann. Med.* **2021**, *53*, 1067–1075. [CrossRef]
96. Lee, Y.-H.; Cho, Y.; Lee, B.-W.; Park, C.-Y.; Lee, D.H.; Cha, B.-S.; Rhee, E.-J. Nonalcoholic Fatty Liver Disease in Diabetes. Part I: Epidemiology and Diagnosis. *Diabetes Metab. J.* **2019**, *43*, 31–45. [CrossRef]
97. Berzigotti, A.; Tsochatzis, E.; Boursier, J.; Castera, L.; Cazzagon, N.; Friedrich-Rust, M.; Petta, S.; Thiele, M. EASL Clinical Practice Guidelines on non-invasive tests for evaluation of liver disease severity and prognosis—2021 update. *J. Hepatol.* **2021**, *75*, 659–689. [CrossRef]
98. European Association for Study of Liver. EASL-ALEH Clinical Practice Guidelines: Non-invasive tests for evaluation of liver disease severity and prognosis. *J. Hepatol.* **2015**, *63*, 237–264. [CrossRef]
99. Long, M.T.; Zhang, X.; Xu, H.; Liu, C.; Corey, K.E.; Chung, R.T.; Loomba, R.; Benjamin, E.J. Hepatic Fibrosis Associates with Multiple Cardiometabolic Disease Risk Factors: The Framingham Heart Study. *Hepatology* **2020**, *73*, 548–559. [CrossRef]
100. You, S.C.; Kim, K.J.; Kim, S.U.; Kim, B.K.; Park, J.Y.; Kim, D.Y.; Ahn, S.H.; Lee, W.J.; Han, K.-H. Factors associated with significant liver fibrosis assessed using transient elastography in general population. *World J. Gastroenterol.* **2015**, *21*, 1158–1166. [CrossRef]
101. Magalhães, R.D.S.; Xavier, S.; Magalhães, J.; Rosa, B.; Marinho, C.; Cotter, J. Transient elastography through controlled attenuated parameter assisting the stratification of cardiovascular disease risk in NAFLD patients. *Clin. Res. Hepatol. Gastroenterol.* **2020**, *45*, 101580. [CrossRef]
102. Kerut, S.E.; Balart, J.T.; Kerut, E.K.; McMullan, M.R. Diagnosis of fatty liver by computed tomography coronary artery calcium score. *Echocardiography* **2017**, *34*, 937–938. [CrossRef]
103. Visseren, F.L.J.; Mach, F.; Smulders, Y.M.; Carballo, D.; Koskinas, K.C.; Bäck, M.; Benetos, A.; Biffi, A.; Boavida, J.-M.; Capodanno, D.; et al. 2021 ESC Guidelines on cardiovascular disease prevention in clinical practice: Developed by the Task Force for cardio-vascular disease prevention in clinical practice with representatives of the European Society of Cardiology and 12 medical societies with the special contribution of the European Association of Preventive Cardiology (EAPC). *Eur. Heart J.* **2021**, *42*, 3227–3337. [CrossRef]
104. Targher, G.; Byrne, C.D.; Tilg, H. NAFLD and increased risk of cardiovascular disease: Clinical associations, pathophysiological mechanisms and pharmacological implications. *Gut* **2020**, *69*, 1691–1705. [CrossRef]
105. Niederseer, D.; Wernly, S.; Bachmayer, S.; Wernly, B.; Bakula, A.; Huber-Schönauer, U.; Semmler, G.; Schmied, C.; Aigner, E.; Datz, C. Diagnosis of Non-Alcoholic Fatty Liver Disease (NAFLD) Is Independently Associated with Cardiovascular Risk in a Large Austrian Screening Cohort. *J. Clin. Med.* **2020**, *9*, 1065. [CrossRef]
106. Van Veelen, A.; van der Sangen, N.M.R.; Delewi, R.; Beijk, M.A.M.; Henriques, J.P.S.; Claessen, B.E.P.M. Detection of Vulnerable Coronary Plaques Using Invasive and Non-Invasive Imaging Modalities. *J. Clin. Med.* **2022**, *11*, 1361. [CrossRef]
107. Xu, X.; Lu, L.; Dong, Q.; Li, X.; Zhang, N.; Xin, Y.; Xuan, S. Research advances in the relationship between nonalcoholic fatty liver disease and atherosclerosis. *Lipids Heal. Dis.* **2015**, *14*, 158. [CrossRef]
108. Caturano, A.; Acierno, C.; Nevola, R.; Pafundi, P.C.; Galiero, R.; Rinaldi, L.; Salvatore, T.; Adinolfi, L.E.; Sasso, F.C. Non-Alcoholic Fatty Liver Disease: From Pathogenesis to Clinical Impact. *Processes* **2021**, *9*, 135. [CrossRef]
109. Kang, S.H.; Cho, Y.; Jeong, S.W.; Kim, S.U.; Lee, J.-W.; Korean NAFLD Study Group. From nonalcoholic fatty liver disease to metabolic-associated fatty liver disease: Big wave or ripple? *Clin. Mol. Hepatol.* **2021**, *27*, 257–269. [CrossRef]
110. Eslam, M.; Sanyal, A.J.; George, J.; on behalf of the International Consensus Panel. MAFLD: A Consensus-Driven Proposed Nomenclature for Metabolic Associated Fatty Liver Disease. *Gastroenterology* **2020**, *158*, 1999–2014.e1991. [CrossRef]
111. Fernandez-Friera, L.; Fuster, V.; López-Melgar, B.; Oliva, B.; García-Ruiz, J.M.; Mendiguren, J.; Bueno, H.; Pocock, S.; Ibanez, B.; Fernández-Ortiz, A.; et al. Normal LDL-Cholesterol Levels Are Associated with Subclinical Atherosclerosis in the Absence of Risk Factors. *J. Am. Coll. Cardiol.* **2017**, *70*, 2979–2991. [CrossRef] [PubMed]
112. Gariani, K.; Jornayvaz, F.R. Pathophysiology of NASH in endocrine diseases. *Endocr. Connect.* **2021**, *10*, R52–R65. [CrossRef] [PubMed]
113. Liu, H.; Lu, H.-Y. Nonalcoholic fatty liver disease and cardiovascular disease. *World J. Gastroenterol.* **2014**, *20*, 8407–8415. [CrossRef] [PubMed]
114. Tang, C.S.; Zhang, H.; Cheung, C.Y.Y.; Xu, M.; Ho, J.C.Y.; Zhou, W.; Cherny, S.S.; Zhang, Y.; Holmen, O.; Au, K.-W.; et al. Exome-wide association analysis reveals novel coding sequence variants associated with lipid traits in Chinese. *Nat. Commun.* **2015**, *6*, 10206. [CrossRef]
115. Francque, S.M.; van der Graaff, D.; Kwanten, W.J. Non-alcoholic fatty liver disease and cardiovascular risk: Pathophysiological mechanisms and implications. *J. Hepatol.* **2016**, *65*, 425–443. [CrossRef]
116. Brouwers, M.C.G.J.; Simons, N.; Stehouwer, C.D.A.; Isaacs, A. Non-alcoholic fatty liver disease and cardiovascular disease: Assessing the evidence for causality. *Diabetologia* **2019**, *63*, 253–260. [CrossRef]
117. Simons, N.; Isaacs, A.; Koek, G.H.; Kuč, S.; Schaper, N.C.; Brouwers, M.C. PNPLA3, TM6SF2, and MBOAT7 Genotypes and Coronary Artery Disease. *Gastroenterology* **2017**, *152*, 912–913. [CrossRef]
118. Hsieh, C.-J.; Wang, P.W.; Hu, T.H. Association of Adiponectin Gene Polymorphism with Nonalcoholic Fatty Liver Disease in Taiwanese Patients with Type 2 Diabetes. *PLoS ONE* **2015**, *10*, e0127521. [CrossRef]
119. Li, X.-L.; Sui, J.-Q.; Lu, L.-L.; Zhang, N.-N.; Xu, X.; Dong, Q.-Y.; Xin, Y.-N.; Xuan, S.-Y. Gene polymorphisms associated with non-alcoholic fatty liver disease and coronary artery disease: A concise review. *Lipids Heal. Dis.* **2016**, *15*, 53. [CrossRef]

120. Dong, M.; Liu, S.; Wang, M.; Wang, Y.; Xin, Y.; Xuan, S. Relationship between AGT rs2493132 polymorphism and the risk of coronary artery disease in patients with NAFLD in the Chinese Han population. *J. Int. Med Res.* **2021**, *49*. [CrossRef]
121. Pulido, M.R.; Diaz-Ruiz, A.; Jiménez-Gómez, Y.; Garcia-Navarro, S.; Gracia-Navarro, F.; Tinahones, F.; López-Miranda, J.; Frühbeck, G.; Vázquez-Martínez, R.; Malagón, M.M. Rab18 Dynamics in Adipocytes in Relation to Lipogenesis, Lipolysis and Obesity. *PLoS ONE* **2011**, *6*, e22931. [CrossRef]
122. Mehta, R.; Otgonsuren, M.; Younoszai, Z.; Allawi, H.; Raybuck, B.; Younossi, Z. Circulating miRNA in patients with non-alcoholic fatty liver disease and coronary artery disease. *BMJ Open Gastroenterol.* **2016**, *3*, e000096. [CrossRef]
123. Cao, Y.-X.; Zhang, H.-W.; Jin, J.-L.; Liu, H.-H.; Zhang, Y.; Xue, R.-X.; Gao, Y.; Guo, Y.-L.; Zhu, C.-G.; Hua, Q.; et al. Prognostic utility of triglyceride-rich lipoprotein-related markers in patients with coronary artery disease. *J. Lipid Res.* **2020**, *61*, 1254–1262. [CrossRef]
124. Dongiovanni, P.; Paolini, E.; Corsini, A.; Sirtori, C.R.; Ruscica, M. Nonalcoholic fatty liver disease or metabolic dysfunction-associated fatty liver disease diagnoses and cardiovascular diseases: From epidemiology to drug approaches. *Eur. J. Clin. Investig.* **2021**, *51*, e13519. [CrossRef]
125. Athyros, V.G.; Tziomalos, K.; Gossios, T.D.; Griva, T.; Anagnostis, P.; Kargiotis, K.; Pagourelias, E.D.; Theocharidou, E.; Karagiannis, A.; Mikhailidis, D.P. Safety and efficacy of long-term statin treatment for cardiovascular events in patients with coronary heart disease and abnormal liver tests in the Greek Atorvastatin and Coronary Heart Disease Evaluation (GREACE) Study: A post-hoc analysis. *Lancet* **2010**, *376*, 1916–1922. [CrossRef]
126. Virtue, S.; Vidal-Puig, A. Adipose tissue expandability, lipotoxicity and the Metabolic Syndrome—An allostatic perspective. *Biochim. Biophys. Acta* **2010**, *1801*, 338–349. [CrossRef]
127. Jeon, W.S.; Park, S.E.; Rhee, E.-J.; Park, C.-Y.; Oh, K.-W.; Park, S.-W.; Lee, W.-Y. Association of Serum Adipocyte-Specific Fatty Acid Binding Protein with Fatty Liver Index as a Predictive Indicator of Nonalcoholic Fatty Liver Disease. *Endocrinol. Metab.* **2013**, *28*, 283–287. [CrossRef]
128. Lee, C.H.; Woo, Y.C.; Chow, W.S.; Cheung, C.Y.Y.; Fong, C.H.Y.; Yuen, M.M.A.; Xu, A.; Tse, H.F.; Lam, K.S.L. Role of Circulating Fibroblast Growth Factor 21 Measurement in Primary Prevention of Coronary Heart Disease Among Chinese Patients with Type 2 Diabetes Mellitus. *J. Am. Hear. Assoc.* **2017**, *6*, e005344. [CrossRef]
129. Gómez-Ambrosi, J.; Gallego-Escuredo, J.M.; Catalán, V.; Rodríguez, A.; Domingo, P.; Moncada, R.; Valentí, V.; Salvador, J.; Giralt, M.; Villarroya, F.; et al. FGF19 and FGF21 serum concentrations in human obesity and type 2 diabetes behave differently after diet- or surgically-induced weight loss. *Clin. Nutr.* **2016**, *36*, 861–868. [CrossRef]
130. Deprince, A.; Haas, J.T.; Staels, B. Dysregulated lipid metabolism links NAFLD to cardiovascular disease. *Mol. Metab.* **2020**, *42*, 101092. [CrossRef]
131. Hao, Y.; Zhou, J.; Zhou, M.; Ma, X.; Lu, Z.; Gao, M.; Pan, X.; Tang, J.; Bao, Y.; Jia, W. Serum Levels of Fibroblast Growth Factor 19 Are Inversely Associated with Coronary Artery Disease in Chinese Individuals. *PLoS ONE* **2013**, *8*, e72345. [CrossRef]
132. Zhou, M.; Learned, R.M.; Rossi, S.J.; DePaoli, A.M.; Tian, H.; Ling, L. Engineered FGF19 eliminates bile acid toxicity and lipotoxicity leading to resolution of steatohepatitis and fibrosis in mice. *Hepatol. Commun.* **2017**, *1*, 1024–1042. [CrossRef]
133. Kasper, P.; Martin, A.; Lang, S.; Kütting, F.; Goeser, T.; Demir, M.; Steffen, H.-M. NAFLD and cardiovascular diseases: A clinical review. *Clin. Res. Cardiol.* **2020**, *110*, 921–937. [CrossRef]
134. Baars, T.; Gieseler, R.K.; Patsalis, P.C.; Canbay, A. Towards harnessing the value of organokine crosstalk to predict the risk for cardiovascular disease in non-alcoholic fatty liver disease. *Metabolism* **2022**, *130*, 155179. [CrossRef]
135. Cheng, Y.; An, B.; Jiang, M.; Xin, Y.; Xuan, S. Association of Tumor Necrosis Factor-alpha Polymorphisms and Risk of Coronary Artery Disease in Patients with Non-alcoholic Fatty Liver Disease. *Zahedan J. Res. Med Sci.* **2015**, *15*, e26818. [CrossRef]
136. Simon, T.G.; Trejo, M.E.P.; McClelland, R.; Bradley, R.; Blaha, M.J.; Zeb, I.; Corey, K.E.; Budoff, M.J.; Chung, R.T. Circulating Interleukin-6 is a biomarker for coronary atherosclerosis in nonalcoholic fatty liver disease: Results from the Multi-Ethnic Study of Atherosclerosis. *Int. J. Cardiol.* **2018**, *259*, 198–204. [CrossRef]
137. Otsuka, F.; Sugiyama, S.; Kojima, S.; Maruyoshi, H.; Funahashi, T.; Sakamoto, T.; Yoshimura, M.; Kimura, K.; Umemura, S.; Ogawa, H. Hypoadiponectinemia is Associated with Impaired Glucose Tolerance and Coronary Artery Disease in Non-Diabetic Men. *Circ. J.* **2007**, *71*, 1703–1709. [CrossRef]
138. Treeprasertsuk, S.; Lopez-Jimenez, F.; Lindor, K.D. Nonalcoholic Fatty Liver Disease and the Coronary Artery Disease. *Am. J. Dig. Dis.* **2010**, *56*, 35–45. [CrossRef]
139. Ridker, P.M.; Everett, B.M.; Thuren, T.; MacFadyen, J.G.; Chang, W.H.; Ballantyne, C.; Fonseca, F.; Nicolau, J.; Koenig, W.; Anker, S.D.; et al. Antiinflammatory Therapy with Canakinumab for Atherosclerotic Disease. *N. Engl. J. Med.* **2017**, *377*, 1119–1131. [CrossRef]
140. Jose, N.; Vasant, P.K.; Kulirankal, K.G. Study of Endothelial Dysfunction in Patients with Non-alcoholic Fatty Liver Disease. *Cureus* **2021**, *13*, e20515. [CrossRef]
141. Yilmaz, Y.; Kurt, R.; Yonal, O.; Polat, N.; Celikel, C.A.; Gurdal, A.; Oflaz, H.; Ozdogan, O.; Imeryuz, N.; Kalayci, C.; et al. Coronary flow reserve is impaired in patients with nonalcoholic fatty liver disease: Association with liver fibrosis. *Atherosclerosis* **2010**, *211*, 182–186. [CrossRef] [PubMed]
142. Keskin, M.; Hayıroğlu, M.; Uzun, A.O.; Güvenç, T.S.; Şahin, S.; Kozan, Ö. Effect of Nonalcoholic Fatty Liver Disease on In-Hospital and Long-Term Outcomes in Patients With ST–Segment Elevation Myocardial Infarction. *Am. J. Cardiol.* **2017**, *120*, 1720–1726. [CrossRef] [PubMed]

143. Persico, M.; Masarone, M.; Damato, A.; Ambrosio, M.; Federico, A.; Rosato, V.; Bucci, T.; Carrizzo, A.; Vecchione, C. Non alcoholic fatty liver disease and eNOS dysfunction in humans. *BMC Gastroenterol.* **2017**, *17*, 35. [CrossRef]
144. Frühbeck, G.; Gómez-Ambrosi, J. Control of body weight: A physiologic and transgenic perspective. *Diabetologia* **2003**, *46*, 143–172. [CrossRef]
145. Fortuño, A.; Rodríguez, A.; Gómez-Ambrosi, J.; Muñiz, P.; Salvador, J.; Díez, J.; Frühbeck, G. Leptin Inhibits Angiotensin II-Induced Intracellular Calcium Increase and Vasoconstriction in the Rat Aorta. *Endocrinology* **2002**, *143*, 3555–3560. [CrossRef]
146. Cernea, S.; Roiban, A.L.; Both, E.; Huțanu, A. Serum leptin and leptin resistance correlations with NAFLD in patients with type 2 diabetes. *Diabetes/Metabolism Res. Rev.* **2018**, *34*, e3050. [CrossRef]
147. Silva, A.C.S.; Miranda, A.S.; Rocha, N.P.; Teixeira, A.L. Renin angiotensin system in liver diseases: Friend or foe? *World J. Gastroenterol.* **2017**, *23*, 3396–3406. [CrossRef]
148. Elsheikh, E.; Younoszai, Z.; Otgonsuren, M.; Hunt, S.; Raybuck, B.; Younossi, Z.M. Markers of endothelial dysfunction in patients with non-alcoholic fatty liver disease and coronary artery disease. *J. Gastroenterol. Hepatol.* **2014**, *29*, 1528–1534. [CrossRef]
149. Dallio, M.; Masarone, M.; Caprio, G.G.; Di Sarno, R.; Tuccillo, C.; Sasso, F.C.; Persico, M.; Loguercio, C.; Federico, A. Endocan Serum Levels in Patients with Non-Alcoholic Fatty Liver Disease with or without Type 2 Diabetes Mellitus: A Pilot Study. *J. Gastrointest. Liver Dis.* **2017**, *26*, 261–268. [CrossRef]
150. Gurel, H.; Genç, H.; Celebi, G.; Sertoglu, E.; Cicek, A.F.; Kayadibi, H.; Ercin, C.N.; Dogru, T. Plasma pentraxin-3 is associated with endothelial dysfunction in non-alcoholic fatty liver disease. *Eur. Rev. Med Pharmacol. Sci.* **2016**, *20*, 4305–4312.
151. Marušić, M.; Paić, M.; Knobloch, M.; Pršo, A.-M.L. NAFLD, Insulin Resistance, and Diabetes Mellitus Type 2. *Can. J. Gastroenterol. Hepatol.* **2021**, *2021*, 6613827. [CrossRef]
152. Sanduzzi Zamparelli, M.; Compare, D.; Coccoli, P.; Rocco, A.; Nardone, O.M.; Marrone, G.; Gasbarrini, A.; Grieco, A.; Nardone, G.; Miele, L. The Metabolic Role of Gut Microbiota in the Development of Nonalcoholic Fatty Liver Disease and Cardiovascular Disease. *Int. J. Mol. Sci.* **2016**, *17*, 1225. [CrossRef]
153. Zhang, Y.; Xu, J.; Wang, X.; Ren, X.; Liu, Y. Changes of intestinal bacterial microbiota in coronary heart disease complicated with nonalcoholic fatty liver disease. *BMC Genom.* **2019**, *20*, 862. [CrossRef]
154. Karlsson, F.H.; Fåk, F.; Nookaew, I.; Tremaroli, V.; Fagerberg, B.; Petranovic, D.; Bäckhed, F.; Nielsen, J. Symptomatic atherosclerosis is associated with an altered gut metagenome. *Nat. Commun.* **2012**, *3*, 1245. [CrossRef]
155. Nguyen, C.C.; Duboc, D.; Rainteau, D.; Sokol, H.; Humbert, L.; Seksik, P.; Bellino, A.; Abdoul, H.; Bouazza, N.; Treluyer, J.-M.; et al. Circulating bile acids concentration is predictive of coronary artery disease in human. *Sci. Rep.* **2021**, *11*, 22661. [CrossRef]
156. Wang, Z.; Tang, W.H.W.; Buffa, J.A.; Fu, X.; Britt, E.B.; Koeth, R.A.; Levison, B.; Fan, Y.; Wu, Y.; Hazen, S.L. Prognostic value of choline and betaine depends on intestinal microbiota-generated metabolite trimethylamine-N-oxide. *Eur. Hear. J.* **2014**, *35*, 904–910. [CrossRef]
157. Roberts, A.B.; Gu, X.; Buffa, J.A.; Hurd, A.G.; Wang, Z.; Zhu, W.; Gupta, N.; Skye, S.M.; Cody, D.B.; Levison, B.S.; et al. Development of a gut microbe–targeted nonlethal therapeutic to inhibit thrombosis potential. *Nat. Med.* **2018**, *24*, 1407–1417. [CrossRef]
158. Lu, F.; Zheng, K.I.; Rios, R.S.; Targher, G.; Byrne, C.D.; Zheng, M. Global epidemiology of lean non-alcoholic fatty liver disease: A systematic review and meta-analysis. *J. Gastroenterol. Hepatol.* **2020**, *35*, 2041–2050. [CrossRef]
159. Zou, B.; Yeo, Y.H.; Nguyen, V.H.; Cheung, R.; Ingelsson, E. Prevalence, characteristics and mortality outcomes of obese, nonobese and lean NAFLD in the United States, 1999–2016. *J. Intern. Med.* **2020**, *288*, 139–151. [CrossRef]
160. Aneni, E.C.; Bittencourt, M.S.; Teng, C.; Cainzos-Achirica, M.; Osondu, C.U.; Soliman, A.; Al-Mallah, M.; Buddoff, M.; Parise, E.R.; Santos, R.D.; et al. The risk of cardiometabolic disorders in lean non-alcoholic fatty liver disease: A longitudinal study. *Am. J. Prev. Cardiol.* **2020**, *4*, 100097. [CrossRef]
161. Semmler, G.; Wernly, S.; Bachmayer, S.; Wernly, B.; Schwenoha, L.; Huber-Schönauer, U.; Stickel, F.; Niederseer, D.; Aigner, E.; Datz, C. Nonalcoholic Fatty Liver Disease in Lean Subjects: Associations with Metabolic Dysregulation and Cardiovascular Risk—A Single-Center Cross-Sectional Study. *Clin. Transl. Gastroenterol.* **2021**, *12*, e00326. [CrossRef]
162. Golabi, P.; Paik, J.; Fukui, N.; Locklear, C.T.; de Avilla, L.; Younossi, Z.M. Patients with Lean Nonalcoholic Fatty Liver Disease Are Metabolically Abnormal and Have a Higher Risk for Mortality. *Clin. Diabetes* **2019**, *37*, 65–72. [CrossRef]
163. Bisaccia, G.; Ricci, F.; Mantini, C.; Tana, C.; Romani, G.L.; Schiavone, C.; Gallina, S. Nonalcoholic fatty liver disease and cardiovascular disease phenotypes. *SAGE Open Med.* **2020**, *8*. [CrossRef]
164. Kumar, R.; Mohan, S. Non-alcoholic Fatty Liver Disease in Lean Subjects: Characteristics and Implications. *J. Clin. Transl. Hepatol.* **2017**, *5*, 216–223. [CrossRef]
165. Lee, C.-H.; Han, K.-D.; Kim, D.H.; Kwak, M.-S. The Repeatedly Elevated Fatty Liver Index Is Associated with Increased Mortality: A Population-Based Cohort Study. *Front. Endocrinol.* **2021**, *12*, 638615. [CrossRef]
166. Yoshitaka, H.; Hamaguchi, M.; Kojima, T.; Fukuda, T.; Ohbora, A.; Fukui, M. Nonoverweight nonalcoholic fatty liver disease and incident cardiovascular disease. *Medicine* **2017**, *96*, e6712. [CrossRef]
167. Honda, Y.; Yoneda, M.; Kessoku, T.; Ogawa, Y.; Tomeno, W.; Imajo, K.; Mawatari, H.; Fujita, K.; Hyogo, H.; Ueno, T.; et al. Characteristics of non-obese non-alcoholic fatty liver disease: Effect of genetic and environmental factors. *Hepatol. Res.* **2016**, *46*, 1011–1018. [CrossRef]
168. Kuchay, M.S.; Martínez-Montoro, J.I.; Choudhary, N.S.; Fernández-García, J.C.; Ramos-Molina, B. Non-Alcoholic Fatty Liver Disease in Lean and Non-Obese Individuals: Current and Future Challenges. *Biomedicines* **2021**, *9*, 1346. [CrossRef]

169. Tang, A.; Ng, C.H.; Phang, P.H.; Chan, K.E.; Chin, Y.H.; Fu, C.E.; Zeng, R.W.; Xiao, J.; Tan, D.J.H.; Quek, J.; et al. Comparative Burden of Metabolic Dysfunction in Lean NAFLD vs. Non-Lean NAFLD—A Systematic Review and Meta-Analysis. *Clin. Gastroenterol. Hepatol.* **2022**. [CrossRef]
170. Kim, Y.; Han, E.; Lee, J.S.; Lee, H.W.; Kim, B.K.; Kim, M.K.; Kim, H.S.; Park, J.Y.; Kim, D.Y.; Ahn, S.H.; et al. Cardiovascular Risk Is Elevated in Lean Subjects with Nonalcoholic Fatty Liver Disease. *Gut Liver* **2022**, *16*, 290–299. [CrossRef]
171. Van Wagner, L.B.; Khan, S.S.; Ning, H.; Siddique, J.; Lewis, C.E.; Carr, J.J.; Vos, M.B.; Speliotes, E.; Terrault, N.A.; Rinella, M.E.; et al. Body mass index trajectories in young adulthood predict non-alcoholic fatty liver disease in middle age: The CARDIA cohort study. *Liver Int.* **2017**, *38*, 706–714. [CrossRef] [PubMed]
172. Sung, K.C.; Ryan, M.C.; Wilson, A.M. The severity of nonalcoholic fatty liver disease is associated with increased cardiovascular risk in a large cohort of non-obese Asian subjects. *Atherosclerosis* **2009**, *203*, 581–586. [CrossRef] [PubMed]

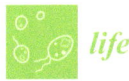

Review

Ischemic Heart Disease and Liver Cirrhosis: Adding Insult to Injury

Irina Gîrleanu [1,2], Anca Trifan [1,2,*], Laura Huiban [1,2], Cristina Muzîca [1,2], Oana Cristina Petrea [1,2], Ana Maria Sîngeap [1,2], Camelia Cojocariu [1,2], Stefan Chiriac [1,2], Tudor Cuciureanu [1,2], Irina Iuliana Costache [1,3] and Carol Stanciu [1,2]

1. Depatment of Internal Medicine, Grigore T. Popa University of Medicine and Pharmacy, 700115 Iaşi, Romania; irina.girleanu@umfiasi.ro (I.G.); huiban.laura@yahoo.com (L.H.); lungu.christina@yahoo.com (C.M.); oana.stoica@umfiasi.ro (O.C.P.); anamaria.singeap@umfiasi.ro (A.M.S.); camelia.cojocariu@umfiasi.ro (C.C.); stefan.chiriac@umfiasi.ro (S.C.); tudor.cuciureanu@umfiasi.ro (T.C.); ii.costache@yahoo.com (I.I.C.); stanciucarol@yahoo.com (C.S.)
2. Institute of Gastroenterology and Hepatology, Saint Spiridon University Hospital, 700115 Iaşi, Romania
3. Cardiology Department, Saint Spiridon University Hospital, 700115 Iaşi, Romania
* Correspondence: anca.trifan@umfiasi.ro; Tel.: +40-762278575

Abstract: The link between heart and liver cirrhosis was recognized decades ago, although much data regarding atherosclerosis and ischemic heart disease are still missing. Ischemic heart disease or coronary artery disease (CAD) and liver cirrhosis could be associated with characteristic epidemiological and pathophysiological features. This connection determines increased rates of morbidity and all-cause mortality in patients with liver cirrhosis. In the era of a metabolic syndrome and non-alcoholic fatty liver disease pandemic, primary prevention and early diagnosis of coronary artery disease could improve the prognosis of liver cirrhosis patients. This review outlines a summary of the literature regarding prevalence, risk assessment and medical and interventional treatment options in this particular population. A collaborative heart–liver team-based approach is imperative for critical management decisions for patients with CAD and liver cirrhosis.

Keywords: coronary artery disease; liver cirrhosis; prevalence; liver transplantation; treatment

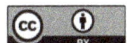

1. Introduction

The association between liver cirrhosis (LC) and coronary artery disease (CAD) is still a matter of debate. Common pathogenic mechanisms (vascular inflammation, endothelial dysfunction, a procoagulant status) were recognized to be associated with developing atherosclerotic lesions in patients with LC [1,2].

Cardiovascular abnormalities in LC are associated with a hyperdynamic hemodynamic status, increased resting cardiac output and a blunt ventricular response to stress, systolic and diastolic dysfunction, along with electrophysiological abnormalities such as QT interval prolongation [3].

LC is characterized by increased oxidative stress and low nitric oxide (NO) bioavailability, resulting in vascular inflammation, endothelial dysfunction, increased production of tissue factor, hypercoagulability and vascular smooth-muscle proliferation [4,5]. To all these factors, hepatic inflammation is superimposed by overexpression of TNF-α, angiotensin II, toll-like receptor 4 and nuclear factor-kB [1]. Portal hypertension is associated with increased gut permeability and pathogen-associated molecular patterns (PAMPs) that activate an immune response and increase systemic inflammation [6]. Alcohol consumption, infections or drug-induced liver injury cause hepatocyte apoptosis with secondary release of damage-associated molecular patterns (DAMPs) with an important role in increasing the inflammatory response [7] (Figure 1).

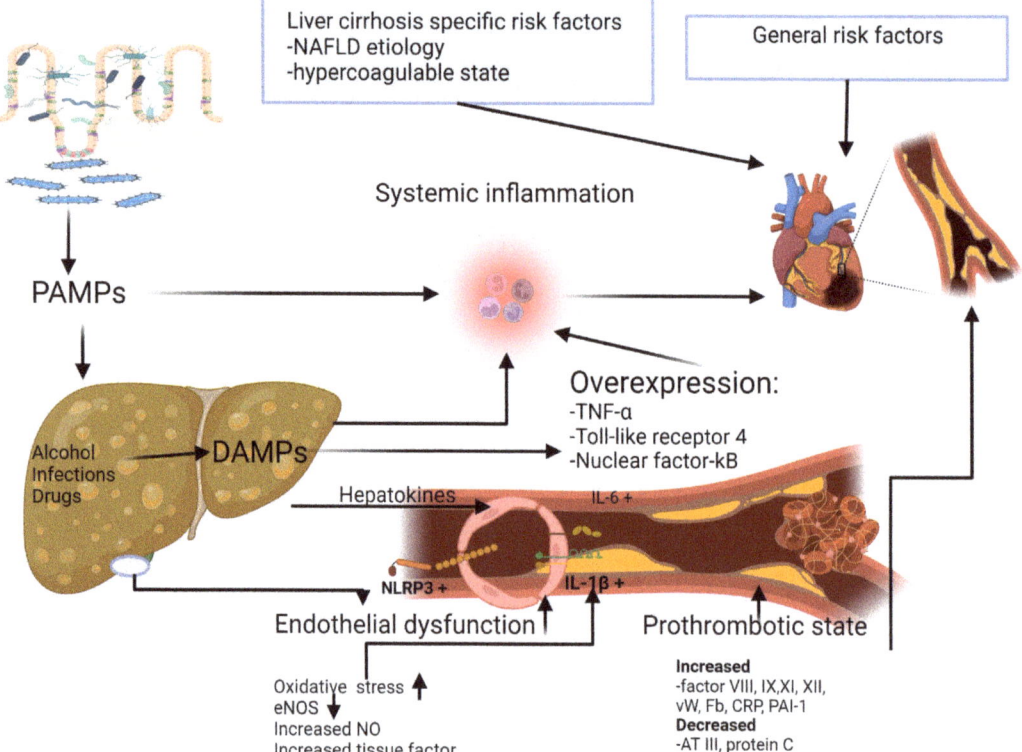

Figure 1. Pathogenic mechanism of coronary artery disease in patients with liver cirrhosis. Abbreviations: ATIII: antithrombin III; CRP: C-reactive protein; DAMPs: damaged-associated molecular patterns; Fb: fibrinogen; IL-6: Interleukin 6; IL-1β: Interleukin 1β; NAFLD: non-alcoholic fatty liver disease; NLRP3: pyrin domain-containing protein 3; NO: nitric oxide; PAI-1: plasminogen activator inhibitor-1; PAMPs: pathogen-associated molecular patterns; TNF-α: tumoral necrosis factor; vW: von Willebrand factor.

Moreover, in cirrhotic patients, increased peripheral NO induces splanchnic vasodilatation. Pulse wave velocity measurement is a non-invasive tool for early atherosclerosis diagnosis in direct relation with intima–media thickness in patients with LC despite splanchnic vasodilatation, confirming the fact that these patients are not protected from developing atherosclerotic lesions [8].

Moreover, the effects of diabetes mellitus (DM), smoking, hypertension and metabolic syndrome, in different combinations, accelerate the process of atherosclerosis and can lead to acute coronary syndrome [3–5]. Additionally, current evidence suggests that when the traditional risk factors for CAD are controlled, cirrhotic patients remain at high risk of developing CAD [8].

Data published until now have demonstrated that the development of CAD in patients with LC is associated with poor prognosis and high mortality rates, including patients on the liver transplant waiting list [9]. Even if important progress has been made regarding early diagnosis and treatment of CAD in recent years, for the cirrhotic population there are still many unresolved issues. Therefore, we aimed to present an updated comprehensive narrative review on the currently available literature related to CAD and LC.

2. Epidemiology, Clinical Presentation and Risk Factors

2.1. Epidemiology of CAD in LC

A few decades ago, patients with liver cirrhosis were considered protected from developing ischemic cardiac disease due to low blood pressure and low cholesterol levels [9]. However, recent data confirmed that CAD are more prevalent in the cirrhotic population compared with the general population [9,10]. The prevalence of CAD in patients with liver cirrhosis ranges between 1.7 and 27%, and it is associated with high mortality during and after liver transplantation surgery [11–15]. This wide prevalence variation could be explained by the heterogeneity of the cirrhotic population and the different diagnostic methods and CAD definitions. Autopsy studies have demonstrated that patients with LC have less advanced atherosclerotic plaques and a low prevalence of calcified atherosclerotic lesions versus non-cirrhotic patients. However, these data were not confirmed by imagistic studies, which confirmed that atherosclerotic lesions are at least as frequent in patients with LC as in general population, especially in the decompensated stage of the disease. The majority of studies evaluating the CAD epidemiology in LC differed in their control groups, and they involved different patients in terms of cardiac symptoms and history, all these representing an important statistical bias. The knowledge of the prevalence of CAD, particularly of anatomically confirmed CAD, in patients with LC is very limited.

Some studies demonstrated a low prevalence (1.7%) of CAD in patients with LC, despite the presence of atherosclerotic risk factors [16,17]. It has to be mentioned that these were retrospective studies, the prevalence of CAD was a secondary endpoint, and most of the patients were diagnosed with viral decompensated LC. When the diagnosis was based on computed tomography (CT) angiography, the prevalence of asymptomatic obstructive CAD was 7.9% in a cohort including the majority of the patients with decompensated viral B liver cirrhosis [10], as was demonstrated in more than 1000 Korean patients.

A recent meta-analysis including almost 13,000 patients concluded that the prevalence of obstructive CAD among patient with LC reached 12.6%, similar to the general population [11], and the highest prevalence was reported in cirrhotic patients aged over 50 years old. Moreover, non-obstructive CAD has a higher rate in patients with LC [10] compared with the general population (30.6% vs. 23.4%, $p = 0.001$). Additionally, acute coronary syndrome had a prevalence of 2.81 per 1000 person-years and was higher in patients with ascites.

2.2. Clinical Presentation of CAD in LC

Liver cirrhosis, especially in the decompensated stage, modifies the clinical presentation and the main symptoms of CAD. Asymptomatic presentation is very common in a cirrhotic population; only a minority of patients with LC who presented with acute myocardial infarction declared chest pain, compared with 72% of patients from the general population [10], although these patients were more likely to report dyspnea, a frequent symptom in patients with LC and grade 2 or 3 ascites or pleural effusion. Thus, recognition of ischemia in patients with LC requires a high index of suspicion, considering that CAD presents atypically in this special population. Chronic coronary syndrome is more difficult to diagnose in patients with LC as most of them have no angina symptoms. They can present with dyspnea on exertion or effort thoracic anterior pain. Differential diagnosis should be made with porto-pulmonary hypertension, pulmonary embolism, pleural effusion, or pneumonia. Special attention should be paid in cirrhotic patients admitted with hemorrhagic complications, as anemia could precipitate an acute coronary syndrome and routine administration of vasoactive treatment—terlipressin—could aggravate the cardiac ischemia.

2.3. Risk Factors for CAD in LC

Risk assessments are based on population studies and are scant for cirrhotic populations. The major cardiovascular risk factors for CAD development are: arterial hypertension, diabetes mellitus, hyperlipidemia, obesity and smoking. DM, obesity and smoking were recognized as risk factors for CAD in patients with LC, along with age greater than 50 years old [9,13,18]. Diabetes mellitus is one of the main cardiovascular risk factors identified in patients with LC, the majority of the patients having asymptomatic CAD, although it is not clearly established if DM is more atherogenic in patients with LC [19]. It was demonstrated that LC is associated with low LDL levels, elevated HDL-2 cholesterol concentration and decreased adipokine levels, all of these leading to improvement in the lipid profile [14].

Controversies still remain regarding the role of heavy alcohol consumption on CAD prevalence. Patel et al. [12] demonstrated that patients diagnosed with alcoholic LC have a lower incidence of severe CAD. In contrast to these findings, Gologorsky et al. [18] found no evidence for low prevalence of CAD in patients with alcoholic LC in a large cohort including almost 6000 patients.

Patients with LC exemplify the shortcomings of risk assessments from population data, as they have low values of arterial pressure and low cholesterol levels. However, these risk prediction scores can be improved by adding liver-specific variables, such as model for end-stage liver disease (MELD) score, albumin level or liver fibrosis scores. Additional risk markers may help to refine atherosclerotic cardiovascular risk (Table 1). Coronary artery calcification can be used to identify CAD in patients with LC, especially in those evaluated for LT. Similarly, the prognostic significance of various circulating biomarkers, such as C-reactive protein, cardiac troponine and natriuretic peptides, may be lower than that of the general population.

Table 1. Risk factors for cardiovascular events.

General Population Risk Factors
Age > 50 years
Smoking
Dyslipidemia
Arterial hypertension
Diabetes mellitus
Family history of CAD
Personal history of CAD
Male sex
Liver-Cirrhosis-Specific Risk Factors
NAFLD etiology
Decompensated liver cirrhosis and hypercoagulable state

Such novel serum biomarkers as matrix metalloprotease 9 (MMP-9), pentraxin 3, growth differentiation factor 15 (GDF-15), myeloperoxidase (MPO) and monocyte chemoattractant protein 1 (MCP-1) were proved to increase CAD risk prediction in a general population. MMP-9, GDF-15 and pentraxin 3 are involved in liver angiogenesis and fibrogenesis processes [20–23]. MCP-1 is an inflammatory chemokine associated with LC complications and mortality [24]. None of these novel biomarkers were evaluated for cardiovascular risk prediction in patients with LC. It has to be mentioned that finding such a biomarker in cirrhotic patients will be very difficult as most of them reflect fibrosis or inflammation, processes highly active in liver cirrhosis. However, it remains to be determined whether incorporation of these biomarkers into clinical care will affect the outcomes of cirrhotic patients. Entirely new cardiovascular risk models may be needed in LC, as the Framingham risk equation underestimates risk in liver transplant recipients, and modified equations have not been validated in this population.

Recently, new data were published regarding the role of non-invasive liver fibrosis scores and the risk of CAD. These studies suggest that advanced liver fibrosis is associated with a high risk of CAD [25], and moreover with complexity of CAD [26].

3. Etiology of Liver Cirrhosis and CAD

There is a well-known association between *non-alcoholic fatty liver disease* (NAFLD) and an increased risk of ischemic heart disease up to 21.6% compared with 5.0% in patients with LC from other etiologies [27]. It was demonstrated that patients with NAFLD have more complex CAD with more than three vessels involved [13], due to poor coronary collateral development [28,29] and vulnerable plaque formation [30,31]. Even if NAFLD has common risk factors with metabolic syndrome and the prevalence of CAD is higher in patients with NAFLD, data regarding the frequency of CAD in patients with NAFLD and advanced fibrosis, including LC, are scant. In a large cohort including patients diagnosed with CAD by coronary angiography and evaluated for NAFLD and fibrosis using transient elastography and controlled attenuation parameters, obstructive CAD was less frequent in patients with advanced liver fibrosis compared with mild fibrosis [32]. Recent studies demonstrated that advanced fibrosis secondary to NAFLD diagnosed by noninvasive serum markers is associated with CAD [2]. On the contrary, in an Asian population, NAFLD liver cirrhosis was associated with a reduced prevalence of CAD [33], confirming that there are still some puzzle pieces missing in the larger picture of NAFLD and CAD. It has not yet been demonstrated that NAFLD is an independent risk factor for CAD in patients with LC; therefore, there are no clear recommendations for screening for CAD in all patients with NAFLD liver cirrhosis.

Data regarding the influence of *chronic alcohol consumption* on the risk of CAD are contradictory. Patel et al. demonstrated in 420 cirrhotic patients that those with alcoholic cirrhosis had a lower incidence of CAD compared with other etiologies of LC [12]. It has to be mentioned that the patients diagnosed with NAFLD liver cirrhosis were not excluded from the control group. Considering that NAFLD is an independent risk factor for CAD in patients with or without metabolic syndrome, the results of this study should be carefully interpreted [34].

The association between *viral hepatitis* and cardiovascular risk is also controversial. Previous studies reported no relationship between viral hepatitis and carotid arteries' atherosclerotic lesions; moreover, viral C etiology was negatively correlated with CAD [35]. On the contrary, recent data have confirmed that virus C infection is associated with increased systemic inflammation, insulin resistance, dyslipidemia, carotidian atherosclerotic plaques and hepatic steatosis [36–38]. Additionally, chronic hepatitis C was associated with an increased epicardial fat thickness and carotid intima–media thickness, and these were in direct positive correlation with LC severity assessed by Child–Pugh class and CAD [39]. Moreover, the antiviral treatment with virological response was associated with a significant decrease in atherosclerotic plaques [40,41].

Primary biliary cholangitis (PBC) is characterized by an increased level of cholesterol and chronic systemic inflammation, although the influence of this dyslipidemia in the development of CAD was not clearly demonstrated. In a retrospective cohort study, Wang et al. demonstrated that only arterial hypertension is an independent risk factor for CAD in patients with PBC [42]. Three large cohorts, including more than 500 cirrhotic patients, also found no relationship between PBC and the CAD development [43–45]. On the contrary, a meta-analysis of only four observational studies demonstrated that PBC is associated with a 57% excess risk of CAD, and patients with PBC should receive appropriate treatment for traditional cardiovascular risk factors [46].

4. CAD Diagnosis in Liver Cirrhosis

Considering the difficulties in the diagnosis of CAD in patients with LC, testing is recommended in symptomatic patients and in those asymptomatic needing moderate to high-risk surgery, including LT. Identifying the best method for CAD screening in patients with LC is still a matter of debate.

For the diagnosis of acute coronary syndrome, the current guidelines should be followed [47], and myocardial infarction should be diagnosed according to the fourth Universal definition of Myocardial Infarction [48]. In patients with chest pain, high-sensitivity troponin level is a reliable marker for myocardial ischemia [49]. In patients with LC, troponin levels may be elevated secondary to myocardial damage unrelated to obstructive CAD [50] as a marker of cirrhotic cardiomyopathy [51] in direct relation to liver disease severity [52].

Coronary angiography is the gold standard for CAD diagnosis, although, in patients with LC, it is an invasive procedure with a high risk of complications: bleeding, acute kidney injury, etc. Considering these particularities, non-invasive tests are preferred for CAD diagnosis in symptomatic cirrhotic patients or those who are asymptomatic undergoing moderate or high-risk surgery. In the setting of acute coronary syndrome, coronary angiography is the main method of diagnosis including in patients with LC.

Cirrhotic patients with acute coronary syndrome, symptomatic angina refractory to treatment, and those asymptomatic with a non-invasive positive test have indication for *invasive coronary angiography* [53]. Transradial access for cardiac catheterization in patients with LC is safer compared with femoral access [54].

The European Association for the Study of the Liver recommends electrocardiogram and echocardiography in all LT candidates, and in those older than 50 years, with multiple cardiovascular risk factors an exercise stress test is indicated [55], although, the American Association for the Study of Liver Disease indicates that all LT candidates should benefit from a stress echocardiography regardless of the cardiovascular risk factors [56].

The non-invasive methods for CAD diagnosis are represented by stress echocardiography, computer tomography angiography (CTA) with coronary artery calcium (CAC) scoring, cardiac magnetic resonance imaging (MRI), and single-photon emission computed tomography myocardial perfusion imaging [19].

Exercise testing is difficult to perform in patients with LC as it is frequently limited by the inability of these patients to reach diagnostic workloads. Second, exercise testing in LC is often limited by baseline electrocardiographic abnormalities and non-selective beta-blocker treatment. Third, most existing data were derived from studies of transplant candidates—the extent to which these data can be generalize to all cirrhotic patients is uncertain. It has to be mentioned that in patients with LC, ST segment depression can be identified in exercise tests in the absence of significant CAD, as a consequence of a disorder in the myocardial microcirculation secondary to vasodilatation mediated by the coronary artery endothelium [57]. Even if exercise stress testing is possible in a patient with LC, its sensitivity is poor.

Other stress tests with other drugs (such as terlipressin and metariminol) or volume challenge still remain in the research field. *Dobutamine stress echocardiography* (DSE) has low specificity as it is less likely for the patients to achieve target heart rate during pharmacological-induced stress [58]. In a study including more than 600 cirrhotic patients, DSE had a sensitivity of only 19% and a specificity of 90% (negative predictive value 84%, positive predictive value 29%) [59]. This low sensitivity is explained by chronotropic incompetence in patients with LC.

Coronary artery calcium score and *computed tomography angiography* (CTA) may offer significant advantages over functional imaging modalities in the setting of liver cirrhosis. In a cohort of 147 cirrhotic patients on the liver transplant waiting list, more than half of the patients were classified in the moderate/high-risk group [17]. Compared with other methods of CAD evaluation in asymptomatic patients with LC, CAC is the most useful predictor and can be used in order to triage the patients for angiography [60]. This method has a 47% positive predictive value and 99% negative predictive value for diagnosis of significant coronary stenosis [19]. CAC measures the total amount of coronary calcium, expressed as Agatston units. Values greater than 400 are associated with severe CAD [61], and could identify the high-risk cirrhotic patients that could benefit from coronary angiography.

In patients with suspected CAD, *stress cardiac MRI* could be used for assessing the myocardial scars and to identify the viable myocardial tissue for revascularization procedures (62). Stress cardiac MRI has a sensitivity of 77% and a specificity of 88% for detecting significant coronary stenosis (>50%) [62], although data for patients with LC are scant, and due to its high cost the utility in routine evaluation of patients with LC is limited.

The diagnosis of CAD in patients with LC could be challenging due to overlapping symptoms, especially in decompensated LC. Chest pain could be secondary to pleuritis, pneumonia or musculoskeletal disorders. Dyspnea has many causes in cirrhotic patients: pleural effusion, porto-pulmonary hypertension, hepato-pulmonary syndrome, pneumonia, pulmonary embolism, large ascites, or anemia. Moreover, in decompensated LC patients, low-voltage ECG is frequent, and transthoracic echocardiographic examination is limited by pleural and pericardial effusion and ascending diaphragms. All these elements concur to a delayed diagnosis of CAD in patients with LC. A diagnostic algorithm is presented in Figure 2.

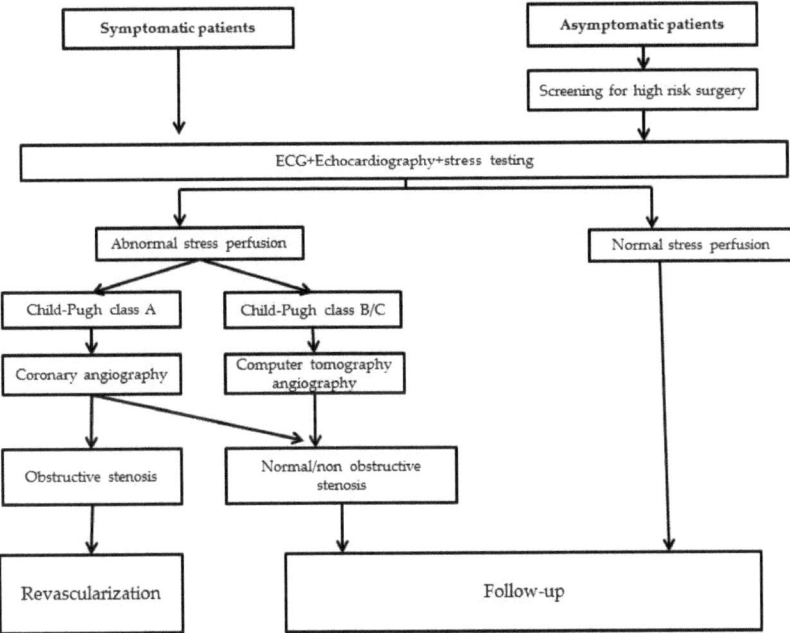

Figure 2. Diagnostic algorithm for patients with LC and CAD.

5. Management of CAD in Liver Cirrhosis

5.1. Medical Therapy

The management of CAD in patients with LC is an unsolved issue. Although medical therapy is the cornerstone of CAD treatment, challenges exist in cirrhotic patients, considering the fact that patients with LC are under-represented in clinical trials and, as such, the evidence to support recommendations is limited.

Such *nonselective beta-blockers* as propranolol and carvedilol are frequently used in patients with LC for variceal bleeding prophylaxis due to their ability to decrease the portal vein pressure. In patients with CAD, the benefit of beta-blocker treatment is well established. It reduces myocardial ischemia and is effective in improving symptoms. Peuter et al. demonstrated that nonselective beta-blockers are associated with a higher decrease in mortality and vascular events than cardioselective receptor blockade in patients with CAD [63], although data evaluating the role of beta-blockers on CAD treatment in patients with LC are lacking.

Antiplatelet therapy could be indicated in patients with LC. Even if this therapy is associated with an increased risk of non-portal hypertension-related bleeding, there is no influence on mortality [64]. Moreover, most of the cirrhotic patients have thrombocytopenia, although platelet aggregation is normal, as was demonstrated by aggregometry methods [65]. Caution should be taken in patients with platelets less than $50 \times 10^9/L$, as those are prone to develop bleeding complications [66].

$P2Y_{12}$ inhibitors block adenosine-diphosphate-induced platelet aggregation. Clopidogrel is an irreversible inhibitor of $P2Y_{12}$ and the liver is the site of metabolic activation. In patients with compensated LC, Child–Pugh class A, clopidogrel pharmacokinetics is not influenced [67]. No dose adjustments should be made in these patients. However, in patients with decompensated LC, Child–Pugh class C, clopidogrel treatment inhibited platelet function with no increase in the side effect rate [65]. Prasugrel, another $P2Y_{12}$ inhibitor, could represent a safe treatment in patients with LC, as it has no hepatic metabolism. Ticagrelor, a reversible $P2Y_{12}$ inhibitor, has hepatic metabolism, being activated by the liver cytochrome 3A4 enzyme, and it is not recommended in patients with Child–Pugh class C liver cirrhosis [68]. Even if Ticagrelor is a reversible $P2Y_{12}$ inhibitor, the effect on platelet inhibition is prolonged with increasing LC severity [69]. Considering all these data, in cirrhotic patients presenting with acute coronary syndrome undergoing PCI, prasugrel is the preferred drug, as it has benefits over ticagrelor in lowering mortality and stroke rate without increasing the bleeding risk [70]. There are only case reports regarding the use of glycoprotein IIb/IIIa inhibitors in patients with LC. Eptifibatide was associated with severe thrombocytopenia in patients with LC and an increased hemorrhagic risk [71].

Dual antiplatelet therapy is recommended for at least 12 months after drug-eluting stent insertion and for at least 1 month after a bare metal stent placement [53]. There are few studies evaluating the safety of this drug association in patients with LC. In a retrospective cohort comparing cirrhotic patients with or without aspirin and clopidogrel treatment, it was demonstrated that the rate of fatal variceal bleedings was very high (12.5% vs. 6.3%), concluding that this treatment should be restricted to cirrhotic patients without esophageal varices [72]. In studies performed on national databases, it was demonstrated that patients with LC have a higher risk of bleeding complications on dual antiplatelet therapy and an individualized approach is needed [73,74].

Controversy surrounds the use of *statins* in patients with LC. There are no studies confirming the benefits of statins in reducing major vascular events in patients with LC, although statins can be safely used in patients with LC. Recent studies confirmed that simvastatin decreases portal pressure [75]. Statins decrease hepatic fibrogenesis, protect from severe LC complications and even reduce the risk of hepatocellular carcinoma by improving inflammation and endothelial dysfunction [76]. It has to be mentioned that data on the use of statins in patients with decompensated LC are very limited.

Considering all these data, Patel et al. [77] demonstrated that aspirin and statins are safe in patients with decompensated LC, and they can be indicated in patients that associate CAD when the benefits of cardiovascular events prevention outweigh the risk of bleeding.

Angiotensin-converting-enzyme inhibitors, angiotensin receptor blockers and direct renin inhibitors are not indicated in patients with LC, especially in those in the decompensated stage of the disease due to the effect of vasodilation, which could increase the risk of acute kidney injury, including hepato-renal syndrome, and predispose the patients to electrolyte disturbances. The risk of hyperkaliemia in cirrhotic patients treated with angiotensin-converting-enzyme inhibitors is 5.2-fold greater compared with that in patients without LC [78]. Patients with LC have an activation of the renin angiotensin aldosterone system and of the sympathetic nervous system, causing renal vasoconstriction, impaired renal perfusion and increased sodium retention. ACE inhibitors or sartans can further impair glomerular filtration due to reduced filtration pressure, and they should be used very cautiously in cirrhotic patients [79,80].

There is little information regarding the safety of other specific anti-angina drugs in patients with LC. *Ranolazine* inhibits the late inward sodium current and has as a side effect QTc prolongation. *Ivabradine* combined with carvedilol could improve diastolic dysfunction and survival rate in patients with liver cirrhosis [81], also decreasing the complication rate.

5.2. Revascularization in Patients with CAD and Liver Cirrhosis

The choice of medical therapy alone or revascularization with percutaneous coronary intervention (PCI) or coronary artery bypass (CABG) in symptomatic patients with LC is controversial. In the absence of dedicated clinical trials, cirrhotic patients presenting with acute coronary syndrome undergo the same invasive approach as those with normal liver function.

5.2.1. Percutaneous Coronary Intervention (PCI)

Mortality in patients with CAD and LC is higher than in the general population, although the mortality rates in this population increased during the last decade [82]. PCI in patients with LC is associated with a higher procedural risk, more frequent cardiogenic shock, cardiac arrest and gastrointestinal bleeding, along with a fivefold increase in acute kidney injury compared with general population [83].

An observational study evaluating the trends in PCI evolution between 2003 and 2016 in the United States demonstrated that PCI procedures increased among patients with LC and decreased in the general population [84]. These data could be explained by a better recognition of cardiovascular risk factors associated with early primary prevention methods in the general population and the lack of a precise cardiovascular score in a cirrhotic population. In this large study, the rates of vascular complications were similar in patients undergoing PCI with or without LC.

A large retrospective cohort including cirrhotic patients with LC undergoing PCI demonstrated that this procedure is associated with high bleeding complications and mortality, especially when bare-metal stents were used [83] compared with the general population. It has to be mentioned that 77% of the procedures were performed on an emergent basis and 15% for ST-elevation myocardial infarction presentation, although no data on the severity of LC were reported. Bare-metal stents were preferred in patients with LC due to short-term use of dual antiplatelet drugs, even if the data published did not demonstrate that bare-metal stents are associated with a lower bleeding risk compared with drug-eluting stents in patients with LC [83]. The long-term safety of PCI in patients with LC was evaluated in a cohort of 64 patients, with the majority in the decompensated stage of the disease. This study demonstrated that cirrhotic patients with CAD diagnosed before liver transplantation have an increased mortality after liver transplantation, as these patients have multivessel CAD. One of the largest retrospective studies including patients with LC and CAD demonstrated that the mortality rate was not influenced by PCI, suggesting that the revascularization in this special population is not associated with a major benefit in terms of survival, given the high rate of liver-related mortality [85]. Long-term data confirmed that the rate of adverse events is higher in cirrhotic patients undergoing PCI for CAD, with a severe bleeding rate of 23% and a rate of acute kidney rate of 26%, of whom patients needed renal replacement, compared with the group that received medical treatment. After 1 year of follow-up, the bleeding rate was doubled in patients receiving PCI [86]. The highest rate of complication was demonstrated in patients with decompensated LC, especially ascites and hepatic encephalopathy, before PCI [86]. Considering all these data, the benefit of this procedure, in asymptomatic decompensated cirrhotic patients is still under debate.

There had been a preferential approach of opting for bare-metal stents in patients with LC because of earlier endothelialization and shorter dual antiplatelet therapy duration times. However, several clinical trials have demonstrated the superior outcomes of second-generation drug-eluting stents compared with bare-metal stents [84–88]. Coronary artery stenting and dual antiplatelet therapy are associated with an independent risk of variceal bleeding [72]. A history of variceal bleeding or presence of varies confers an increased risk, and primary or secondary prophylaxis of variceal bleeding is recommended prior to cardiac catheterization.

5.2.2. Coronary Artery Bypass Grafting (CABG)

Cardiac surgery is associated with a high risk of mortality in patients with LC, with an overall mortality rate of 26% [89]. Two large patients cohorts, the first one including patients evaluated between 1998 and 2004, and the second including those admitted between 2002 and 2014, demonstrated that coronary artery bypass grafting procedures in patients with LC increased, although they were associated with high morbidity and mortality risk [90,91], even if there is a tendency of decreasing in recent years. Bleeding complications were the most frequent cause of morbidity after CABG, and the patients in a decompensated stage of LC were more prone to developing complications and had increased in-hospital mortality. The highest mortality risk was identified in patients with a MELD score > 13 and Child–Pugh class more than 7 points [92], and these patients could benefit more from other methods for revascularization.

The waiting period from CABG and liver transplantation is still a matter of debate. This period varies between 12 h and 18 days. The data published until now conclude that we have to wait more than 10 days until liver transplantation after CABG [92].

Considering all these data, LC should be included in the cardiac risk assessment, and the decisions regarding the best option should include a combination between liver disease severity models and cardiovascular risk scores.

6. Conclusions

Patients with LC and CAD constitute a high-risk population with unique epidemiological and pathophysiological characteristics. Considering the increasing prevalence of alcoholism, diabetes mellitus, obesity and non-alcoholic liver disease, the prevalence of CAD in LC is on the rise. The prognostic factors for CAD in LC have to be clarified, along with the role of screening programs and the most appropriate interventional preventive regimes. Data on the safety and efficacy of antiplatelet drugs in LC patients are derived from observational studies in patients with mild to moderate LC, and we have limited data on patients with severe decompensated LC. Additionally, the optimal duration of dual antiplatelet therapy in LC patients still remains to be defined, along with the limits of interventional revascularization procedures.

The data we have until now confirm the utility of non-invasive methods of diagnosis, and the safety and efficacy of beta-blockers and statins in patients with LC and CAD. Treatment decisions should balance between bleeding and thrombotic risks, especially in Child–Pugh C cirrhotic patients.

A heart–liver team-based approach is imperative for critical management decisions for this patient population, and clinicians need to become more aware of the association between CAD and LC.

Author Contributions: All authors participated in discussion; writing and/or editing of the manuscript have made significant contribution to this manuscript. All authors have read and approved the final version submitted. All authors accept responsibility for its content. I.G., A.T., C.C., I.I.C. and C.S. participated in the design of the review, collected the data, analysis and interpretation, manuscript preparation and revision, and drafted the manuscript, and approved the final version of the final draft submitted. L.H., C.S., C.M., S.C., T.C., I.G., A.M.S. and O.C.P. performed acquisition of data and contributed to the drafting of the manuscript. I.G., C.C., A.M.S., O.C.P., C.S., I.I.C. and T.C. contributed to the interpretation of data. All authors have read and agreed to the published version of the manuscript.

Funding: This research received no external funding.

Institutional Review Board Statement: The study did not require ethical approval.

Conflicts of Interest: The authors declare no conflict of interest.

References

1. Vairappan, B. Endothelial dysfunction in cirrhosis: Role of inflammation and oxidative stress. *World. J. Hepatol.* **2015**, *7*, 443. [CrossRef] [PubMed]
2. Chen, L.; Jing, X.; Wu, C.; Zeng, Y.; Xie, Y.; Wang, M.; Chen, W.; Hu, X.; Zhou, Y.; Cai, X. Nonalcoholic Fatty Liver Disease-Associated Liver Fibrosis Is Linked with the Severity of Coronary Artery Disease Mediated by Systemic Inflammation. *Dis. Markers* **2021**, *2021*, 6591784. [CrossRef] [PubMed]
3. El Hadi, H.; Di Vincenzo, A.; Vettor, R.; Rossato, M. Relationship between Heart Disease and Liver Disease: A Two-Way Street. *Cells* **2020**, *9*, 567. [CrossRef] [PubMed]
4. Lluch, P.; Torondel, B.; Medina, P.; Segarra, G.; del Olmo, J.A.; Serra, M.A.; Rodrigo, J.M. Plasma concentrations of nitric oxide and asymmetric dimethylarginine in human alcoholic cirrhosis. *J. Hepatol.* **2004**, *41*, 55–59. [CrossRef] [PubMed]
5. Deanfield, J.E.; Halcox, J.P.; Rabelink, T.J. Endothelial Function and Dysfunction: Testing and Clinical Relevance. *Circulation* **2007**, *115*, 1285–1295. [CrossRef]
6. Albillos, A.; Lario, M.; Álvarez-Mon, M. Cirrhosis-associated immune dysfunction: Distinctive features and clinical relevance. *J. Hepatol.* **2014**, *61*, 1385–1396. [CrossRef]
7. Han, H.; Desert, R.; Das, S.; Song, Z.; Athavale, D.; Ge, X.; Nieto, N. Danger signals in liver injury and restoration of homeostasis. *J. Hepatol.* **2020**, *73*, 933–951. [CrossRef]
8. Noda, Y.; Nomura, M.; Nakaya, Y.; Bando, S.; Ito, S. Relationship between liver cirrhosis and arteriosclerosis: Evaluation by pulse wave velocity, carotid arterial echotomography and autonomic nervous activity. *Geriatr. Gerontol. Int.* **2007**, *7*, 72–79. [CrossRef]
9. Lin, S.-Y.; Lin, C.-L.; Lin, C.-C.; Wang, I.-K.; Hsu, W.-H.; Kao, C.-H. Risk of acute coronary syndrome and peripheral arterial disease in chronic liver disease and cirrhosis: A nationwide population-based study. *Atherosclerosis* **2018**, *270*, 154–159. [CrossRef]
10. An, J.; Shim, J.H.; Kim, S.-O.; Lee, D.; Kim, K.M.; Lim, Y.-S.; Lee, H.C.; Chung, Y.-H.; Lee, Y.S. Prevalence and Prediction of Coronary Artery Disease in Patients With Liver Cirrhosis: A Registry-Based Matched Case–Control Study. *Circulation* **2014**, *130*, 1353–1362. [CrossRef]
11. Zhao, J.; Li, N.; Sun, H.; Liang, C. The prevalence of coronary artery disease in patients with liver cirrhosis: A meta-analysis. *Eur. J. Gastroenterol. Hepatol.* **2018**, *30*, 118–120. [CrossRef]
12. Patel, S.; Kiefer, T.L.; Ahmed, A.; Ali, Z.A.; Tremmel, J.A.; Lee, D.P.; Yeung, A.C.; Fearon, W.F. Comparison of the frequency of coronary artery disease in alcohol-related versus non-alcohol-related endstage liver disease. *Am. J. Cardiol.* **2011**, *108*, 1552–1555. [CrossRef]
13. Patel, S.S.; Nabi, E.; Guzman, L.; Abbate, A.; Bhati, C.; Stravitz, R.T.; Reichman, T.; Matherly, S.C.; Driscoll, C.; Lee, H.; et al. Coronary artery disease in decompensated patients undergoing liver transplantation evaluation. *Liver Transpl.* **2018**, *24*, 333–342. [CrossRef]
14. Patel, S.; Siddiqui, M.B.; Chandrakumaran, A.; Rodriguez, V.A.; Faridnia, M.; Roman, J.H.; Zhang, E.; Patrone, M.V.; Kakiyama, G.; Walker, C.; et al. Progression to Cirrhosis Leads to Improvement in Atherogenic Milieu. *Dig. Dis. Sci.* **2021**, *66*, 263–272. [CrossRef]
15. Azarbal, B.; Poommipanit, P.; Arbit, B.; Hage, A.; Patel, J.; Kittleson, M.; Kar, S.; Kaldas, F.M.; Busuttil, R.W. Feasibility and safety of percutaneous coronary intervention in patients with end-stage liver disease referred for liver transplantation. *Liver Transpl.* **2011**, *17*, 809–813. [CrossRef]
16. Berzigotti, A.; Bonfiglioli, A.; Muscari, A.; Bianchi, G.; LiBassi, S.; Bernardi, M.; Zoli, M. Reduced prevalence of ischemic events and abnormal supraortic flow patterns in patients with liver cirrhosis. *Liver Int.* **2005**, *25*, 331–336. [CrossRef]
17. McAvoy, N.C.; Kochar, N.; McKillop, G.; Newby, D.E.; Hayes, P.C. Prevalence of coronary artery calcification in patients undergoing assessment for orthotopic liver transplantation: Prevalence of Coronary Artery Calcification. *Liver Transpl.* **2008**, *14*, 1725–1731. [CrossRef]
18. Gologorsky, E.; Pretto, E.A.; Fukazawa, K. Coronary artery disease and its risk factors in patients presenting for liver transplantation. *J. Clin. Anesth.* **2013**, *25*, 618–623. [CrossRef]
19. Dangl, M.; Eisenberg, T.; Grant, J.K.; Vincent, L.; Colombo, R.; Sancassani, R.; Braghiroli, J.; Martin, P.; Vianna, R.; Nicolau-Raducu, R.; et al. A comprehensive review of coronary artery disease in patients with end-stage liver disease. *Transpl. Rev.* **2022**, *36*, 100709. [CrossRef]
20. Tamarappoo, B.K.; Lin, A.; Commandeur, F.; McElhinney, P.A.; Cadet, S.; Goeller, M.; Razipour, A.; Chen, X.; Gransar, H.; Cantu, S.; et al. Machine learning integration of circulating and imaging biomarkers for explainable patient-specific prediction of cardiac events: A prospective study. *Atherosclerosis* **2021**, *318*, 76–82. [CrossRef]
21. Huang, H.; Ho, H.; Chang, C.; Chuang, C.; Pun, C.K.; Lee, F.; Huang, Y.; Hou, M.; Hsu, S. Matrix metalloproteinase-9 inhibition or deletion attenuates portal hypertension in rodents. *J. Cell. Mol. Med.* **2021**, *25*, 10073–10087. [CrossRef]
22. Balin, Ş.Ö.; Çabalak, M.; Tartar, A.S.; Kazancı, Ü.; Telo, S.; Demirdağ, K.; Akbulut, A. Pentraxin-3: A Novel Marker for Indicating Liver Fibrosis in Chronic Hepatitis B Patients? *Turk. J. Gastroenterol.* **2021**, *32*, 581–585. [CrossRef]
23. Prystupa, A.; Kiciński, P.; Luchowska-Kocot, D.; Błażewicz, A.; Niedziałek, J.; Mizerski, G.; Jojczuk, M.; Ochal, A.; Sak, J.J.; Załuska, W. Association between Serum Selenium Concentrations and Levels of Proinflammatory and Profibrotic Cytokines-Interleukin-6 and Growth Differentiation Factor-15, in Patients with Alcoholic Liver Cirrhosis. *Int. J. Environ. Res. Public Health* **2017**, *14*, E437. [CrossRef]

24. Graupera, I.; Solà, E.; Fabrellas, N.; Moreira, R.; Solé, C.; Huelin, P.; de la Prada, G.; Pose, E.; Ariza, X.; Risso, A.; et al. Urine Monocyte Chemoattractant Protein-1 Is an Independent Predictive Factor of Hospital Readmission and Survival in Cirrhosis. *PLoS ONE* **2016**, *11*, e0157371. [CrossRef]
25. Lee, J.; Kim, H.S.; Cho, Y.K.; Kim, E.H.; Lee, M.J.; Bae, I.Y.; Jung, C.H.; Park, J.-Y.; Kim, H.-K.; Lee, W.J. Association between noninvasive assessment of liver fibrosis and coronary artery calcification progression in patients with nonalcoholic fatty liver disease. *Sci. Rep.* **2020**, *10*, 18323. [CrossRef]
26. Turan, Y. The Nonalcoholic Fatty Liver Disease Fibrosis Score Is Related to Epicardial Fat Thickness and Complexity of Coronary Artery Disease. *Angiology* **2020**, *71*, 77–82. [CrossRef]
27. Kadayifci, A.; Tan, V.; Ursell, P.C.; Merriman, R.B.; Bass, N.M. Clinical and pathologic risk factors for atherosclerosis in cirrhosis: A comparison between NASH-related cirrhosis and cirrhosis due to other aetiologies. *J. Hepatol.* **2008**, *49*, 595–599. [CrossRef]
28. Arslan, U.; Kocaoğlu, İ.; Balcı, M.; Duyuler, S.; Korkmaz, A. The association between impaired collateral circulation and non-alcoholic fatty liver in patients with severe coronary artery disease. *J. Cardiol.* **2012**, *60*, 210–214. [CrossRef]
29. Ağaç, M.T.; Korkmaz, L.; Çavuşoğlu, G.; Karadeniz, A.G.; Ağaç, S.; Bektas, H.; Erkan, H.; Varol, M.O.; Vatan, M.B.; Acar, Z.; et al. Association Between Nonalcoholic Fatty Liver Disease and Coronary Artery Disease Complexity in Patients With Acute Coronary Syndrome: A Pilot Study. *Angiology* **2013**, *64*, 604–608. [CrossRef]
30. Akabame, S.; Hamaguchi, M.; Tomiyasu, K.; Tanaka, M.; Kobayashi-Takenaka, Y.; Nakano, K.; Oda, Y.; Yoshikawa, T. Evaluation of Vulnerable Coronary Plaques and Non-Alcoholic Fatty Liver Disease (NAFLD) by 64-Detector Multislice Computed Tomography (MSCT). *Circ. J.* **2007**, *72*, 618–625. [CrossRef]
31. Kazankov, K.; Munk, K.; Øvrehus, K.A.; Jensen, J.M.; Siggaard, C.B.; Grønbaek, H.; Nørgaard, B.L.; Vilstrup, H. High burden of coronary atherosclerosis in patients with cirrhosis. *Eur. J. Clin. Invest.* **2017**, *47*, 565–573. [CrossRef] [PubMed]
32. Friedrich-Rust, M.; Schoelzel, F.; Maier, S.; Seeger, F.; Rey, J.; Fichtlscherer, S.; Herrmann, E.; Zeuzem, S.; Bojunga, J. Severity of coronary artery disease is associated with non-alcoholic fatty liver dis-ease: A single-blinded prospective mono-center study. *PLoS ONE* **2017**, *12*, e0186720. [CrossRef] [PubMed]
33. Tsai, M.-C.; Yang, T.-W.; Wang, C.-C.; Wang, Y.-T.; Sung, W.-W.; Tseng, M.-H.; Lin, C.-C. Favorable clinical outcome of nonalcoholic liver cirrhosis patients with coronary artery disease: A population-based study. *World J. Gastroenterol.* **2018**, *24*, 3547–3555. [CrossRef] [PubMed]
34. Chiriac, S.; Stanciu, C.; Girleanu, I.; Cojocariu, C.; Sfarti, C.; Singeap, A.-M.; Cuciureanu, T.; Huiban, L.; Muzica, C.M.; Zenovia, S.; et al. Nonalcoholic Fatty Liver Disease and Cardiovascular Diseases: The Heart of the Matter. *Can. J. Gastroenterol. Hepatol.* **2021**, *2021*, 6696857. [CrossRef]
35. Kalaitzakis, E.; Rosengren, A.; Skommevik, T.; Björnsson, E. Coronary Artery Disease in Patients with Liver Cirrhosis. *Dig. Dis. Sci.* **2010**, *55*, 467–475. [CrossRef]
36. Alyan, O.; Kacmaz, F.; Ozdemir, O.; Deveci, B.; Astan, R.; Celebi, A.S.; Ilkay, E. Hepatitis C Infection is Associated With Increased Coronary Artery Atherosclerosis Defined by Modified Reardon Severity Score System. *Circ. J.* **2008**, *72*, 1960–1965. [CrossRef]
37. Dai, C.-Y.; Yeh, M.-L.; Huang, C.-F.; Hou, C.-H.; Hsieh, M.-Y.; Huang, J.-F.; Lin, I.-L.; Lin, Z.-Y.; Chen, S.-C.; Wang, L.-Y.; et al. Chronic hepatitis C infection is associated with insulin resistance and lipid profiles: Metabolic profiles and hepatitis C. *J. Gastroenterol. Hepatol.* **2015**, *30*, 879–884. [CrossRef]
38. Cuciureanu, T.; Chiriac, S.; Chiorescu, M.; Gîrleanu, I.; Trifan, A. Chronic hepatitis C virus infection: A new modifiable cardio-metabolic risk factor? *Clujul Med.* **2017**, *90*, 251–255. [CrossRef]
39. Barakat, A.A.E.-K.; Nasr, F.M.; Metwaly, A.A.; Morsy, S.; Eldamarawy, M. Atherosclerosis in chronic hepatitis C virus patients with and without liver cirrhosis. *Egypt. Heart J.* **2017**, *69*, 139–147. [CrossRef]
40. Adinolfi, L.E.; Rinaldi, L.; Nevola, R. Chronic hepatitis C, atherosclerosis and cardiovascular disease: What impact of direct-acting antiviral treatments? *World J. Gastroenterol.* **2018**, *24*, 4617–4621. [CrossRef]
41. Roguljic, H.; Nincevic, V.; Bojanic, K.; Kuna, L.; Smolic, R.; Vcev, A.; Primorac, D.; Vceva, A.; Wu, G.Y.; Smolic, M. Impact of DAA Treatment on Cardiovascular Disease Risk in Chronic HCV Infection: An Update. *Front. Pharmacol.* **2021**, *12*, 678546. [CrossRef]
42. Wang, C.; Zhao, P.; Liu, W. Risk of incident coronary artery disease in patients with primary biliary cirrhosis. *Int. J. Clin. Exp. Med.* **2014**, *7*, 2921–2924.
43. Longo, M.; Crosignani, A.; Battezzati, P.M.; Giussani, S.C.; Invernizzi, P.; Zuin, M.; Podda, M. Hyperlipidaemic state and cardiovascular risk in primary biliary cirrhosis. *Gut* **2002**, *51*, 265–269. [CrossRef]
44. Crippin, J.S.; Lindor, K.D.; Jorgensen, R.; Kottke, B.A.; Harrison, J.M.; Murtaugh, P.A.; Dickson, E.R. Hypercholesterolemia and atherosclerosis in primary biliary cirrhosis: What is the risk? *Hepatology* **1992**, *15*, 858–862. [CrossRef]
45. Van Dam, G.M.; Gips, C.H. Primary Biliary Cirrhosis in The Netherlands: An Analysis of Associated Diseases, Cardiovascular Risk, and Malignancies on the Basis of Mortality Figures. *Scand. J. Gastroenterol.* **1997**, *32*, 77–83. [CrossRef]
46. Ungprasert, P.; Wijarnpreecha, K.; Ahuja, W.; Spanuchart, I.; Thongprayoon, C. Coronary artery disease in primary biliary cirrhosis: A systematic review and meta-analysis of observational studies: CAD in PBC. *Hepatol. Res.* **2015**, *45*, 1055–1061. [CrossRef]
47. Collet, J.-P.; Thiele, H.; Barbato, E.; Barthélémy, O.; Bauersachs, J.; Bhatt, D.L.; Dendale, P.; Dorobantu, M.; Edvardsen, T.; Folliguet, T.; et al. 2020 ESC Guidelines for the management of acute coronary syndromes in patients presenting without persistent ST-segment elevation. *Eur. Heart J.* **2021**, *42*, 1289–1367. [CrossRef]

48. Thygesen, K.; Alpert, J.S.; Jaffe, A.S.; Chaitman, B.R.; Bax, J.J.; Morrow, D.A.; White, H.D.; ESC Scientific Document Group. Fourth universal definition of myocardial infarction (2018). *Eur. Heart J.* **2019**, *40*, 237–269. [CrossRef]
49. Thygesen, K.; Mair, J.; Katus, H.; Plebani, M.; Venge, P.; Collinson, P.; Lindahl, B.; Giannitsis, E.; Hasin, Y.; Galvani, M.; et al. Recommendations for the use of cardiac troponin measurement in acute cardiac care. *Eur. Heart J.* **2010**, *31*, 2197–2204. [CrossRef]
50. Shimoni, Z.; Arbuzov, R.; Froom, P. Troponin Testing in Patients Without Chest Pain or Electrocardiographic Ischemic Changes. *Am. J. Med.* **2017**, *130*, 1205–1210. [CrossRef]
51. Zardi, E.M.; Abbate, A.; Zardi, D.M.; Dobrina, A.; Margiotta, D.; Van Tassel, B.W.; Afeltra, A.; Sanyal, A.J. Cirrhotic Cardiomyopathy. *J. Am. Coll. Cardiol.* **2010**, *56*, 539–549. [CrossRef]
52. Wiese, S.; Mortensen, C.; Gøtze, J.P.; Christensen, E.; Andersen, O.; Bendtsen, F.; Møller, S. Cardiac and proinflammatory markers predict prognosis in cirrhosis. *Liver Int.* **2014**, *34*, e19–e30. [CrossRef]
53. Lawton, J.S.; Tamis-Holland, J.E.; Bangalore, S.; Bates, E.R.; Beckie, T.M.; Bischoff, J.M.; Bittl, J.A.; Cohen, M.G.; DiMaio, J.M.; Don, C.W.; et al. 2021 ACC/AHA/SCAI Guideline for Coronary Artery Revascularization. *J. Am. Coll. Cardiol.* **2022**, *79*, e21–e129. [CrossRef]
54. Jacobs, E.; Singh, V.; Damluji, A.; Shah, N.R.; Warsch, J.L.; Ghanta, R.; Martin, P.; Alfonso, C.E.; Martinez, C.A.; Moscucci, M.; et al. Safety of transradial cardiac catheterization in patients with end-stage liver disease: Transradial catheterization in ESLD. *Catheter. Cardiovasc. Interv.* **2014**, *83*, 360–366. [CrossRef]
55. European Association for the Study of the Liver. EASL Clinical Practice Guidelines: Liver transplantation. *J. Hepatol.* **2016**, *64*, 433–485. [CrossRef]
56. Martin, P.; DiMartini, A.; Feng, S.; Brown, R.; Fallon, M. Evaluation for liver transplantation in adults: 2013 practice guideline. *Hepatology* **2014**, *59*, 1144–1165. [CrossRef]
57. Mori, T.; Nomura, M.; Hori, A.; Kondo, N.; Bando, S.; Ito, S. Mechanism of ST segment depression during exercise tests in patients with liver cirrhosis. *J. Med. Invest.* **2007**, *54*, 109–115. [CrossRef]
58. Harinstein, M.E.; Flaherty, J.D.; Ansari, A.H.; Robin, J.; Davidson, C.J.; Rossi, J.S.; Flamm, S.L.; Blei, A.T.; Bonow, R.O.; Abecassis, M.; et al. Predictive Value of Dobutamine Stress Echocardiography for Coronary Artery Disease Detection in Liver Transplant Candidates: DSE in Liver Transplant Candidates. *Am. J. Transplant.* **2008**, *8*, 1523–1528. [CrossRef]
59. Doytchinova, A.T.; Feigenbaum, T.D.; Pondicherry-Harish, R.C.; Sepanski, P.; Green-Hess, D.; Feigenbaum, H.; Sawada, S.G. Diagnostic Performance of Dobutamine Stress Echocardiography in End-Stage Liver Disease. *JACC Cardiovasc. Imaging* **2019**, *12*, 2115–2122. [CrossRef]
60. Bhatti, S.; Lizaola-Mayo, B.; Al-Shoha, M.; Garcia-Saenz-de-Sicilia, M.; Habash, F.; Ayoub, K.; Karr, M.; Ahmed, Z.; Borja-Cacho, D.; Duarte-Rojo, A. Use of Computed Tomography Coronary Calcium Score for Coronary Artery Disease Risk Stratification During Liver Transplant Evaluation. *J. Clin. Exp. Hepatol.* **2022**, *12*, 319–328. [CrossRef]
61. Greenland, P.; Blaha, M.J.; Budoff, M.J.; Erbel, R.; Watson, K.E. Coronary Calcium Score and Cardiovascular Risk. *J. Am. Coll. Cardiol.* **2018**, *72*, 434–447. [CrossRef] [PubMed]
62. Klem, I.; Heitner, J.F.; Shah, D.J.; Sketch, M.H.; Behar, V.; Weinsaft, J.; Cawley, P.; Parker, M.; Elliott, M.; Judd, R.M.; et al. Improved Detection of Coronary Artery Disease by Stress Perfusion Cardiovascular Magnetic Resonance With the Use of Delayed Enhancement Infarction Imaging. *J. Am. Coll. Cardiol.* **2006**, *47*, 1630–1638. [CrossRef] [PubMed]
63. de Peuter, O.R.; Lussana, F.; Peters, R.J.G.; Büller, H.R.; Kamphuisen, P.W. A systematic review of selective and non-selective beta blockers for prevention of vascular events in patients with acute coronary syndrome or heart failure. *Neth. J. Med.* **2009**, *67*, 284–294. [PubMed]
64. Krill, T.; Brown, G.; Weideman, R.A.; Cipher, D.J.; Spechler, S.J.; Brilakis, E.; Feagins, L.A. Patients with cirrhosis who have coronary artery disease treated with cardiac stents have high rates of gastrointestinal bleeding, but no increased mortality. *Aliment. Pharmacol. Ther.* **2017**, *46*, 183–192. [CrossRef]
65. Trankle, C.R.; Vo, C.; Martin, E.; Puckett, L.; Siddiqui, M.S.; Brophy, D.F.; Stravitz, T.; Guzman, L.A. Clopidogrel Responsiveness in Patients With Decompensated Cirrhosis of the Liver Undergoing Pre-Transplant PCI. *JACC Cardiovasc. Interv.* **2020**, *13*, 661–663. [CrossRef]
66. Ostojic, Z.; Ostojic, A.; Bulum, J.; Mrzljak, A. Safety and efficacy of dual antiplatelet therapy after percutaneous coronary interventions in patients with end-stage liver disease. *World J. Cardiol.* **2021**, *13*, 599–607. [CrossRef]
67. Slugg, P.H.; Much, D.R.; Smith, W.B.; Vargas, R.; Nichola, P.; Necciari, J. Cirrhosis Does Not Affect the Pharmacokinetics and Pharmacodynamics of Clopidogrel. *J. Clin. Pharmacol.* **2000**, *40*, 396–401. [CrossRef]
68. Wood, A.; Eghtesad, B.; Menon, K.V.N.; Fares, M.; Tong, M.Z.-Y.; Sharma, V.; Lopez, R.; Modaresi Esfeh, J. Safety and Outcomes of Combined Liver Transplantation and Cardiac Surgery in Cirrhosis. *Ann. Thorac. Surg.* **2021**, *111*, 62–68. [CrossRef]
69. Zhang, M.; You, X.; Ke, M.; Jiao, Z.; Wu, H.; Huang, P.; Lin, C. Prediction of Ticagrelor and its Active Metabolite in Liver Cirrhosis Populations Using a Physiologically Based Pharmacokinetic Model Involving Pharmacodynamics. *J. Pharm. Sci.* **2019**, *108*, 2781–2790. [CrossRef]
70. Ahmed, T.; Grigorian, A.Y.; Messerli, A.W. Management of Acute Coronary Syndrome in Patients with Liver Cirrhosis. *Am. J. Cardiovasc. Drugs* **2022**, *22*, 55–67. [CrossRef]
71. Weinreich, M.; Mendoza, D.; Pettei, T.; Grayver, E. Eptifibatide and Cirrhosis: Rethinking GPIIb-IIIa Inhibitors for Acute Coronary Syndrome in the Setting of Liver Dysfunction. *Cardiol. Res.* **2014**, *5*, 191–194. [CrossRef]

72. Russo, M.W.; Pierson, J.; Narang, T.; Montegudo, A.; Eskind, L.; Gulati, S. Coronary Artery Stents and Antiplatelet Therapy in Patients With Cirrhosis. *J. Clin. Gastroenterol.* **2012**, *46*, 339–344. [CrossRef]
73. Lu, D.Y.; Saybolt, M.D.; Kiss, D.H.; Matthai, W.H.; Forde, K.A.; Giri, J.; Wilensky, R.L. One-Year Outcomes of Percutaneous Coronary Intervention in Patients with End-Stage Liver Disease. *Clin. Med. Insights Cardiol.* **2020**, *14*, 117954682090149. [CrossRef]
74. Wu, V.C.-C.; Chen, S.-W.; Chou, A.-H.; Ting, P.-C.; Chang, C.-H.; Wu, M.; Hsieh, M.-J.; Wang, C.-Y.; Chang, S.-H.; Lin, M.-S.; et al. Dual antiplatelet therapy in patients with cirrhosis and acute myocardial infarction—A 13-year nationwide cohort study. *PLoS ONE* **2019**, *14*, e0223380. [CrossRef]
75. Muñoz, A.E.; Pollarsky, F.D.; Marino, M.; Cartier, M.; Vázquez, H.; Salgado, P.; Romero, G. Addition of statins to the standard treatment in patients with cirrhosis: Safety and efficacy. *World J. Gastroenterol.* **2021**, *27*, 4639–4652. [CrossRef]
76. VanWagner, L.B. Aspirin and statin use for management of atherosclerotic cardiovascular disease in liver transplant candidates: Are we missing the mark?: Vanwagner. *Liver Transpl.* **2018**, *24*, 865–867. [CrossRef]
77. Patel, S.S.; Guzman, L.A.; Lin, F.-P.; Pence, T.; Reichman, T.; John, B.; Celi, F.S.; Liptrap, E.; Bhati, C.; Siddiqui, M.S. Utilization of aspirin and statin in management of coronary artery disease in patients with cirrhosis undergoing liver transplant evaluation. *Liver Transpl.* **2018**, *24*, 872–880. [CrossRef]
78. Amir, O.; Hassan, Y.; Sarriff, A.; Awaisu, A.; Abd. Aziz, N.; Ismail, O. Incidence of risk factors for developing hyperkalemia when using ACE inhibitors in cardiovascular diseases. *Pharm. World Sci.* **2009**, *31*, 387–393. [CrossRef]
79. Sacerdoti, D.; Bolognesi, M.; Merkel, C.; Angeli, P.; Gatta, A. Renal vasoconstriction in cirrhosis evaluated by duplex Doppler ultrasonography. *Hepatology* **1993**, *17*, 219–224.
80. Franz, C.C.; Egger, S.; Born, C.; Rätz Bravo, A.E.; Krähenbühl, S. Potential drug-drug interactions and adverse drug reactions in patients with liver cirrhosis. *Eur. J. Clin. Pharmacol.* **2012**, *68*, 179–188. [CrossRef]
81. Premkumar, M.; Rangegowda, D.; Vyas, T.; Khumuckham, J.S.; Shasthry, S.M.; Thomas, S.S.; Goyal, R.; Kumar, G.; Sarin, S.K. Carvedilol Combined With Ivabradine Improves Left Ventricular Diastolic Dysfunction, Clinical Progression, and Survival in Cirrhosis. *J. Clin. Gastroenterol.* **2020**, *54*, 561–568. [CrossRef] [PubMed]
82. Abougergi, M.S.; Karagozian, R.; Grace, N.D.; Saltzman, J.R.; Qamar, A.A. ST Elevation Myocardial Infarction Mortality Among Patients With Liver Cirrhosis: A Nationwide Analysis Across a Decade. *J. Clin. Gastroenterol.* **2015**, *49*, 778–783. [CrossRef] [PubMed]
83. Singh, V.; Patel, N.J.; Rodriguez, A.P.; Shantha, G.; Arora, S.; Deshmukh, A.; Cohen, M.G.; Grines, C.; De Marchena, E.; Badheka, A.; et al. Percutaneous Coronary Intervention in Patients With End-Stage Liver Disease. *Am. J. Cardiol.* **2016**, *117*, 1729–1734. [CrossRef] [PubMed]
84. Alqahtani, F.; Balla, S.; AlHajji, M.; Chaudhary, F.; Albeiruti, R.; Kawsara, A.; Alkhouli, M. Temporal trends in the utilization and outcomes of percutaneous coronary interventions in patients with liver cirrhosis. *Catheter. Cardiovasc. Interv.* **2020**, *96*, 802–810. [CrossRef]
85. Marui, A.; Kimura, T.; Tanaka, S.; Miwa, S.; Yamazaki, K.; Minakata, K.; Nakata, T.; Ikeda, T.; Furukawa, Y.; Kita, T.; et al. Coronary Revascularization in Patients With Liver Cirrhosis. *Ann. Thorac. Surg.* **2011**, *91*, 1393–1399. [CrossRef]
86. Lu, D.Y.; Steitieh, D.; Feldman, D.N.; Cheung, J.W.; Wong, S.C.; Halazun, H.; Halazun, K.J.; Amin, N.; Wang, J.; Chae, J.; et al. Impact Of Cirrhosis On 90-Day Outcomes After Percutaneous Coronary Intervention (from A Nationwide Database). *Am. J. Cardiol.* **2020**, *125*, 1295–1304. [CrossRef]
87. Urban, P.; Meredith, I.T.; Abizaid, A.; Pocock, S.J.; Carrié, D.; Naber, C.; Lipiecki, J.; Richardt, G.; Iñiguez, A.; Brunel, P.; et al. Polymer-free Drug-Coated Coronary Stents in Patients at High Bleeding Risk. *N. Engl. J. Med.* **2015**, *373*, 2038–2047. [CrossRef]
88. Windecker, S.; Latib, A.; Kedhi, E.; Kirtane, A.J.; Kandzari, D.E.; Mehran, R.; Price, M.J.; Abizaid, A.; Simon, D.I.; Worthley, S.G.; et al. Polymer-based or Polymer-free Stents in Patients at High Bleeding Risk. *N. Engl. J. Med.* **2020**, *382*, 1208–1218. [CrossRef]
89. Murata, M.; Kato, T.S.; Kuwaki, K.; Yamamoto, T.; Dohi, S.; Amano, A. Preoperative hepatic dysfunction could predict postoperative mortality and morbidity in patients undergoing cardiac surgery: Utilization of the MELD scoring system. *Int. J. Cardiol.* **2016**, *203*, 682–689. [CrossRef]
90. Shaheen, A.A.M.; Kaplan, G.G.; Hubbard, J.N.; Myers, R.P. Morbidity and mortality following coronary artery bypass graft surgery in patients with cirrhosis: A population-based study. *Liver Int.* **2009**, *29*, 1141–1151. [CrossRef]
91. Singh, V.; Savani, G.T.; Mendirichaga, R.; Jonnalagadda, A.K.; Cohen, M.G.; Palacios, I.F. Frequency of Complications Including Death from Coronary Artery Bypass Grafting in Patients With Hepatic Cirrhosis. *Am. J. Cardiol.* **2018**, *122*, 1853–1861. [CrossRef]
92. Imam, A.; Karatas, C.; Mecit, N.; Kalayoglu, M.; Kanmaz, T. Cardiac Intervention Before Liver Transplantation. *Transplant. Proc.* **2021**, *53*, 1622–1625. [CrossRef]

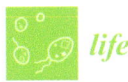

Review

Ischemic Heart Disease in Patients with Inflammatory Bowel Disease: Risk Factors, Mechanisms and Prevention

Alina Ecaterina Jucan [1], Otilia Gavrilescu [1,2,*], Mihaela Dranga [1,2,*], Iolanda Valentina Popa [2], Bogdan Mircea Mihai [1,2], Cristina Cijevschi Prelipcean [1] and Cătălina Mihai [1,2]

1. Saint Spiridon County Hospital, 700111 Iași, Romania; alina-ecaterina_ghiata@email.umfiasi.ro (A.E.J.); bogdan.mihai@umfiasi.ro (B.M.M.); cristina.cijevschi.prelipcean@umfiasi.ro (C.C.P.); catalina.mihai@umfiasi.ro (C.M.)
2. Faculty of Medicine, University of Medicine and Pharmacy "Grigore T. Popa", 700115 Iași, Romania; iolanda-valentina.g.popa@umfiasi.ro
* Correspondence: otilianedelciuc@yahoo.com (O.G.); mihaela_dra@yahoo.com (M.D.)

Abstract: According to new research, a possible association between inflammatory bowel disease (IBD) and an increased risk of ischemic heart disease (IHD) has been demonstrated, but this concern is still debatable. The purpose of this review is to investigate the link between IHD and IBD, as well as identify further research pathways that could help develop clinical recommendations for the management of IHD risk in IBD patients. There is growing evidence suggesting that disruption of the intestinal mucosal barrier in IBD is associated with the translocation of microbial lipopolysaccharides (LPS) and other endotoxins into the bloodstream, which might induce a pro-inflammatory cytokines response that can lead to endothelial dysfunction, atherosclerosis and acute cardiovascular events. Therefore, it is considered that the long-term inflammation process in IBD patients, similar to other chronic inflammatory diseases, may lead to IHD risk. The main cardiovascular risk factors, including high blood pressure, dyslipidemia, diabetes, smoking, and obesity, should be checked in all patients with IBD, and followed by strategies to reduce and manage early aggression. IBD activity is an important risk factor for acute cardiovascular events, and optimizing therapy for IBD patients should be followed as recommended in current guidelines, especially during active flares. Large long-term prospective studies, new biomarkers and scores are warranted to an optimal management of IHD risk in IBD patients.

Keywords: ischemic heart disease; inflammatory bowel disease; ulcerative colitis; Crohn's disease; myocardial infarction; coronary artery disease; cardiovascular risk

Citation: Jucan, A.E.; Gavrilescu, O.; Dranga, M.; Popa, I.V.; Mihai, B.M.; Prelipcean, C.C.; Mihai, C. Ischemic Heart Disease in Patients with Inflammatory Bowel Disease: Risk Factors, Mechanisms and Prevention. *Life* **2022**, *12*, 1113. https://doi.org/10.3390/life12081113

Academic Editor: Gary Tse

Received: 21 June 2022
Accepted: 22 July 2022
Published: 24 July 2022

Publisher's Note: MDPI stays neutral with regard to jurisdictional claims in published maps and institutional affiliations.

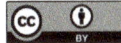

Copyright: © 2022 by the authors. Licensee MDPI, Basel, Switzerland. This article is an open access article distributed under the terms and conditions of the Creative Commons Attribution (CC BY) license (https://creativecommons.org/licenses/by/4.0/).

1. Introduction

Inflammatory bowel disease (IBD) is a recurrent chronic idiopathic inflammatory condition of the gastrointestinal tract. Various factors are involved in its pathogenesis, such as genetic susceptibility of the host, and it is precipitated by environmental and microbial factors [1]. Crohn's disease (CD) and ulcerative colitis (UC) are the two major subtypes of IBD, characterized by chronic intestinal inflammation, while the most common symptoms are frequent diarrhea, often with blood and pus in stools, abdominal pain and cramping, fever, and weight loss [2]. The incidence and prevalence of IBD are still increasing worldwide. Besides of the primary gastrointestinal complications of IBD, a broad-spectrum of extra-intestinal manifestations and IBD complications have also been outlined due to persistent long-standing systemic inflammation [3,4].

Ischemic heart disease (IHD) is still the leading global cause of death worldwide; there is a general concern to identify patients with cardiovascular risk factors and to apply preventive measures.

The state of chronic inflammation in IBD can lead to endothelial dysfunction and platelet aggregation, confers a higher risk of developing atherosclerosis and coronary artery disease, and thereby a higher risk of acute coronary events [5]. IBD patients have been highlighted to have increased carotid intimal thickness, endothelial dysfunction, and wall stiffness, mainly due to increased circulating inflammatory cytokines [6]. Thus, several inflammatory mediators such as high C-reactive protein (CRP) and circulating pro-inflammatory markers such as tumor necrosis factor-α (TNF-α) and interleukins are involved in the pathogenesis of IBD, as well as in atherosclerosis [7]. Increased levels of the aforementioned inflammatory mediators, together with increased burden of traditional cardiovascular disease risk factors in the general population, drive a higher risk of IHD in IBD patients [8].

Multiple large population studies have shown a positive association between IBD and IHD, especially in women and young patients, but the data remain controversial [9,10]. The pathophysiological mechanisms behind this phenomenon have not been fully understood. We speculate that the difference between IBD and non-IBD men regarding IHD risk becomes estompated due to higher prevalence of traditional cardiovascular risk factors in men compared to women. Furthermore, higher risk of acute arterial events observed in younger IBD patients may reflect the different impact of inflammation across age groups. The use of contraceptive pills and higher CRP levels among women could also be a contributory factor.

2. Epidemiological Links between IBD and IHD

We searched PubMed utilizing the keywords: "inflammatory bowel disease", "IBD", "guidelines", "treatment plan", "ischemic heart disease", and "diagnosis" in all possible combinations. We extracted information regarding diagnosis, management, and treatment linking the two diseases, IBD and IHD. This review aims to summarize the current knowledge related to IBD and IHD with respect to its pathophysiology and risk factors in order to promote further research that can improve understanding and help develop clinical practice guidelines for prevention and management of IHD in patients with IBD.

Epidemiology

Large cohort studies evaluated the link between IBD and risk of IHD (Table 1) and found conflicting results.

Although some retrospective cohort studies did not find significant associations [11,15,18,23], the meta-analysis [13,14,19] found a positive correlation between IBD and IHD. In a meta-analysis conducted in 2017 by Feng et al. [19] were included 10 cohort studies investigating the risk of developing IHD in IBD. Researchers noticed an elevated risk of developing IHD in IBD patients compared to matched controls without IBD (RR = 1.244). Data found women, young age (<50 years), short-term follow-up (<5 years) may be at high IHD risk [19]. A large population trial conducted by Panhwar et al. in the United States of America in 2019 [22], involved a large database over 29 million patients from 26 different healthcare systems nationwide. A higher prevalence of acute MI was observed in both patients with UC and CD, as compared to non-IBD patients (the frequency of MI- UC 6.7% vs. CD 8.8% vs. non-IBD 3.3%, odds ratio [OR] for UC 2.09 [2.04–2.13] and CD 2.79 [2.74–2.85]), but the risk of having an acute cardiovascular event was highest in younger IBD patients (30–34 years old) and decreased with age (OR 12.05 [11.16–13.01]). The reasons for this issue have not been fully established – the higher CRP concentrations and the use of contraceptive pills among women could be decisive [22].

On the other hand, various studies have shown that the risk of myocardial injury mortality is lower among patients diagnosed with IBD when compared with non-IBD patients [21,23]. This can be attributed to the protective role of currently therapy of IBD based on 5-ASA, thiopurines and biologic therapy used in this patient group as part of their treatment. Salicylic acid shows anti-inflammatory and anti-oxidant properties, which may suggest a cardio-protective effect of 5-ASA when used prolonged, and a decreased risk of IHD compared to patients who have never received 5-ASA [12]. TNF-α blockers present reliable anti-inflammatory properties, and a number of studies are now available to report their protective effect on the risk of IHD in patients treated with anti-TNF drugs [24].

Table 1. Studies evaluating the risk of ischemic heart disease in inflammatory bowel disease patients.

Author	Year of Publication	Type of Study	Study Showing the Association between IBD and IHD	Conclusion
Osterman et al. [11]	2011	Retrospective cohort study	No	IBD patients did not appear to be at elevated risk of early MI when compared with patients from general practice.
Rungoe et al. [12]	2013	Cohort study	Positive	People diagnosed with IBD were compared with IBD-free individuals during 1997–2009 ($n = 28,833$). The risk of IHD was highest in the first year after IBD diagnosis (IRR = 2.13). The risk of IHD was 1.22 during 1–13 years of follow-up after IBD diagnosis.
Kristensen et al. [9]	2013	Cohort study	Positive	IBD patients had an increased total risk of MI (RR, 1.17 [95% confidence interval 1.05–1.31]). During periods of persistent IBD activity the RRs of MI increased to 1.49 (1.16–1.93). In remission periods, the risk of MI was similar to controls.
Fumery et al. [13]	2014	Meta-analysis	Positive	The study found an increased risk of IHD (RR, 1.23; 95% CI, 0.94–1.62). Cardiovascular mortality in patients with IBD compared to general population was not increased.
Singh et al. [14]	2014	Meta-analysis	Positive	There has been a modest increase in the risk of CV morbidity due to IHD, particularly in women.
Ruisi et al. [15]	2015	Cohort study	No	The study did not show an association with IBD and premature CV events in a cohort of 300 patients with IBD without traditional risk factors for CV disease.
Close et al. [16]	2015	Retrospective cohort study	Positive	A higher proportion of IBD patients were diagnosed with IHD: 2220 (11.6%) compared with 6504 (8.6%) of controls. Most IHD diagnoses predated the diagnosis of IBD. Patients with UC had a higher risk of IHD (unadjusted HR 1.3 (95% CI 1.1–1.5), $p < 0.001$) or MI (unadjusted HR 1.4 (95% CI 1.1–1.6), $p = 0.004$).
McAuliffe et al. [17]	2015	Retrospective cohort study	Positive	Patients with moderate to severe IBD had increased rates of MI vs. patients with mild IBD.
Barnes et al. [18]	2016	Retrospective cross-sectional study	No	Patients with IBD demonstrated lower rates of acute MI than in the general population (1.3% vs. 3.1%, $p < 0.001$).

Table 1. *Cont.*

Author	Year of Publication	Type of Study	Study Showing the Association between IBD and IHD	Conclusion
Feng et al. [19]	2017	Meta-analysis	Positive	Increased risk of IHD in IBD patients (RR, 1.244; 95% CI, 1.142–1.355). Increased risk in CD (RR, 1.243; 95% CI, 1.042–1.482) compared to UC (RR, 1.206; 95% CI, 1.170–1.242).
Le Gall et al. [20]	2018	Cohort Study	Positive	Occurrence of AAE (acute coronary syndrome). Disease activity may increase the risk of AAE.
Sun et al. [21]	2018	Meta-analysis	Positive	Higher risk of MI in women with IBD than in men; inflammation seems to play a more important role in CV disease in women than in men.
Kirchgesner et al. [10]	2018	Cohort study	Positive	IBD patients are at increased risk of AAE—SIR 1.35, with the highest risk in young patients.
Panhwar et al. [22]	2019	Cohort study	Positive	The prevalence of MI was higher in patients with UC and CD than in patients without IBD (UC 6.7% vs. CD 8.8% vs. non-IBD 3.3%). The relative risk of MI was associated with a higher rate in younger patients, and decreased with age.
Sinh et al. [23]	2021	Retrospective cross-sectional study	No	The study showed no difference between in-hospital mortality in patients with MI with or without UC (7.75% vs. 7.05%; $p = 0.25$) or in patients with MI with or without CD (6.50% vs. 6.59%; $p = 0.87$). Patients with MI with IBD had a longer length of stay.

Abbreviations: IBD—inflammatory bowel disease; MI—myocardial infarction; RR—rate ratio; UC—ulcerative colitis; CD—Crohn's disease; IHD—ischemic heart disease; CV—cardiovascular; SIR—standardised incidence ratio; AAE—acute arterial events.

The retrospective study conducted by Barnes et al. showed that patients with IBD were less likely to be admitted to hospital for acute myocardial injury compared to general population (1.3% vs. 3.2%; $p < 0.001$); in the adjusted analysis of risk factors for IHD, the OR was 0.54 for patients with IBD hospitalized for MI [18]. In 2021, another interesting study published by Sinh et al. aimed to investigate the MI outcomes in 2,629,161 patients, of which 3784 with CD and 3607 with UC. It showed that IBD did not impact in-hospital mortality due to MI-UC (odds ratio [OR], 1.12; 95% CI 0.98–1.29) and CD (OR 0.99; 95% CI 0.86–1.15). However, patients diagnosed with UC had higher total hospitalization costs compared to patients with MI without IBD [23].

Despite the fact that more recent attention has been paid to the possible links between IHD and IBD, some issues remain uncertain and the results are still unclear. Nevertheless, clinicians need to consider screening for IHD in all patients with IBD with a particular focus on women with IBD and younger adults (under the 50 years of age), who appear to be at the highest risk of developing an acute myocardial injury.

3. Risk Factors for IHD in IBD Patients

3.1. Traditional Cardiovascular Risk Factors

Traditional cardiovascular risk factors associated with IHD are obesity, type 2 diabetes mellitus (DM), hypertension, hyperlipidemia, smoking, and stress [25]. Some of them (Western lifestyles, chronic stress, tobacco in CD) are present in both diseases.

Classically, patients with IBD are considered underweight due to malnutrition. However, with the increasing prevalence of obesity in the general population and the emergence of innovative therapies that control and maintain remission in IBD, the prevalence of obesity can reach 40% of patients with IBD [26]. Obesity increases thromboembolic risk, the risk of surgery in UC, the perianal damage, and the need for hospitalization in CD [27]. However, Hu's [28] meta-analysis demonstrates that obese patients with IBD have a better evolution compared to non-obese patients, with a lower probability of hospitalization, surgery, and corticosteroid therapy.

Large population studies show an increased risk of type 2 DM in patients with IBD, independent of corticosteroid use [29]. There are few studies that prospectively follow the evolution of IBD in patients with DM. Published data suggest increased inflammatory activity, increased resource requirements, decreased QoL, increased risk of complications, infections, and higher mortality in diabetic patients with IBD [30].

Both metabolic syndrome and IBD have an increasing incidence and prevalence, as a consequence of lifestyle changes, with the widespread adoption of the "Western" type. The association of IBD with metabolic syndrome is not accidental, as there are common etiopathogenic links between the two diseases: inflammation, abnormal immune response, disorders in the endocrine function of adipose tissue, intestinal dysbiosis [31].

In a recent study, Golovics et al. identified older age, female gender, hyperlipidemia, and hypertension ($p < 0.001$ for each) as risk factors for developing MI in both CD and UC in the logistic-regression-based prevalence models. DM has also been labelled as an additional risk factor for MI in both CD and UC [32]. In a large database, Panhwar et al. examined the risk of MI in patients with or without IBD, and noted that traditional cardiovascular risk factors were more common among patients with both UC and CDIBD and MI [22]. On the other hand, the association between IBD and the high risk of MI persisted despite adjustments for traditional cardiovascular risk factors, thus suggesting that IBD may represent an independent risk factor for developing MI [22].

The study conducted by Correia et al. [33] revealed that a high percentage of women that used oral contraceptive pills (OCPs) had an elevated risk of MI. The use of hormonal contraception is associated with the risk of developing acute cardiovascular events, correlated to the pro-inflammatory state of IBD. This could possibly explain the increased risk of acute coronary syndrome in young women with IBD.

3.2. Risk Factors Related to IBD

3.2.1. Increased IHD with Disease Activity

Disease activity may have an independent impact on the risk of acute arterial events in patients with IBD. Le Gall, et al. [20] demonstrated that clinically active IBD was significantly associated with an increased risk of acute ischemic events in patients with IBD (Odds ratio (OR): 12.3, 95%CI: 2.8 ± 53.6). The disease activity was evaluated trough indirect markers, including hospitalizations, surgical treatments, and exposure therapies. Additionally, as reported in the Danish study, the risk of cardiovascular events is highest during active flares; this risk decreases during times of remission [9]. Periods of active flares (defined as 3-month periods before and after IBD-related hospitalization or surgery) were independently associated with an elevated risk of cardiovascular events in patients with CD (HR 1.74, 95% CI 1.44–2.09) and patients with UC (HR 1.87, 95% CI 1.58–2.22) [10]. Card et al. conducted a cohort analysis of the association between IBD, disease activity and the risk of MI, stroke and cardiovascular mortality. Although they did not find a significant increase in vascular events in patients with IBD in general, the study demonstrated that the incidence of the events correlated with a higher disease activity [34]. Furthermore, Agca et al. revealed in their study that cardiovascular events occur especially during disease flares in undertreated patients [35].

The activation of the coagulation cascade and proinflammatory cytokines as a consequence of active intestinal inflammation may be a factor that contributes to the occurrence of acute arterial events [36]. Disease activity should be regarded as a modifiable risk factor for cardiovascular events, and aggressive control of inflammation might reduce the risk of thrombosis in patients with IBD.

3.2.2. IBD Treatment

Corticosteroids are used in the management of acute flares of IBD, and as mentioned above, several studies have demonstrated an increased risk of IHD in acute flares and the fulminant and active stages of IBD. There are inconsistent data on whether corticosteroids have an increased cardiovascular risk in IBD patients, and thus it is difficult to decipher whether the increase in cardiovascular events during this time period is due to the direct effect of steroids or the uncontrolled disease activity. The adverse effects of long-term steroid use in IBD patients were studied by Lewis et al. in their cohort study [37]. CD patients had increased mortality with prolonged steroid use as compared with anti-TNF use; that was mainly related to major cardiovascular events (nonfatal MI, nonfatal stroke, and need for vascularization) [37]. Furthermore, in their article, Close et al. revealed that patients with UC had a higher incidence of IHD and MI with steroid use [16].

In the study conducted by Jaaouani et al. [38] the use of aminosalicylates, immune modifiers, and biologic therapies did not affect acute coronary syndrome events. However, exposure to anti-TNFs is associated with a decreased risk of acute arterial events in patients with IBD, particularly in men with CD [39]. A study conducted by Paschou et al. [40] revealed a decrease in insulin levels and homeostatic model assessment for insulin resistance index in patients with IBD after receiving treatment with biological therapy for a period of six months. Data suggest that clinical treatment can promote not only controlling intestinal inflammation, but also controlling risk factors for cardiovascular disease, resulting in the reduction of the overall risk of cardiovascular events in the long term [41]. However, prospective studies are needed to prove these effects in the general IBD population. With the advent of new drugs that enable better control of inflammatory activity and the establishment of treatment strategies with defined therapeutic targets, a reduction and a better control of the cardiovascular risk in IBD population is expected.

4. Inflammation—The Main Pathogenic Links between IBD and IHD

It is known that inflammation has been involved in the pathogenesis of atherosclerosis and coronary artery disease. Elevated markers of inflammation are associated with increased cardiovascular risk in all patients, with or without an inflammatory disorder [42].

IBD is associated with deregulation and increase in various cytokines [43]. Pro-inflammatory markers like homocysteine and CRP, which are known to be increased in patients with cardiovascular disease, are also found in chronic systemic inflammation in conditions like IBD [35]. CRP is a predictor of cardiovascular events and may contribute to atherogenesis [44]. The serum CRP level greater than 5mg/L during one year or in the previous 3 years were all associated with an higher risk of acute ischemic event (OR: 3.2, 95%CI: 1.2 ± 8.5) [20]. It has been established that its concentration increases in an active phase of IBD, thus proving that the cardiovascular risk is higher when CRP concentrations are increased.

As mentioned in Figure 1, other representatives pro-inflammatory mediators involved in IBD are tumor necrosis factor alpha (TNF-α), immunoglobulins (IgG, IgM), interleukin-6 (IL-6), interleukin-1 (IL-1), and vascular endothelial growth factor (VEGF). Notably, TNF-α is a proatherogenic cytokine [45] because blockade of TNF-α with biological therapy (infliximab, adalimumab) diminished severity of UC or CD [46] and enhanced the endothelial dysfunction in IBD patients [47]. VEGF, which is known to promote vessel formation, may contribute to IBD by increasing angiogenesis and inflammation [48]. Activation of these cytokines can increase oxidative stress, endothelial dysfunction, and macrophage accumulation, which can also stimulate atherosclerotic plaque formation [49]. Chronic inflammation promotes structural and functional changes of the endothelium. It has been acknowledged that the disrupted intestinal mucosal barrier in IBD facilitates the translocation of microbial lipopolysaccharides (LPS) and other endotoxins into circulation, inducing expression of pro-inflammatory cytokines [50], which may contribute to endothelial damage, atherosclerosis, and cardiovascular events. The mechanism that highlights this link has not been well established, but the state of chronic inflammation is considered to have a significant contribution for both IBD and IHD progression [51]. Other probable mechanisms involved could be arterial stiffening and coronary microcirculatory dysfunction [52]. In recent research, which included 17 studies with 558 UC patients, and 693 CD patients, the correlation between arterial stiffness and IBD was explored, and showed that the strength of the association of arterial stiffness between UC and CD was similar [53]. The association between IBD and arterial stiffness enhanced the hypothesis of systemic inflammation, possibly playing a role in the pathogenesis of arterial stiffness, which is widely recognized as a crucial intermediate process of CVD [53]. Furthermore, the dysfunctional endothelial system in patients with UC and CD has been observed as the markers of endothelial function.

At the molecular level, it has been showed that the increased expression of Toll-like receptors 2 and 4 (TLR2 and 4) in inflammatory cells likely mediate the damaging signaling events triggered by LPS and other microbial toxins, and in fact, elevated levels of TLR2 and 4 have been observed in atherosclerotic plaques [49].

In addition, under conditions of chronic inflammation, phenotypical changes in vascular smooth muscle occur, as well as medial calcification and reduced elasticity of vessels [49].

More than that, changes in nutrition and absorption, next to inflammation, can lead to lipid alterations.

Chronic systemic inflammation has been shown to be implicated in all phases of IHD, from vascular endothelial dysfunction to the onset and rupture of atherosclerotic plaque [54]. Increased permeability is clearly present in IBD, and could be a hypothesis leading to abnormal absorption of bacteria and toxic substances from the intestinal microbiota, which drives, as a consequence, both enteric and systemic inflammatory reactions and the diffusion in the bloodstream of bacterial endotoxins [55]. Inflammatory cytokines and modified lipoproteins are also largely responsible for the increased production of reactive oxygen species, which increases the expression of cell adhesion molecules by stimulating leukocyte migration to the subendothelial space, a key component in initiating and maintaining the atherosclerotic process [56,57].

Nevertheless, chronic inflammation, characteristic for IBD and associated with increased concentrations of pro-inflammatory cytokine represent the essential factor associated with the severity of IBD.

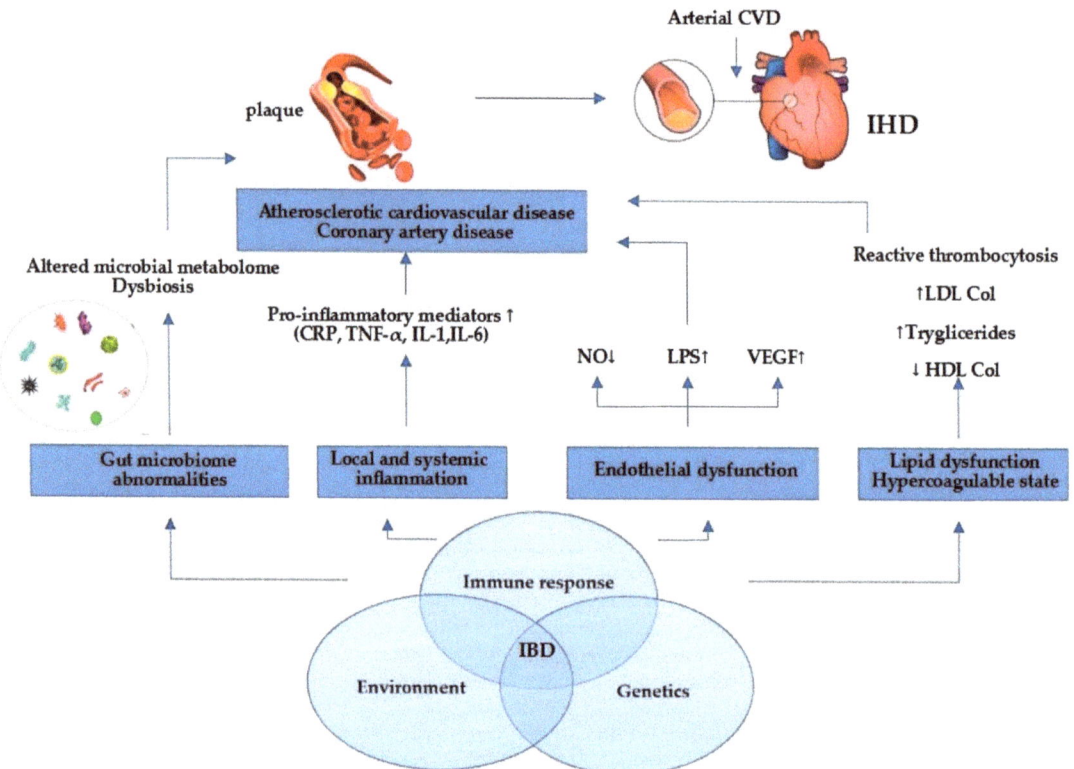

Figure 1. Link between IBD and IHD. Elevated pro-inflammatory mediators promote atherosclerotic plaque formation and cardiovascular events through endothelial dysfunction, gut microbiome abnormalities, pro-inflammatory state, and lipid dysfunction. Abbreviations: NO = nitric oxide; LPS = lipopolysaccharide; VEGF = vascular endothelial growth factor; LDL = low-density lipoprotein; HDL = high-density lipoprotein; CRP = C-reactive protein; TNF-α = tumor necrosis factor alpha; IL-1 = interleukin-1; IL-6 = interleukin-6; CVD = cardiovascular disease; IHD = ischemic heart disease.

5. Proposed Strategies for IHD Prevention among IBD Patients

5.1. Traditional Cardiovascular Risk Factors Modification in IBD Patients

Cardiovascular prevention should be started soon after the diagnosis of IBD as the highest risk is in the first years of evolution [58,59]. Optimal management involves the multidisciplinary team, together with the patient, according to evidence-based interventions, in order to reduce the risk of IHD [60]. All patients with IBD should be screened for cardiovascular risk factors identification; their presence requires aggressive management. Screening includes lifestyle habits, smoking status, body mass index, blood pressure, glucose, and lipid profile [61]. Stratification of cardiovascular risk in IBD patients is a challenge, as the scores used in the general population are difficult to translate into a young population. Complete tobacco cessation is key.

The statins' role in cardiovascular prevention in IBD patients is not fully understood. Patients with IBD typically have normal lipid levels, although some studies have reported alterations in lipid profile, especially HDL-cholesterol [5]. In addition to the lipid-lowering and stabilizing effect of atheroma plaque, statins also have anti-inflammatory properties [62]. The study conducted by Lochhead et al. revealed that statin treatment may have a protective role in the onset of CD, regardless of age, sex, comorbidities, or type of statin [63].

However, until further high-quality prospective research focusing on the role of statins in IBD progression should be performed, the role of statins in preventing IBD is still limited, conflicting, and has important limitations [63]. Until then, statins will be used according to the same rules as in the general population, with the mention that the presence of IBD is an enhancer for initiating therapy.

5.2. Disease Activity Control

Inflammation is the main trigger in IHD development in IBD patients. Cardiovascular disease especially occurs during disease flares in undertreated patients. Therefore, it is necessary to optimize the management of IBD, especially during active flares. IBD therapy not only controls intestinal inflammation, but also has the potential to prevent cardiovascular events in these patients [64]. Aminosalicylates and anti-TNF agents may decrease cardiovascular risk, while corticosteroids increase it [10]. Deep remission is an ultimate treatment goal in the management of patients. New treatment drug options may provide expectations for long-term remission with lower relapse rates.

The main guidelines recommendations regarding the management of IHD risk in IBD patients are resumed in Table 2.

Table 2. Guidelines statements regarding IHD risk in IBD patients.

Guideline	Recommendation
ECCO, 2015 [65] The First European Evidence-based Consensus on Extra-intestinal Manifestations in Inflammatory Bowel Disease.	• The risks of IHD, cerebrovascular accident, and mesenteric ischaemia are modestly increased in IBD, particularly in women • Systemic inflammation predisposes to premature atherosclerosis • Cardiovascular mortality has not been shown to be increased in IBD

International consensus on the prevention of venous and arterial thrombotic events in patients with inflammatory bowel disease, 2021 [66].	• Epidemiology
	   - It is an increased risk of arterial thrombosis in young patients
	   - IBD female patients have an increased risk of stroke and IHD compared to males
	• Traditional cardiovascular risk factors should be screened and controlled in all IBD patients
	• The risk of both arterial and venous thrombotic events is increased during IBD flares. Disease activity control is one of the main factors of cardiovascular protection
	• IBD Therapy
	   - 5-ASA (long term administration) and Anti-TNF agents decrease the risk of arterial thrombosis and IHD
	   - Steroids increase both arterial and venous thrombotic events in IBD patients

2019 ESC Guidelines for the diagnosis and management of chronic coronary syndromes [67].	• Lifestyle changes, smoking cessation, maintaining an optimal body weight, a healthy diet, and regular exercise are the most important measures in preventing cardiovascular risk. • Patients with IBD, along with those with other inflammatory conditions (systemic lupus erythematosus, rheumatoid arthritis) and neoplasms have an additional cardiovascular risk; they require aggressive screening, prevention and management measures
2019 ACC/AHA guidelines [68].	• For initiating or intensifying statin therapy in adults with borderline and intermediate-risk for atherosclerotic cardiovascular disease, inflammatory diseases are "risk-enhancing" clinical factors

Abbreviations: ECCO—European Crohn's and Colitis Organisation; IHD—Ischemic heart disease; IBD—Inflammatory bowel disease; 5-ASA—5-aminosalicylic acid; ESC—European Society of Cardiology; Anti-TNF—Anti-Tumor Necrosis Factor; ACC/AHA—American College of Cardiology/American Heart Association.

6. Conclusions

Systemic inflammation in IBD patients leads to oxidative stress and elevated levels of inflammatory cytokines such as TNF-α, leading to phenotypic changes in smooth muscle cells that culminate in atherosclerosis and CVD. The significance of IBD in causing atherosclerosis, ischemic heart disease and myocardial infarction is currently being recognized.

Patients with IBD are at increased risk of IHD—particularly women and young patients with IBD flare. The management of IBD patients should focus on a multidisciplinary, team-based approach to preventive care, remission of IBD disease activity, and aggressive reduction of cardiovascular risk factors, and thus gastroenterologists and cardiologists should work together to screen for cardiovascular risk factors and optimize anti-inflammatory treatment in IBD patients. Future prospective studies are needed to understand common etiopathogenic mechanisms, to find biomarkers and scores for patient stratification, and to establish optimal management.

Author Contributions: Conceptualization, C.M. and A.E.J.; methodology, C.M.; software, O.G.; validation, C.C.P., C.M. and M.D.; formal analysis, M.D.; investigation, A.E.J.; resources, C.C.P.; data curation, A.E.J.; writing—original draft preparation, A.E.J.; writing—review and editing, C.M.; visualization, B.M.M.; supervision, I.V.P.; project administration, O.G.; and funding acquisition, C.M. All authors contributed equally to the elaboration and writing of the manuscript. All authors have read and agreed to the published version of the manuscript.

Funding: This research received no external funding.

Institutional Review Board Statement: Not applicable.

Informed Consent Statement: Not applicable.

Data Availability Statement: Not applicable.

Conflicts of Interest: The authors declare no conflict of interest.

References

1. Weissman, S.; Sinh, P.; Mehta, T.I.; Thaker, R.K.; Derman, A.; Heiberger, C.; Qureshi, N.; Amrutiya, V.; Atoot, A.; Dave, M.; et al. Atherosclerotic cardiovascular disease in inflammatory bowel disease: The role of chronic inflammation. *World J. Gastrointest. Pathophysiol.* **2020**, *11*, 104–113. [CrossRef] [PubMed]
2. Seyedian, S.S.; Nokhostin, F.; Malamir, M.D. A review of the diagnosis, prevention, and treatment methods of inflammatory bowel disease. *J. Med. Life* **2019**, *12*, 113–122. [CrossRef] [PubMed]
3. Herzog, D.; Fournier, N.; Buehr, P.; Rueger, V.; Koller, R.; Heyland, K.; Nydegger, A.; Spalinger, J.; Schibli, S.; Petit, L.M.; et al. Age at disease onset of inflammatory bowel disease is associated with later extraintestinal manifestations and complications. *Eur. J. Gastroenterol. Hepatol.* **2018**, *30*, 598–607. [CrossRef] [PubMed]
4. Hedin, C.R.H.; Vavricka, S.R.; Stagg, A.J.; Schoepfer, A.; Raine, T.; Puig, L.; Rieder, F. The pathogenesis of extraintestinal manifestations: Implications for IBD research, diagnosis, and therapy. *J. Crohn's Colitis* **2019**, *13*, 541–554. [CrossRef]
5. Cainzos-Achirica, M.; Glassner, K.; Zawahir, H.S.; Dey, A.K.; Agrawal, T.; Quigley, E.; Abraham, B.P.; Acquah, I.; Yahya, T.; Mehta, N.N.; et al. Inflammatory Bowel Disease and Atherosclerotic Cardiovascular Disease: JACC Review Topic of the Week. *J. Am. Coll. Cardiol.* **2020**, *76*, 2895–2905. [CrossRef]
6. Zanoli, L.; Boutouyrie, P.; Fatuzzo, P.; Granata, A.; Lentini, P.; Öztürk, K.; Cappello, M.; Theocharidou, E.; Tuttolomondo, A.; Pinto, A.; et al. Inflammation and Aortic Stiffness: An Individual Participant Data Meta-Analysis in Patients With Inflammatory Bowel Disease. *J. Am. Heart Assoc.* **2017**, *6*, e007003. [CrossRef] [PubMed]
7. Bigeh, A.; Sanchez, A.; Maestas, C.; Gulati, M. Inflammatory bowel disease and the risk for cardiovascular disease: Does all inflammation lead to heart disease? *Trends Cardiovasc. Med.* **2020**, *30*, 463–469. [CrossRef]
8. Mitchell, N.E.; Harrison, N.; Junga, Z.; Singla, M. Heart Under Attack: Cardiac Manifestations of Inflammatory Bowel Disease. *Inflamm. Bowel Dis.* **2018**, *24*, 2322–2326. [CrossRef]
9. Kristensen, S.L.; Ahlehoff, O.; Lindhardsen, J.; Erichsen, R.; Jensen, G.V.; Torp-Pedersen, C.; Nielsen, O.H.; Gislason, G.H.; Hansen, P.R. Disease activity in inflammatory bowel disease is associated with increased risk of myocardial infarction, stroke and cardiovascular death—A Danish nationwide cohort study. *PLoS ONE* **2013**, *8*, e56944. [CrossRef]
10. Kirchgesner, J.; Beaugerie, L.; Carrat, F.; Andersen, N.N.; Jess, T.; Schwarzinger, M. BERENICE study group. Increased risk of acute arterial events in young patients and severely active IBD: A nationwide French cohort study. *Gut* **2018**, *67*, 1261–1268. [CrossRef]

11. Osterman, M.T.; Yang, Y.X.; Brensinger, C.; Forde, K.A.; Lichtenstein, G.R.; Lewis, J.D. No increased risk of myocardial infarction among patients with ulcerative colitis or Crohn's disease. *Clin. Gastroenterol. Hepatol.* **2011**, *9*, 875–880. [CrossRef] [PubMed]
12. Rungoe, C.; Basit, S.; Ranthe, M.F.; Wohlfahrt, J.; Langholz, E.; Jess, T. Risk of ischaemic heart disease in patients with inflammatory bowel disease: A nationwide Danish cohort study. *Gut* **2013**, *62*, 689–694. [CrossRef] [PubMed]
13. Fumery, M.; Xiaocang, C.; Dauchet, L.; Gower-Rousseau, C.; Peyrin-Biroulet, L.; Colombel, J.F. Thromboembolic events and cardiovascular mortality in inflammatory bowel diseases: A meta-analysis of observational studies. *J. Crohn's Colitis* **2014**, *8*, 469–479. [CrossRef] [PubMed]
14. Singh, S.; Singh, H.; Loftus, E.V.; Pardi, D.S. Risk of cerebrovascular accidents and ischemic heart disease in patients with inflammatory bowel disease: A systematic review and meta-analysis. *Clin. Gastroenterol. Hepatol.* **2014**, *12*, 382–393. [CrossRef]
15. Ruisi, P.; Makaryus, J.N.; Ruisi, M.; Makaryus, A.N. Inflammatory bowel disease as a risk factor for premature coronary artery disease. *J. Clin. Med. Res.* **2015**, *7*, 257–261. [CrossRef]
16. Close, H.; Mason, J.M.; Wilson, D.W.; Hungin, A.P.; Jones, R.; Rubin, G. Risk of Ischaemic Heart Disease in Patients with Inflammatory Bowel Disease: Cohort Study Using the General Practice Research Database. *PLoS ONE* **2015**, *10*, e0139745. [CrossRef]
17. McAuliffe, M.E.; Lanes, S.; Leach, T.; Parikh, A.; Faich, G.; Porter, J.; Holick, C.; Esposito, D.; Zhao, Y.; Fox, I. Occurrence of adverse events among patients with inflammatory bowel disease in the Health Core Integrated Research Database. *Curr. Med. Res. Opin.* **2015**, *31*, 1655–1664. [CrossRef]
18. Barnes, E.L.; Beery, R.M.; Schulman, A.R.; McCarthy, E.P.; Korzenik, J.R.; Winter, R.W. Hospitalizations for Acute Myocardial Infarction Are Decreased Among Patients with Inflammatory Bowel Disease Using a Nationwide Inpatient Database. *Inflamm. Bowel Dis.* **2016**, *22*, 2229–2237. [CrossRef]
19. Feng, W.; Chen, G.; Cai, D.; Zhao, S.; Cheng, J.; Shen, H. Inflammatory Bowel Disease and Risk of Ischemic Heart Disease: An Updated Meta-Analysis of Cohort Studies. *J. Am. Heart Assoc.* **2017**, *6*, e005892. [CrossRef]
20. Le Gall, G.; Kirchgesner, J.; Bejaoui, M.; Landman, C.; Nion-Larmurier, I.; Bourrier, A.; Sokol, H.; Seksik, P.; Beaugerie, L. Clinical activity is an independent risk factor of ischemic heart and cerebrovascular arterial disease in patients with inflammatory bowel disease. *PLoS ONE* **2018**, *13*, e0201991. [CrossRef]
21. Sun, H.H.; Tian, F. Inflammatory bowel disease and cardiovascular disease incidence and mortality: A meta-analysis. *Eur. J. Prev. Cardiol.* **2018**, *25*, 1623–1631. [CrossRef] [PubMed]
22. Panhwar, M.S.; Mansoor, E.; Al-Kindi, S.G.; Sinh, P.; Katz, J.; Oliveira, G.H.; Cooper, G.S.; Ginwalla, M. Risk of myocardial infarction in inflammatory bowel disease: A population-based national study. *Inflamm. Bowel Dis.* **2019**, *25*, 1080–1087. [CrossRef] [PubMed]
23. Sinh, P.; Tabibian, J.H.; Biyani, P.S.; Mehta, K.; Mansoor, E.; Loftus, E.V.; Dave, M. Inflammatory Bowel Disease Does Not Impact Mortality but Increases Length of Hospitalization in Patients with Acute Myocardial Infarction. *Dig. Dis. Sci.* **2021**, *66*, 4169–4177. [CrossRef] [PubMed]
24. Atzeni, F.; Nucera, V.; Galloway, J.; Zoltán, S.; Nurmohamed, M. Cardiovascular risk in ankylosing spondylitis and the effect of anti-TNF drugs: A narrative review. *Expert Opin. Biol. Ther.* **2020**, *20*, 517–524. [CrossRef]
25. Katta, N.; Loethen, T.; Lavie, C.J.; Alpert, M.A. Obesity and Coronary Heart Disease: Epidemiology, Pathology, and Coronary Artery Imaging. *Curr. Probl. Cardiol.* **2021**, *46*, 100655. [CrossRef]
26. Singh, S.; Dulai, P.S.; Zarrinpar, A.; Ramamoorthy, S.; Sandborn, W.J. Obesity in IBD: Epidemiology, pathogenesis, disease course and treatment outcomes. *Nat. Rev. Gastroenterol. Hepatol.* **2017**, *14*, 110–121. [CrossRef]
27. Seminerio, J.L.; Koutroubakis, I.E.; Ramos-Rivers, C.; Hashash, J.G.; Dudekula, A.; Regueiro, M.; Baidoo, L.; Barrie, A.; Swoger, J.; Schwartz, M.; et al. Impact of Obesity on the Management and Clinical Course of Patients with Inflammatory Bowel Disease. *Inflamm. Bowel Dis.* **2015**, *21*, 2857–2863. [CrossRef]
28. Hu, Q.; Ren, J.; Li, G.; Wu, X.; Li, J. The Impact of Obesity on the Clinical Course of Inflammatory Bowel Disease: A Meta-Analysis. *Med. Sci. Monit. Int. Med. J. Exp. Clin. Res.* **2017**, *23*, 2599–2606. [CrossRef]
29. Jess, T.; Jensen, B.W.; Andersson, M.; Villumsen, M.; Allin, K.H. Inflammatory Bowel Diseases Increase Risk of Type 2 Diabetes in a Nationwide Cohort Study. *Clin. Gastroenterol. Hepatol. Off. Clin. Pract. J. Am. Gastroenterol. Assoc.* **2020**, *18*, 881–888.e1. [CrossRef]
30. Kumar, A.; Teslova, T.; Taub, E.; Miller, J.D.; Lukin, D.J. Comorbid Diabetes in Inflammatory Bowel Disease Predicts Adverse Disease-Related Outcomes and Infectious Complications. *Dig. Dis. Sci.* **2021**, *66*, 2005–2013. [CrossRef]
31. Michalak, A.; Mosińska, P.; Fichna, J. Common links between metabolic syndrome and inflammatory bowel disease: Current overview and future perspectives. *Pharmacol. Rep. PR* **2016**, *68*, 837–846. [CrossRef]
32. Golovics, P.A.; Verdon, C.; Wetwittayakhlang, P.; Filliter, C.; Gonczi, L.; Hahn, G.D.; Wild, G.E.; Afif, W.; Bitton, A.; Bessissow, T.; et al. Increased Prevalence of Myocardial Infarction and Stable Stroke Proportions in Patients with Inflammatory Bowel Diseases in Quebec in 1996–2015. *J. Clin. Med.* **2022**, *11*, 686. [CrossRef] [PubMed]
33. Correia, P.; Machado, S.; Meyer, I.; Amiguet, M.; Eskandari, A.; Michel, P. Ischemic stroke on hormonal contraceptives: Characteristics, mechanisms and outcome. *Eur. Stroke J.* **2021**, *6*, 205–212. [CrossRef]
34. Card, T.R.; Zittan, E.; Nguyen, G.C.; Grainge, M.J. Disease activity in inflammatory bowel disease is associated with arterial vascular disease. *Inflamm. Bowel Dis.* **2021**, *27*, 629–638. [CrossRef] [PubMed]

35. Agca, R.; Smulders, Y.; Nurmohamed, M. Cardiovascular disease risk in immune-mediated inflammatory diseases: Recommendations for clinical practice. *Heart* **2022**, *108*, 73–79. [CrossRef] [PubMed]
36. Sleutjes, J.; van Lennep, J.; van der Woude, C.J.; de Vries, A.C. Thromboembolic and atherosclerotic cardiovascular events in inflammatory bowel disease: Epidemiology, pathogenesis and clinical management. *Ther. Adv. Gastroenterol.* **2021**, *14*, 17562848211032126. [CrossRef] [PubMed]
37. Lewis, J.D.; Scott, F.I.; Brensinger, C.M.; Roy, J.A.; Osterman, M.T.; Mamtani, R.; Bewtra, M.; Chen, L.; Yun, H.; Xie, F.; et al. Increased mortality rates with prolonged corticosteroid therapy when compared with antitumor necrosis factor-α-directed therapy for inflammatory bowel disease. *Am. J. Gastroenterol.* **2018**, *113*, 405–417. [CrossRef]
38. Jaaouani, A.; Ismaiel, A.; Popa, S.-L.; Dumitrascu, D.L. Acute Coronary Syndromes and Inflammatory Bowel Disease: The Gut–Heart Connection. *J. Clin. Med.* **2021**, *10*, 4710. [CrossRef]
39. Kirchgesner, J.; Nyboe Andersen, N.; Carrat, F.; Jess, T.; Beaugerie, L.; BERENICE Study Group. Risk of acute arterial events associated with treatment of inflammatory bowel diseases: Nationwide French cohort study. *Gut* **2020**, *69*, 852–858. [CrossRef]
40. Paschou, S.A.; Kothonas, F.; Lafkas, A.; Myroforidis, A.; Loi, V.; Terzi, T.; Karagianni, O.; Poulou, A.; Goumas, K.; Vryonidou, A. Favorable effect of anti-TNF therapy on insulin sensitivity in nonobese, nondiabetic patients with inflammatory bowel disease. *Int. J. Endocrinol.* **2018**, *2018*, 6712901. [CrossRef]
41. Lamb, C.A.; Kennedy, N.A.; Raine, T.; Hendy, P.A.; Smith, P.J.; Limdi, J.K.; Hayee, B.; Lomer, M.; Parkes, G.C.; Selinger, C.; et al. British Society of Gastroenterology consensus guidelines on the management of inflammatory bowel disease in adults. *Gut* **2019**, *68* (Suppl. S3), s1–s106. [CrossRef] [PubMed]
42. Soysal, P.; Arik, F.; Smith, L.; Jackson, S.E.; Isik, A.T. Inflammation, frailty and cardiovascular disease. *Adv. Exp. Med. Biol.* **2020**, *1216*, 55–64. [CrossRef] [PubMed]
43. Leppkes, M.; Neurath, M.F. Cytokines in inflammatory bowel diseases—Update 2020. *Pharmacol. Res.* **2020**, *158*, 104835. [CrossRef] [PubMed]
44. Wang, A.; Liu, J.; Li, C.; Gao, J.; Li, X.; Chen, S.; Wu, S.; Ding, H.; Fan, H.; Hou, S. Cumulative exposure to high-sensitivity C-reactive protein predicts the risk of cardiovascular disease. *J. Am. Heart Assoc.* **2017**, *6*, e005610. [CrossRef]
45. Tousoulis, D.; Oikonomou, E.; Economou, E.K.; Crea, F.; Kaski, J.C. Inflammatory cytokines in atherosclerosis: Current therapeutic approaches. *Eur. Heart J.* **2016**, *37*, 1723–1732. [CrossRef]
46. Fallon, K.A.; Fiocchi, C. Current Therapy in Inflammatory Bowel Disease: Why and How We Need to Change? *EMJ Innov.* **2021**, *6*, 40–49. [CrossRef]
47. Cibor, D.; Domagala-Rodacka, R.; Rodacki, T.; Jurczyszyn, A.; Mach, T.; Owczarek, D. Endothelial dysfunction in inflammatory bowel diseases: Pathogenesis, assessment and implications. *World J. Gastroenterol.* **2016**, *22*, 1067–1077. [CrossRef]
48. Alkim, C.; Alkim, H.; Koksal, A.R.; Boga, S.; Sen, I. Angiogenesis in Inflammatory Bowel Disease. *Int. J. Inflamm.* **2015**, *2015*, 970890. [CrossRef]
49. Wu, P.; Jia, F.; Zhang, B.; Zhang, P. Risk of cardiovascular disease in inflammatory bowel disease. *Exp. Ther. Med.* **2017**, *13*, 395–400. [CrossRef]
50. Ghosh, S.S.; Wang, J.; Yannie, P.J.; Ghosh, S. Intestinal Barrier Dysfunction, LPS Translocation, and Disease Development. *J. Endocr. Soc.* **2020**, *4*, bvz039. [CrossRef]
51. Kamperidis, N.; Kamperidis, V.; Zegkos, T.; Kostourou, I.; Nikolaidou, O.; Arebi, N.; Karvounis, H. Atherosclerosis and Inflammatory Bowel Disease-Shared Pathogenesis and Implications for Treatment. *Angiology* **2021**, *72*, 303–314. [CrossRef] [PubMed]
52. Kakuta, K.; Dohi, K.; Yamamoto, T.; Fujimoto, N.; Shimoyama, T.; Umegae, S.; Ito, M. Coronary Microvascular Dysfunction Restored After Surgery in Inflammatory Bowel Disease: A Prospective Observational Study. *J. Am. Heart Assoc.* **2021**, *10*, e019125. [CrossRef] [PubMed]
53. Lu, Q.; Shi, R.; Mao, T.; Wang, Z.; Sun, Z.; Tan, X.; Wang, Y.; Li, J. Arterial Stiffness in Inflammatory Bowel Disease: An Updated Systematic Review and Meta-Analysis. *Turk. J. Gastroenterol. Off. J. Turk. Soc. Gastroenterol.* **2021**, *32*, 422–430. [CrossRef] [PubMed]
54. Pepe, M.; Carulli, E.; Forleo, C.; Moscarelli, M.; Di Cillo, O.; Bortone, A.S.; Nestola, P.L.; Biondi-Zoccai, G.; Giordano, A.; Favale, S. Inflammatory Bowel Disease and Acute Coronary Syndromes: From Pathogenesis to the Fine Line Between Bleeding and Ischemic Risk. *Inflamm. Bowel Dis.* **2021**, *27*, 725–731. [CrossRef]
55. Vanuytsel, T.; Tack, J.; Farre, R. The Role of Intestinal Permeability in Gastrointestinal Disorders and Current Methods of Evaluation. *Front. Nutr.* **2021**, *8*, 717925. [CrossRef]
56. Steyers, C.M., III; Miller, F.J., Jr. Endothelial Dysfunction in Chronic Inflammatory Diseases. *Int. J. Mol. Sci.* **2014**, *15*, 11324–11349. [CrossRef]
57. Lorey, M.B.; Öörni, K.; Kovanen, P.T. Modified Lipoproteins Induce Arterial Wall Inflammation During Atherogenesis. *Front. Cardiovasc. Med.* **2022**, *9*, 841545. [CrossRef]
58. Biondi, R.B.; Salmazo, P.S.; Bazan, S.; Hueb, J.C.; de Paiva, S.; Sassaki, L.Y. Cardiovascular Risk in Individuals with Inflammatory Bowel Disease. *Clin. Exp. Gastroenterol.* **2020**, *13*, 107–113. [CrossRef]
59. Lee, M.T.; Mahtta, D.; Chen, L.; Hussain, A.; Al Rifai, M.; Sinh, P.; Khalid, U.; Nasir, K.; Ballantyne, C.M.; Petersen, L.A.; et al. Premature Atherosclerotic Cardiovascular Disease Risk Among Patients with Inflammatory Bowel Disease. *Am. J. Med.* **2021**, *134*, 1047–1051.e2. [CrossRef]

60. Dineen-Griffin, S.; Garcia-Cardenas, V.; Williams, K.; Benrimoj, S.I. Helping patients help themselves: A systematic review of self-management support strategies in primary health care practice. *PLoS ONE* **2019**, *14*, e0220116. [CrossRef]
61. Wu, H.; Hu, T.; Hao, H.; Hill, A.M.; Xu, C.; Liu, Z. Inflammatory bowel disease and cardiovascular diseases: A concise review. *Eur. Heart J. Open* **2022**, *2*, oeab029. [CrossRef]
62. Harris, S.K.; Roos, M.G.; Landry, G.J. Statin use in patients with peripheral arterial disease. *J. Vasc. Surg.* **2016**, *64*, 1881–1888. [CrossRef] [PubMed]
63. Lochhead, P.; Khalili, H.; Sachs, M.C.; Chan, A.T.; Olén, O.; Ludvigsson, J.F. Association Between Statin Use and Inflammatory Bowel Diseases: Results from a Swedish, Nationwide, Population-based Case-control Study. *J. Crohn's Colitis* **2021**, *15*, 757–765. [CrossRef]
64. Czubkowski, P.; Osiecki, M.; Szymańska, E.; Kierkuś, J. The risk of cardiovascular complications in inflammatory bowel disease. *Clin. Exp. Med.* **2020**, *20*, 481–491. [CrossRef] [PubMed]
65. Harbord, M.; Annese, V.; Vavricka, S.R.; Allez, M.; Barreiro-de Acosta, M.; Boberg, K.M.; Burisch, J.; De Vos, M.; De Vries, A.M.; Dick, A.D.; et al. European Crohn's and Colitis Organisation. The First European Evidence-based Consensus on Extra-intestinal Manifestations in Inflammatory Bowel Disease. *J. Crohn's Colitis* **2016**, *10*, 239–254. [CrossRef] [PubMed]
66. Olivera, P.A.; Zuily, S.; Kotze, G.K.; Regnault, V.; Al Awadhi, S.; Bossuyt, P.; Gearry, R.B.; Ghosh, S.; Kobayashi, T.; Lacolley, P.; et al. International consensus on the prevention of venous and arterial thrombotic events in patients with inflammatory bowel disease. *Nat. Rev. Gastroenterol. Hepatol.* **2018**, *18*, 857–873. [CrossRef] [PubMed]
67. Knuuti, J.; Wijns, W.; Saraste, A.; Capodanno, D.; Barbato, E.; Funck-Brentano, C.; Prescott, E.; Storey, R.F.; Deaton, C.; Cuisset, T.; et al. ESC Scientific Document Group. 2019 ESC Guidelines for the diagnosis and management of chronic coronary syndromes. *Eur. Heart J.* **2020**, *41*, 407–477. [CrossRef]
68. Arnett, D.K.; Blumenthal, R.S.; Albert, M.A.; Buroker, A.B.; Goldberger, Z.D.; Hahn, E.J.; Himmelfarb, C.D.; Khera, A.; Lloyd-Jones, D.; McEvoy, J.W.; et al. 2019 ACC/AHA Guideline on the Primary Prevention of Cardiovascular Disease: Executive Summary: A Report of the American College of Cardiology/American Heart Association Task Force on Clinical Practice Guidelines. *J. Am. Coll. Cardiol.* **2019**, *74*, 1376–1414. [CrossRef]

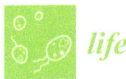

Review

A Real Pandora's Box in Pandemic Times: A Narrative Review on the Acute Cardiac Injury Due to COVID-19

Amalia-Stefana Timpau [1,2,†], Radu-Stefan Miftode [2,*], Daniela Leca [1,†], Razvan Timpau [3], Ionela-Larisa Miftode [1], Antoniu Octavian Petris [2], Irina Iuliana Costache [2,*], Ovidiu Mitu [2], Ana Nicolae [2,†], Alexandru Oancea [2], Alexandru Jigoranu [2], Cristina Gabriela Tuchilus [4] and Egidia-Gabriela Miftode [1]

1. Department of Infectious Diseases (Internal Medicine II), Faculty of Medicine, University of Medicine and Pharmacy "Gr. T. Popa", 700115 Iasi, Romania; amalia-stefana-v-darie@d.umfiasi.ro (A.-S.T.); lecadaniela@ymail.com (D.L.); ionela-larisa.miftode@umfiasi.ro (I.-L.M.); egidia.miftode@umfiasi.ro (E.-G.M.)
2. Department of Internal Medicine I (Cardiology), Faculty of Medicine, University of Medicine and Pharmacy "Gr. T. Popa", 700115 Iasi, Romania; antoniu.petris@umfiasi.ro (A.O.P.); ovidiu.mitu@umfiasi.ro (O.M.); nicolaeana2001@yahoo.com (A.N.); oancea.alexandru-florinel@email.umfiasi.ro (A.O.); jigoranu.raul-alexandru@email.umfiasi.ro (A.J.)
3. Department of Radiology and Medical Imaging, St. Spiridon Emergency Hospital, 700115 Iasi, Romania; razvan-timpau@email.umfiasi.ro
4. Department of Preventive Medicine and Interdisciplinarity (Microbiology), Faculty of Medicine, University of Medicine and Pharmacy "Gr. T. Popa", 700115 Iasi, Romania; cristina.tuchilus@umfiasi.ro
* Correspondence: radu-stefan.miftode@umfiasi.ro (R.-S.M.); irina.costache@umfiasi.ro (I.I.C.)
† These authors contributed equally to this work.

Abstract: The intricate relationship between severe acute respiratory syndrome coronavirus 2 (SARS-CoV-2) and the cardiovascular system is an extensively studied pandemic topic, as there is an ever-increasing amount of evidence that reports a high prevalence of acute cardiac injury in the context of viral infection. In patients with Coronavirus disease 2019, COVID-19, a significant increase in serum levels of cardiac troponin or other various biomarkers was observed, suggesting acute cardiac injury, thus predicting both a severe course of the disease and a poor outcome. Pathogenesis of acute cardiac injury is not yet completely elucidated, though several mechanisms are allegedly involved, such as a direct cardiomyocyte injury, oxygen supply-demand inequity caused by hypoxia, several active myocardial depressant factors during sepsis, and endothelial dysfunction due to the hyperinflammatory status. Moreover, the increased levels of plasma cytokines and catecholamines and a significantly enhanced prothrombotic environment may lead to the destabilization and rupture of atheroma plaques, subsequently triggering an acute coronary syndrome. In the present review, we focus on describing the epidemiology, pathogenesis, and role of biomarkers in the diagnosis and prognosis of patients with acute cardiac injury in the setting of the COVID-19 pandemic. We also explore some novel therapeutic strategies involving immunomodulatory therapy, as well as their role in preventing a severe form of the disease, with both the short-term outcome and the long-term cardiovascular sequelae being equally important in patients with SARS-CoV-2 induced acute cardiac injury.

Keywords: myocardial injury; COVID-19; cytokines; biomarkers; heart failure

1. Introduction

The deadliest pandemic in the modern era is currently ongoing and is caused by severe acute respiratory syndrome-coronavirus-2 (SARS-CoV-2) which is the most recent member of the coronavirus family to emerge this century, after the severe acute respiratory syndrome coronavirus (SARS-CoV) and the Middle East respiratory syndrome coronavirus (MERS-CoV) in the early 2000s [1]. Most respiratory infections usually evolve with mild to moderate symptoms, but coronaviruses drew attention that viral pneumonia may also

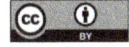

progress to severe forms further complicated with multiple organ failure [2,3]. Several studies analyzed the short- and mid-term impact of cardiovascular complications, highlighting that acute cardiac injury in patients with a confirmed diagnosis of Coronavirus disease 2019 (COVID-19) represents significant associated morbidity [4–7]. Moreover, additional research investigating the long-term sequelae of COVID-19 indicates a substantial risk of cardiovascular complications, particularly heart failure (HF) and atrial fibrillation, even in patients not requiring hospitalization during the acute phase of the viral infection [8].

Diagnosis of acute cardiac injury is outlined using the cardiac troponin (cTn) assay above the 99th percentile as the upper reference limit. Myocardial injury is considered acute if the dynamic cTn concentration exceeds the biological variation limits [9]. However, one should consider that a personal history of cardiovascular disease and elevated levels of cTn are factors of poor prognosis, being significantly associated with an increased risk of mortality in patients hospitalized with COVID-19. Specifically, two meta-analyses reported an 8 to 21-fold higher risk of fatal events in patients with SARS-CoV-2-related acute cardiac injury [10,11]. A plethora of studies show that approximately one in every three patients with COVID-19 will develop a certain phenotype of myocardial injury [7,12,13], the risk being significantly higher in patients with previously diagnosed chronic coronary heart disease [14]. Additional supporting evidence concerning acute cardiac injury due to coronavirus infection was provided by a large meta-analysis performed by Abate et al. which reported an alarming 22.3% prevalence of myocardial injury in patients who tested positive for SARS-CoV-2 [10].

Despite the increased risk of myocardial infarction associated with COVID-19, starting with the onset of the pandemic, various literature data paradoxically reported an up to 50% reduction in hospitalization rates due to this cardiovascular pathology. This might be either a consequence of patients unwilling to risk exposure to a SARS-CoV-2 infection or due to the significant reduction in available hospital beds for "non-COVID-19" patients [15,16]. Furthermore, a restraint for percutaneous coronary intervention (PCI) procedures was observed particularly in patients with a confirmed or just even suspected COVID-19 diagnosis. Non-infected patients received primary PCI as a conventional approach, while in patients positive for SARS-CoV-2, the strategy focused on fibrinolysis in a higher number of cases, as the latter represents a therapeutic option that involves a lower interaction and, subsequently, lower exposure to viral particles [17,18].

The possible occurrence of cardiovascular complications in SARS-CoV-2 infection, the risk factors and specific symptoms of myocardial injury, and the implementation of adequate investigations and treatment have a profound impact on the patients' prognosis [19]. There is still no management consensus for patients with acute cardiac injury; the constant pandemic-related challenge for clinicians is to continuously balance the benefits of a comprehensive cardiac evaluation and the risk of spreading the infection. Supportive care and an integrative approach to the underlying infectious disease may represent a feasible standard of care in patients with COVID-19-associated acute cardiac injury [20].

In this regard, the present review is conceived to provide an overview on SARS-CoV-2 induced acute cardiac injury, describing the allegedly involved mechanisms, highlighting the contribution of cardiac biomarkers in both the initial diagnostic approach and subsequent follow-up of COVID-19-related acute cardiac injury, as well as pointing out some state-of-the-art data for therapeutic strategies to address it.

2. Cardiovascular Pathophysiology Related to COVID-19 and the Most Common Clinical Phenotypes

2.1. The Pathophysiological Continuum between Infection and Cardiac Injury

Coronaviruses have a specific crown-like surface appearance and a structure made from four structural proteins, known as the spike (S), envelope (E), membrane (M), and nucleocapsid (N) proteins. SARS-CoV-2 enters the cell after the proteolytic cleavage of the S protein followed by its binding to the cell-surface receptor angiotensin 2 conversion enzyme (ACE 2) [21]. The latter is a membrane protein that plays a vital role in the cardiovascular and immune systems and is well expressed in the lung and heart endothelial cells, macrophages, and cardiomyocytes [22]. ACE 2 levels are higher in patients receiving treatment with medications that inhibit the renin-angiotensin-aldosterone system, such as ACE inhibitors or angiotensin receptor blockers [23]. The use of these neurohormonal modulating drugs was controversial in the early stages of the pandemic. Nevertheless, multiple studies conducted during the last two years have demonstrated that is not advisable to interrupt their chronic administration, nor to change the therapeutic class. Basically, the current consensus emphasizes that maintaining the previously prescribed treatment does not adversely affect the course of viral infection and continues to provide cardiac protection at the same time [24–26]. Moreover, ACE 2 has been shown to provide additional protective effects against pulmonary injury in patients with ARDS due to severe forms of COVID-19 [27].

A SARS-CoV-2 infection may both exacerbate pre-existing cardiovascular comorbidities and trigger new ones. HF is among the most frequently reported cardiovascular complications related to COVID-19 infection, being diagnosed in up to 24% of patients, while venous thromboembolism was identified in 21% of cases, followed by dysrhythmias and myocarditis in 17% and 7% of patients, respectively [5,6,27,28]. The main risk factors for SARS-CoV-2-induced acute cardiac injury include smoking, male gender, and comorbidities, including diabetes mellitus, arterial hypertension, and coronary artery disease [10,11]. The imbalance between pro-inflammatory and anti-inflammatory mediators may be responsible for the development of major cardiovascular events [29]. The response to infection is governed by the adequate activity of both the innate and acquired immune systems.

Two major immunity defects are required for the onset of the critical illness in COVID-19 which is frequently associated with myocardial injury. The first is represented by a lack of initial control over the viral clearance, mainly through the innate immune system, while the second resides in the inability to regulate a balanced production of pro- and anti-inflammatory cytokines [2,30]. The innate immune response to viral infection is based on interferon types I and III. On one hand, in SARS-CoV-2 infection, interferon levels were observed to increase only in critical patients, whereas in all other positive cases the immune response was reduced and/or delayed. On the other hand, the response was quicker and more vigorous in patients hospitalized for influenza pneumonia. This particular ability of SARS-CoV-2 to elude the early innate immune response may lead to an insufficient viral clearance, followed by the development of a hyperinflammatory condition, and, in certain categories of patients, the onset of acute respiratory distress syndrome (ARDS) [31,32].

Moreover, the innate immunity may also trigger the adaptive immunity consisting of CD4+ and CD8+ T cell lymphocytes and B lymphocytes that produce neutralizing antibodies. The combined T and B cell responses contribute to SARS-CoV-2 infection resolution and a robust immunity [32]. Cytokines, predominantly produced by macrophages, mast cells, and dendritic cells, but also by B and T lymphocytes, play a central role in coordinating the immune response. A balanced synthesis of cytokines is required for an effective antiviral effect, but their excessive serum levels may cause a cytokine storm with massive collateral damage to vascular structures and alveolar barriers [33].

Cardiac troponin levels have been shown to be linearly correlated with C-reactive protein levels, indicating that acute cardiac injury may be closely related to systemic inflammation [34]. The distinctive pathogenesis of vascular damage is promoted by the presence of the cellular receptor of SARS-CoV-2 on the vascular cell's surface, contributing to endothelial dysfunction [35]. Furthermore, direct infection of the endothelial lining may lead to vasculitis and apoptosis. As a result, the exposed subendothelial surface facilitates platelet aggregation in an attempt to repair the vascular damage. However, even in the absence of direct endothelial invasion, high levels of inflammatory cytokines have the ability to impair the endothelial function by increasing the number of adhesion molecules, thus promoting thrombogenic processes [36–38]. Coagulopathic events include thrombin generation, platelet consumption, and increased levels of fibrinogen and the Von Willebrand factor [39]. Viral coagulopathy is manifested by venous thrombosis, usually further complicated with venous thromboembolism but also by arterial thrombosis, most commonly found in myocardial or cerebral territories. Parenteral anticoagulants, such as unfractionated heparin and low molecular weight heparins, are routinely used in the treatment of patients admitted with moderate-to-severe COVID-19, while direct oral anticoagulants are predominantly used in the ambulatory management of patients presenting a mild form of the disease [40].

2.2. Acute Coronary Syndromes in the COVID-19 Pandemic: The "Perfect" Cardio-Inflammatory Symbiosis

The interplay between atherosclerotic disease and inflammation has been well-described, starting with the formation of atheroma plaque up to its erosion and rupture, with the subsequent occurrence of an acute coronary syndrome [41]. Total occlusion of a coronary artery induced by an eroded, vulnerable atherosclerotic plaque and the overlying thrombus formation might be a consequence of a hyperinflammatory environment along with the prothrombotic state induced by SARS-CoV-2 infection. This mechanism represents the basic pathophysiological substrate of ST-elevation myocardial infarction (STEMI) but also accounts for approximately 25% of cases admitted with non-ST-elevation myocardial infarction (NSTEMI) [42,43]. The real epidemiological impact of COVID-19 in patients with cardiac ischemia is mirrored by the worrisome incidence rates of myocardial infarction among SARS-CoV-2 positive cases, ranging from 1.1% to 8.9% [44,45]. The risk of developing myocardial infarction is significantly higher in the early stages of the infection, with a 5-fold increase in risk during the first 14 days of COVID-19, compared to the pre-illness period [46].

Those high figures can be explained, at least partially, by certain similarities concerning the inflammatory pathways operating both in COVID-19 and atherosclerosis. Even before the COVID-19 pandemic, the American Heart Association (AHA) suggested that viral infections could destabilize the atherosclerotic plaques, and various collagenolytic enzymes, such as matrix metalloproteinases (MMP), were becoming associated with increased plaque vulnerability [47,48]. Those MMPs can be activated by a plethora of cytokines (e.g., TNF-alpha, INF-γ, IL-1, and IL-6), thus diminishing the cohesion of the atherosclerotic plaque and consecutively increasing the risk of acute coronary syndromes [48,49]. Based on these observations, the COVID-19 pandemic again turned the spotlight on statins' pleiotropic effects, primarily based on their anti-inflammatory response, doubled by the amelioration of the endothelial function. The plaque stabilization occurs via the enhanced calcification and thickening of the fibrous cap, with inflammation playing a central role. The large JUPITER study even highlighted that patients treated with rosuvastatin presented decreased serum levels of C-reactive protein and a reduced apparition of major cardiovascular events, compared to the placebo group [50,51], while a large Swedish study claimed that previous chronic treatment with statins exhibited a modest preventive therapeutic effect on COVID-19 mortality [52]. The continuation and/or initiation of statins in COVID-19 patients may also be beneficial from the perspective of the lipid profile, as hypercholesterolemia is associated with an increased susceptibility to SARS-CoV-2 infection. It was demonstrated that high cholesterol levels are associated not only with increased density of ACE2 receptors on host cell membranes but also with a more effective interaction between the viral spike protein and the ACE2 receptors [53].

In addition, significant platelet activation occurs during the systemic inflammation associated with SARS-CoV-2 infection. This phenomenon is induced by the binding of pro-inflammatory interleukins to the platelet surface receptors, and by reducing the availability of endothelial nitric oxide. At the same time, neutrophils express adhesion molecules favoring platelet aggregation. These mechanisms, together with endothelial injury, facilitate the interaction between the platelets and the endothelial cells, thus aggravating the thromboinflammatory pathways, representing a hallmark for COVID-19 [54].

Even if mortality caused by acute myocardial infarction has reached its lowest level in the era of PCI, it still remains associated with considerable morbidity. Restoring adequate myocardial reperfusion in a timely manner limits the area of the infarction and significantly improves the outcome, regardless of the associated pathologies [55]. However, contradictorily, the resumption of blood flow to the ischemic area may lead to additional myocardial damage, a phenomenon known as reperfusion myocardial injury. This paradoxical mechanism may be responsible for the loss of up to 50% of viable myocardium and elevated cytokine levels, in addition, biochemical and metabolic changes caused by hypoxia play a core role in its occurrence [56]. A cohort study including patients over the age of 65 showed that more than three-quarters (76%) of patients who survived a first acute myocardial infarction developed HF in the next 5 years [57]. Despite modern reperfusion strategies and neurohormonal blocking therapies, the incidence of HF remains unacceptably high and there is an urgent need for better management in order to improve both survival and quality of life after myocardial infarction. However, abnormally activated immune responses during infection with SARS-CoV-2 lead to a suboptimal myocardial repair with a higher incidence of HF [58].

Type 2 myocardial infarction is caused by the imbalance between a deficient myocardial oxygen supply and an increased metabolic demand, due to specific cardiac and non-cardiac pathological conditions.

A variable association of some commonly met mechanisms in COVID-19 patients seems relevant in this context:

(1) Previously stable coronary artery disease that limits myocardial perfusion;
(2) Endothelial dysfunction in the coronary microcirculation;
(3) Significantly increased arterial hypertension resulting from elevated circulating levels of Angiotensin II and catecholamines;
(4) Hypoxemia due to acute respiratory distress syndrome (ARDS) or in situ pulmonary vascular thrombosis. In the case of sepsis, pulmonary injury, and respiratory failure, significant increases in biomarkers of overload and myocardial injury can be noticed [12,59].

Moreover, infections in general, and COVID-19-associated pneumonia in particular, can unbalance the thin equilibrium between myocardial O_2 supply and consumption. The increase in the physiological demand for O_2 caused by systemic infection can be so significant that this imbalance occurs even in the absence of angiography-relevant atherosclerotic plaques. Several studies emphasized this pathway as the main mechanism of COVID-related acute cardiac injury. Essentially, vasodilation represents the main pathophysiological mechanism of the response of the cardiovascular system to sepsis. In addition, hypotension is the natural consequence of vasodilation, which can even progress to hemodynamic collapse, thus inducing or aggravating coronary hypoperfusion with subsequent acute myocardial injury through a reduced O_2 supply [60]. At the same time, in the context of sepsis, reflex tachycardia increases the myocardial oxygen demand. Of course, the presence of atheroma plaques is a risk factor for the unfavorable evolution in patients with sepsis, increasing the risk of acute myocardial injury [61,62], but COVID-19 is also highly associated with non-atherosclerotic coronary perfusion impairment, such as spasm of the coronary arteries, dissection of the coronary wall, microthrombosis in the context of the hypercoagulant state, or vasculitis-like injury of the coronary vessels [63,64]. Regardless of the intimate mechanism of COVID-19-related myocardial infarction with non-obstructive coronary arteries, the patients' prognosis is poor, with high mortality rates mainly due to the increased prevalence of severe comorbidities, such as ARDS, obesity, or congenital thrombophilia [64,65].

Under these circumstances, it is difficult to clearly differentiate between patients with acute coronary syndromes, such as unstable angina or NSTEMI, and those with acute myocarditis or myocardial injury caused exclusively by metabolic imbalances in the context of fever, tachycardia, or hypoxemia due to ARDS [59]. Those patients require an integrative diagnostic and therapeutic approach, focusing not only on SARS-CoV-2 infection and the major associated cardiovascular pathology but also on the frequently coexisting factors of poor prognosis.

2.3. Heart Failure in COVID-19 Patients: Different Pathways, Same Target

Patients admitted for COVID-19 may develop either an acute decompensation of a chronic, previously stable HF or a de-novo acute HF as an immediate consequence of acute cardiac injury [66]. Pathogenesis of COVID-19 cardiomyopathy is intimately related to inflammatory cytokines, referring here to diastolic dysfunction and increased myocardial stiffness mediated by interleukin-6 (IL-6), negative inotropic effects exerted by interleukin-1β (IL-1β), or myocardial fibrosis induced by IL-1β and tumor necrosis factor alfa (TNF-α). Even higher levels of those biomarkers are detected during cytokine storms in the severe forms of SARS-CoV-2 infection [67–69]. A significantly increased incidence of acute HF was reported in patients deceased due to severe COVID-19, as compared to their survivor counterparts [70]. Moreover, the in-hospital mortality rate in patients presenting both acute HF and COVID-19 was extremely high, reaching up to 44.1% at the peak of the pandemic. Beyond the acute phase, COVID-19 may be responsible for HF as a long-term cardiovascular complication, but further clinical studies are required [66].

2.4. Myocarditis in COVID-19: Between Certainties and Controversies

The correlation between human coronaviruses and myocarditis is well-established [71]. Concerning SARS-CoV-2 infection, three pathophysiological mechanisms may contribute to myocarditis occurrence in patients with COVID-19. Firstly, it is worth mentioning the direct viral cardiomyocytes' invasion with subsequent injury accompanied by various immune mechanisms such as T cell-mediated cytotoxicity and cytokines' negative inotropic effects. Additionally, the autoimmune mechanisms triggered as a response to the release of cryptic antigens from cardiomyocytes following SARS-CoV-2-induced lesions could also enhance the development of myocarditis [72–74]. A very recent extensive study, including more than 100,000 subjects diagnosed with COVID-19, showed a 2 to 3-fold higher risk of myocarditis among infected patients [75], while the net prevalence of myocarditis among cases that required hospitalization was 2.4 per 1000 admissions [76]. Importantly, myocarditis was far more prevalent among non-vaccinated young males, compared to their non-vaccinated counterparts [77].

There is also evidence to support the hypothesis of molecular mimicry [78]. Necropsy studies that included endomyocardial biopsy suggest that direct viral toxicity is not the main mechanism of myocardial injury, as current evidence indicates that viral presence in the heart tissue is not necessarily associated with myocarditis [79]. Local myocardial inflammation, as well as severe systemic inflammation, can be a direct cause of myocardial injury in COVID-19 cases. It is already known that patients with sepsis-associated cardiomyopathy have an exacerbated inflammatory status that is characterized by elevated circulating levels of several cytokines, including the previously-mentioned IL-6 and TNF-α [59]. In vitro exposure to IL-6 has reduced the cardiomyocyte contractility, while recombinant TNF-α administration decreased the ejection fraction of the left ventricle in experimental models. Mechanisms of these myocytotoxic effects include the modulation of calcium channels' flows and nitric oxide synthesis which are thought to play a major role in depressing myocardial function in sepsis [59,80,81]. The reversible acute cardiac dysfunction occurring in the context of a septic environment is known as sepsis-induced cardiomyopathy (SICM). Immune response to infection leads to mitochondrial dysfunction, disruption of contractile apparatus by altering calcium balance, and myocyte apoptosis [82,83]. Increased levels of cTn detected in SICM may also appear as a consequence of myocardial edema [84].

However, it remains unclear to what extent myocarditis is caused by direct viral myocardial damage or is just a consequence of systemic inflammation.

2.5. Stress Cardiomyopathy: An Additional Trigger

The incidence of stress cardiomyopathy (also known as tako-tsubo cardiomyopathy) during the COVID-19 pandemic appears to follow an increasing trend, with psychological distress and anxiety having a core role in its onset. Incriminated mechanisms include the sympathetic activation causing catecholamine-induced myocardial stunning and microvascular dysfunction that is transient and more frequently observed in elderly women [85]. It is worth mentioning that a study showed that this hypercatholaminergic condition due to cytokine storm in critical patients (from ICU departments) induces a significantly increased blood pressure, compared to non-critical patients (145 mmHg vs. 122 mmHg; $p < 0.001$); interestingly, this hypertensive pattern in patients with severe forms of COVID-19 is actually associated with an improved prognosis, a lower need for inotropic support, and a decreased risk of developing cardiogenic shock or multiple organ dysfunction [86].

2.6. Right Ventricular Failure: A Key Element in the Hemodynamics of COVID-19 Patients

The right ventricle (RV) represents an essential component in the hemodynamic homeostasis of patients with COVID-19, an acute RV dysfunction being considered a factor of poor prognosis. Several mechanisms have a complementary role in RV injury [87,88]:

- Pulmonary hypertension induced by vasoactive mediators;
- Pulmonary vasoconstriction due to hypoxemia;
- Vascular remodeling;
- Microthrombi in pulmonary vessels due to inflammatory cytokines;
- Mechanical compression due to atelectasis, interstitial edema, or associated pleural effusion.

Moreover, in ICU-admitted patients due to a severe course of COVID-19, persistent ventilation with elevated positive expiratory pressures leads to a significantly increased RV afterload, thus inducing additional mechanical strain in a cavity with rather thin walls and further reducing an already impaired cardiac output [88]. This pathophysiological chain of events is clearly expressed by the rise of serum concentrations for several biomarkers, such as NT-proBNP, ST2, or GDF-15 molecules, that express various mechanisms suggestive not only of myocardial dysfunction but also of inflammation or oxidative stress, conditions that are commonly found in infected patients [89–91].

3. Biomarkers in the Diagnosis and Prognosis of Acute Myocardial Injury Due to COVID-19: Classic Approach, Novel Challenge

3.1. Cardiac Troponins

Despite the fact that diagnostic utility and performance of cTn in coronary heart disease are well known [92], the constantly reported high levels of cTn in COVID-19 patients triggered confusion among clinicians since the beginning of the pandemic [73,93–96]. A sudden cTn elevation may be suggestive of STEMI/N-STEMI, type 2 myocardial infarction, myocarditis, stress cardiomyopathy, sepsis-induced cardiomyopathy, or non-ischemic myocardial injury, each of these pathologies having different therapeutic approaches (Figure 1). A modest rise in cTn levels is seen in patients with mild and moderate forms of COVID-19, without influencing the clinical outcome [97]. The rise of cTn serum levels in patients who succumb to SARS-CoV-2 infection shows a particular pattern as compared to the concentration dynamics that characterize acute coronary syndromes (ACS). In COVID-19, there is a steady upward trend of cTn serum levels while ACS is generally observed as a very typical abrupt rise [98]. Nevertheless, a cTn elevation can also be detected in certain non-cardiac conditions, such as systemic inflammatory response syndrome, sepsis, pulmonary embolism, critical illness, or end-stage renal disease [99]. In fact, no overt ischemia is found in as many as 60% of cases where an acute cardiac injury is identified [12]. Therefore, a prompt differential diagnosis and a timely intervention in patients with SARS-CoV-2-related acute cardiac injury are mandatory [10].

In terms of prognosis, several meta-analyses reported that high serum levels of this biomarker are significantly correlated with increased mortality risk [10,98]. The ability of cTn concentration at admission to predict in-hospital mortality was outlined by an area under a curve greater than 0.90 (ROC analysis) [3,98,100]. In addition to being directly associated with major cardiovascular events, elevated cTn levels are also related to an increased risk of respiratory, hepatic, and renal impairment [101]. Serial measurements of cTn levels in patients with high initial values detected at admission are recommended either to confirm or to exclude myocardial infarction [102]. Taking into account the frequently elevated cTn serum levels, the question of whether it should be routinely assessed in COVID-19 pneumonia was raised. However, the American College of Cardiology stated in a recent review that clinicians are advised to measure cTn only in selected cases, either in patients with preexisting cardiovascular comorbidities or in clinical circumstances highly suggestive of ischemic etiology [103].

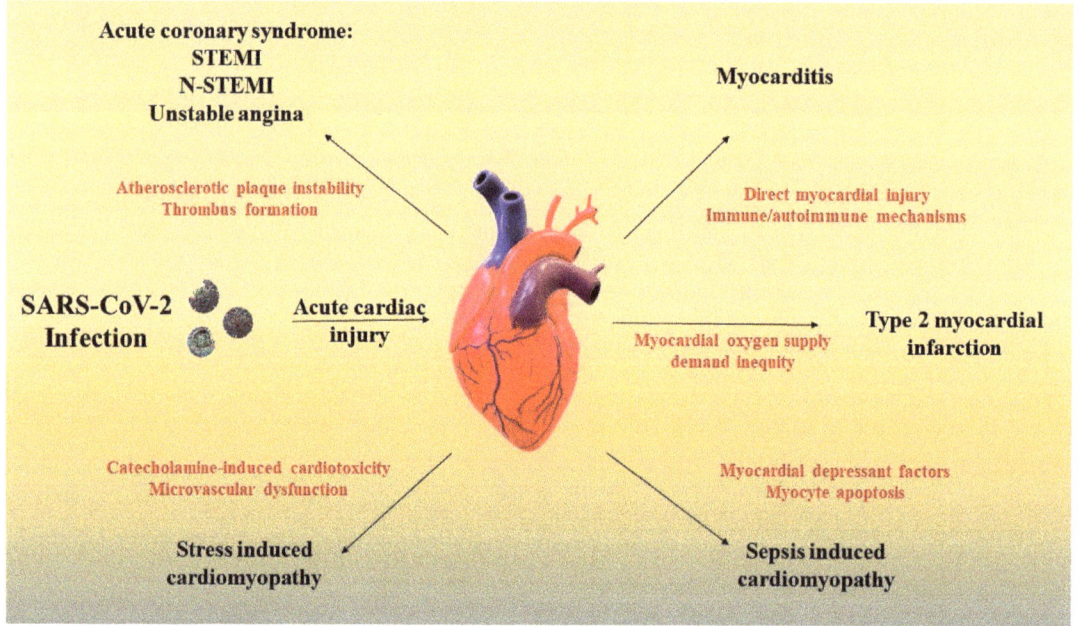

Figure 1. Potential pathophysiological mechanisms of SARS-CoV-2 induced acute cardiac injury; acute coronary syndromes occur by destabilization and rupture of atheroma plaques with the consequent formation of a thrombus that causes occlusion of the artery responsible for heart attack [41]. Myocarditis can occur through direct myocardial injury and immune or autoimmune mechanisms [72–74]. Type 2 myocardial infarction occurs due to an imbalance between the need and supply of oxygen [12]. Sepsis-induced cardiomyopathy occurs due to myocytic apoptosis and cardiodepressant factors [82,83]. Stress-induced cardiomyopathy occurs through the cardiotoxic effect of catecholamines and is secondary to microvascular dysfunction [85]. Legend: STEMI: ST-elevation myocardial infarction; and N-STEMI: non-ST-elevation myocardial infarction.

3.2. The Interleukins

The interleukin-1 family comprises 11 cytokines with core roles in innate and adaptive immunity [104]. IL-1β represents the "apical" cytokine of the innate immune system, as it regulates cytokine and chemokine synthesis, and self-catalyzes its own production. In the acute inflammatory response phase to viral infection, an early increase in serum IL-1β and TNF-α levels are observed within the first 30 min, followed by a rise in IL-6 levels [105]. While IL-1β and TNF-α levels may drop within 24–48 h, elevated IL-6 levels persist for a longer period over the course of the infection [48]. Despite its short half-life, as an upstream cytokine, IL-1β may contribute to CRS development, inducing IL-6 production, leading to macrophage activation and pyroptosis, and caspase-1-dependent host cell death mediated by inflammatory cytokines [104,106–108]. The pathological consequence of pyroptosis is represented by endothelial cell inflammation with subsequent endothelial dysfunction and is potentially the initial step in the continuum of myocardial injury [39].

In acute myocardial infarction, IL-1 plays multiple roles in the injury, repair, and remodeling processes, as depicted in Figure 2 [109]. Infarcted cardiomyocytes cause the release of IL-1α, epithelial injury stimulates the release of IL-1β, while monocytes are a source of IL-1β in acute coronary syndromes [110,111]. The inflammatory reaction that is normally involved in the clearance of dead cells and matrix detritus, could also extend the area of myocardial damage. Consequently, an auto-inflammatory loop is induced, as IL-1 recruits and activates more innate immune cells [43,111]. Stopping this inflammatory reaction is not a passive process, requiring anti-inflammatory mediators such as IL-10 and Transforming Growth Factor (TGF)-β which inactivate mononuclear cells and inhibit the transcription of IL-1, as well as other pro-resolving lipid mediators [43,109,112]. In ACS, elevated IL-1β levels are associated with diastolic dysfunction and remodeling [110,113]. Patients with more severe forms of COVID-19 might be at high risk, as it was demonstrated that elevated levels of IL-6 and high IL-1β levels are correlated with a poor prognosis in the setting of ACS [110,114].

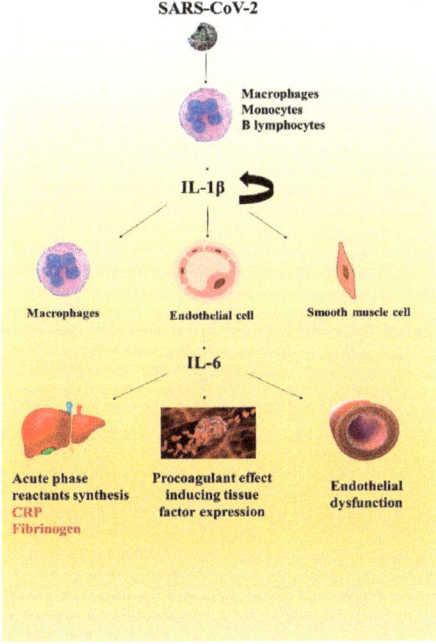

Figure 2. The inflammatory cascade during SARS-CoV-2 infection. IL-1β is synthesized by macrophages, monocytes, and B lymphocytes, and has the ability to self-induce its production and stimulate the synthesis of IL-6 in macrophages, endothelial cells, and smooth muscle cells [12,96,97]. Further, IL-6 determines the liver synthesis of acute phase reactants and exerts a pro-coagulant effect by inducing tissue factor synthesis, also causing endothelial dysfunction by increasing vascular permeability [108–110]. Legend: IL-1β: Interleukin 1β; IL-6: Interleukin-6; and CRP: C reactive protein.

Interleukin-6 family members, such as IL-6, IL-11, IL-30, IL-31, OSM, LIF, CNTF, CT-1, CT-2, and CLC, have an important role in heart disease pathogenesis as they exhibit pro-inflammatory, anti-inflammatory, and proatherogenic effects using different trans-signaling pathways [115]. IL-6 is synthesized by T lymphocytes, macrophages, and adipocytes, as well as by cardiovascular system structures such as endothelial cells, vascular smooth muscle cells, or ischemic cardiomyocytes [116]. It promotes inflammation through two signaling pathways, the *cis*-signaling pathway that uses the membrane IL-6 receptor and the *trans*-signaling pathway utilizing the soluble IL-6 receptor. The latter mechanism is utilized for activating and promoting inflammation in cells without the membrane receptor for IL-6 (e.g., endothelial cells) [117,118]. Increased IL-6 levels are essential for regulating the immune response, inducing the hepatic synthesis of acute phase biomarkers, and activating immune system cells and intercellular signaling. Through these mechanisms, IL-6 actively contributes to host defense, initiating the healing process of tissue injury [119]. By inducing the tissue factor expression on endothelial cells, this pro-inflammatory cytokine may also contribute to the occurrence of thrombotic complications [120].

IL-6 also plays a role in hematopoiesis, neurogenesis, and liver regeneration [121–123]. On one hand, it exhibits a short-term, prompt pro-inflammatory response for combating SARS-CoV-2 infection, thus having a protective effect [124]. On the other hand, the continuous synthesis of IL-6 has deleterious consequences, contributing to the development of inflammatory and autoimmune diseases [125]. The polymorphism of IL-6 is also observed at the cardiac level when its dual role is initially protective by limiting myocyte injury during acute myocardial infarction. In contrast, persistently elevated IL-6 levels in patients with acute myocardial infarction are associated with low left ventricular ejection fraction and HF [124,126].

IL-6 is involved in the development of ischemia-reperfusion injury, its deficiency having beneficial effects on infarct size, independently of IL-1β, TNFα levels, or neutrophil influx [127]. A meta-analysis conducted by Yang et al. has shown that the severity of acute coronary syndromes significantly correlates with IL-6 levels [128]. High IL-6 levels are associated with a decreased ejection fraction and a larger infarct size at the 4-month follow-up visit after STEMI [129]. Furthermore, in the ACS setting, IL-6 outperformed the accuracy of CRP in predicting long-term cardiovascular death [130]. The molecular mechanisms by which IL-6 causes cardiomyocytes' apoptosis and remodeling-related ischemia-reperfusion deserve a deeper insight. Nguyen et al. report high levels of IL-6 being a predictor of cardiovascular complications in COVID-19 patients [67] (Table 1). Persistently high levels of IL-6 during the recovery phase of the infection may contribute to impaired left ventricular function. Moreover, high levels of cTn suggesting ongoing myocardial injury were detected in these patients [131].

Table 1. Biomarkers suggesting acute cardiac injury in COVID-19.

IL-1β	High levels are associated with a hypercoagulable state and thrombotic events, worsening the prognosis [68]
IL-6	Elevated levels correlate with the occurrence of major adverse cardiac events and/or mortality risk [67]
IL-10	Increases ACE 2 expression and may promote endothelial cell infection and vasculitis [132]
TNF-α	Positively correlated with acute cardiac injury, disease severity, and high mortality rates in ICU patients [69]
IFN-γ	Elevated levels detected in cytokine storm cause multiple organ dysfunction [133]
CRP	Independent predictor of very high cardiac troponin levels, associated with high rates of all-cause mortality [134]
Troponin	High levels indicate a risk of death 8 to 21 times higher [10,11]
D-dimers	COVID-19-associated coagulopathy, biologically expressed through increased D-dimer and prolonged PT is a predictor of myocardial injury and poor prognosis [135]
NT-proBNP	Prognostic value similar to troponin in survival rates [136]
ST2	Superior prognostic value compared to NT-proBNP [88,137]

Interleukin 10 (IL-10) is an anti-inflammatory cytokine synthesized by various immune cells, including macrophages and lymphocytes. It exerts its anti-inflammatory effects by activating T lymphocytes and by directly inhibiting the innate immune-related functions of dendritic cells and macrophages [138]. In patients with SARS-CoV-2 infection, an early, substantial rise of IL-10 was observed, along with IL-6 as a disease severity predictor. Increased levels of IL-10 may be a consequence of the attempt to reduce the inflammatory response, thus preventing the cytokine storm [139].

Nevertheless, simultaneously high levels of IL-10 and pro-inflammatory cytokines, as well as the correlation with disease severity, may be explained either by the inability of the cytokine to reduce inflammation or by a dysregulated function [140–142]. Controversial evidence supporting the potential pro-inflammatory role of IL-10 outside of COVID-19 indicates that hyperactivation of CD8+ T cells and their functional exhaustion of this biomarker may contribute to the interplay of the cytokine storm [143]. The protective effect of IL-10 has been demonstrated in animal studies, with low levels being correlated with extensive atherosclerotic lesions, doubled by a higher risk of plaque rupture [144]. IL-10 wields an anti-atherogenic role from the initiation of plaque formation by modulating lipid metabolism in macrophages [119]. However, in human subjects, IL-10 levels are highly variable, being elevated, decreased, or stationary in patients with stable coronary artery disease or unstable angina, as compared to controls [145–147].

Furthermore, controversies persist also concerning IL-10's prognosis value; in patients with ACS, high IL-10 serum levels may be related to either an improved or worsened outcome [132,148,149]. Administration of recombinant IL-10 has been proposed by some authors for the therapeutic management of ARDS in COVID-19, but clinical evidence has shown that it might be detrimental as it promotes T cell exhaustion [34,141]. Further clinical studies are required in order to elucidate all of its functions and outline the complete profile of IL-10.

3.3. Tumor Necrosis Factor Alfa (TNF-α)

TNF-α is a pro-inflammatory cytokine promoting the SARS-CoV-2 interaction with ACE 2 and taking part in cytokine releasing syndrome (CRS) together with IL-1, IL-6, and IL-10. It is an important cytokine of the innate immune system, inhibiting viral replication and carcinogenesis [101]. Song et al. reported that plasma levels of TNF-α, IL-6, and CRP are positively correlated with acute cardiac injury [69].

3.4. D-Dimers

Assessing the inflammatory status in the evaluation of coagulant status is important since ubiquitous coagulation abnormalities are found in critically-ill patients. D-dimer levels have shown the same pattern as cTn in patients with severe forms of the disease, increasing progressively as patients' clinical status worsened [150]. The high affinity of SARS-CoV-2 for endothelial cells might induce apoptosis of vascular cells with the enhanced release of prothrombotic molecules, thereby triggering not only a local but also a systemic coagulopathy that may affect the pulmonary vessels as well as coronary arteries, with the subsequent microthrombi formation and extensive cardiopulmonary injury [38,151]. Accordingly, D-dimer serum levels represent an accurate predictor for mortality in COVID-19 pneumonia as it was demonstrated that these molecules may also reflect certain phenomena that are associated with illness severity, such as extravascular fibrinolysis, interstitial pulmonary edema, and lung injury in COVID-19 patients without venous thromboembolism [152]. Concerning optimal cut-off values indicative of a poor prognosis, literature data reported figures ranging from 1.5 to 2.1 mg/L [153,154].

3.5. C-Reactive Protein (CRP)

A surge in serum levels of CRP is a consistent finding in infectious pathology, with COVID-19 as no exception. CRP is a non-specific, liver-synthesized, acute-phase protein that is related to essential inflammatory and immune processes, such as apoptosis, phagocytosis, NO release, the complement pathway, and regulates cytokine production, such as IL-6 or TNF-α [155]. Moreover, extensive literature data highlighted that elevated CRP serum levels are independent predictors of mortality not only in COVID-19 [71] but also in patients with cardiovascular pathology, particularly related to atherothrombosis, thus outlining CRP as a dual, cardio-inflammatory biomarker, and a useful prognosis tool in the pandemic, given its routine, widespread measurement in clinical practice [156,157].

The use of high-sensitivity assays (hs-CRP) enhances its ability to identify severe forms of the disease in the early stages, as several data reported that especially high CRP levels occur in severe cases compared to non-severe ones, and higher concentrations being reported in COVID-19 patients who developed shock, ARDS, or acute cardiac injury [158,159]

Interestingly, a very recent study by Lionte et al. highlighted that elevated hs-CRP was associated with a poor prognosis in non-critically ill patients with COVID-19, thus further supporting the hypothesis of a sustained, both pulmonary and systemic impact, of SARS-CoV-2 related inflammation [160].

Another potentially useful prognosis tool is represented by the dynamic assessment of hs-CRP. The CRP velocity refers to the variation of this biomarker's serum levels after seriated measurements; recent results already demonstrate the correlation between increasing hs-CRP and a poorer LVEF following an acute myocardial infarction [161], the same pattern observed in the case of COVID-19's outcome, as reported in an extensive meta-analysis [162].

CRP has also been used as a therapeutic target in a small number of patients with respiratory failure and severe pulmonary infiltrates. After selective apheresis of CRP, an improvement in the radiological appearance was observed, suggesting that performing this technique immediately after admission could significantly reduce pulmonary injuries [163]. Two studies have established that patients with CRP values above 41.8 mg/L and 41.4 mg/L, respectively, have a higher risk of progressing to a severe form of the disease [164,165]. In patients already diagnosed with a severe form of COVID-19, our research team recently identified a high-risk CRP concentration cut-off; a value above 23 mg/L is associated with a negative vital prognosis [70].

3.6. N-Terminal Pro-Brain Natriuretic Peptide (NT-proBNP)

NT-proBNP is a "classical" biomarker in HF, being correlated with both elevated left ventricular filling pressures and systolic dysfunction [166]. In SARS-CoV-2 infection, the dynamic changes of NT-proBNP, CRP, and cTn concentrations are basically related to the extent of the inflammatory response, tissue injury, and functional impairment. Guo et al. reported higher levels of natriuretic peptides in severe forms of COVID-19 pneumonia, especially in deceased patients [26], while De Falco et al. showed that the prognosis value of NT-proBNP is similar to cTn, specifically for mortality risk stratification [136].

However, it is difficult to strictly correlate the presence of COVID-19 with the cardiovascular lesions evolving with increased biomarkers. Multiple studies have shown that elevated serum levels of cTn or NT-proBNP are similarly associated with a poor prognosis in a plethora of potentially COVID-19-related pathologies, such as pneumonia, septic shock, or acute respiratory distress syndrome [88,167,168]. For example, patients with pneumonia who had elevated concentrations of NT-proBNP were more prone to be admitted to ICU wards, regardless of the presence of cardiac dysfunction. There is growing evidence supporting the hypothesis of hypoxia-induced vasoconstriction that ultimately leads to pulmonary hypertension, which in turn may increase parietal RV stress in patients with extensive pulmonary lesions, thereby causing an increased NT-proBNP release from cardiomyocytes, a very plausible mechanism in the context of COVID-19 [168–170]. An additional inducer of myocardial parietal stress may be the widespread use of vasopressors in patients with septic shock, while acute kidney injury in severely ill patients may alter the clearance of NT-proBNP, leading to a false, non-cardiac increase in these biomarkers [88,170]. Other COVID-19-related causes for an increased NT-proBNP include oxidative stress, arrhythmias due to disease, per se, or due to its specific medications, and microvascular ischemia due to a demand-supply mismatch [82]. The importance of this mosaic characterized by high sensitivity and low specificity resides in the persistently strong correlation between NT-proBNP and mortality rates in severe COVID-19 patients, even after the exclusion of cases presenting HF [171].

Under these pandemic circumstances, it is essential to investigate a biomarker capable of detecting subclinical myocardial injury at an early stage in COVID-19 patients. For example, the soluble isoform of ST2 (sST2) is a very promising cardiac biomarker, not only for initial assessment but also for the long-term prognosis of patients with HF and COVID-19.

3.7. ST2

ST2 is a member of the extensive interleukin 1 (IL-1)/Toll-like receptor (TLR) family, more commonly known as interleukin 1 receptor-like 1 (IL1RL-1). Different cardiovascular effects of the ST2 molecule have been observed, depending on the isoform under which it is expressed: a transmembrane receptor form (ST2L) and a circulating, soluble, receptor form (sST2) that can be assessed in serum using various ELISA-based kits [88,137,168]. The ST2L also represents the receptor for IL-33, exercising cardioprotective actions through binding, such as inhibiting myocardial fibrosis, limiting ventricular hypertrophy, and preventing early apoptosis. On the other hand, the sequestration of IL-33 in the bloodstream by the decoy sST2 isoform prevents the occurrence of these positive effects, also representing the substrate of its high serum levels in patients with HF or with other myocardial injuries.

The diagnostic and prognostic role of ST2 in cardiovascular pathology has been validated by numerous studies, especially in patients with acute HF, as it is considered a reliable marker of fibrosis, ventricular wall strain, and increased filling pressures, also accurately predicting re-hospitalizations and fatal events [168,172–174].

The potential role of ST2 as a dual cardio-inflammatory biomarker was highlighted by some authors that observed abnormally elevated levels of sST2 in patients who tested positive for SARS-CoV-2 infection without presenting cardiovascular comorbidities [175]. Very interestingly, there is additional evidence reporting even a superior concentration of ST2 among COVID-19 patients compared to chronic, clinically stable HF [176,177].

The IL-33/ST2 axis also represents an essential pathway for pulmonary lesion and lung disease progression. IL-33 is an alarmin-type cytokine whose gene is overexpressed under stressful local conditions, such as an infection leading to alveolar injury or necrosis. As opposed to the positive effect at the myocardial level, the interaction between IL-33 and ST2L promotes inflammation by inducing the TGF β-mediated differentiation of T-cells and the increased secretion and release of pro-inflammatory cytokines or chemokines (e.g., IL-6, IL-1β, TNFα, IL-8, IL-4, IL-5, and IL-13), with a subsequent persistence and even amplification of inflammation's deleterious consequences. Therefore, the detection of high serum levels of sST2, the "decoy" receptor isoform, may suggest a regulatory mechanism for limiting inflammation and for preventing further inflammatory cell inflow and consecutive tissue damage [178]. Moreover, the IL-33/ST2 axis plays an important role in pulmonary fibrosis, as shown in two experimental models in which mice treated with a profibrotic substance exhibited a linear increase in IL-33 expression, an aspect explained by the alleged activation of fibroblasts by inflammatory cytokines triggered by the interaction between IL-33 and ST2L [179,180].

Based on these findings, it is reasonable to assume that COVID-19 may drastically activate the IL-33/ST2 system in a way similar to that observed for other inflammatory markers, directly affecting patients' outcomes via sST2's negative cardiovascular impact, such as pro-hypertrophic and pro-apoptotic effects [178,181].

Cytokine releasing syndrome (CRS) refers to a severely unregulated immune response to infection. The hallmark of CRS is represented by the proliferation and activation of lymphocytes and macrophages, followed by a significantly increased release of cytokines [182]. As previously mentioned, the cytokine superfamily comprises interleukins, chemokines, tumor necrosis factors, interferons, transforming growth factors, and colony-stimulating factors [96]. The upstream cytokine IL-1β induces IL-6 synthesis which increases vascular permeability, causing myocardial interstitial edema [183] and decreased myocardial contractility [184]. Cardiotoxicity, in the setting of CRS, is clinically expressed by left ventricular dysfunction, hypotension, and even cardiogenic shock [185]. Elevated levels of IL-6 in hospitalized patients with COVID-19 are directly correlated with high levels of cTn. These findings support the potential role of IL-6 in SARS-CoV-2-related acute cardiac injury during cytokine storms [34].

The COVID-19 pandemic turned the spotlight on the routine determination of cardiac biomarkers in SARS-CoV-2 infected patients. Multiple studies already confirmed that cTn, NT-proBNP, ST2, IL-6, IL-10, IL-1, and TNF-α represent relevant biomarkers that are useful for risk stratification in patients with acute cardiac injury due to COVID-19 pneumonia [88]. Moreover, given the well-established relationship between inflammation and atherosclerosis, a reasonable approach would consist of an assessment of subclinical markers of atherosclerosis, such as carotid intima-media thickness, pulse wave velocity, and ankle-brachial index, which are readily determined and well correlated with multiple cardiovascular risk scores, such as SCORE or Framingham [186]. Keeping in mind the socioeconomic challenges associated with the pandemic and the increased prevalence of cardiovascular comorbidities among admitted patients, we consider that judicious use of all these available diagnostic and prognostic biomarkers may facilitate the identification of individuals with a high-risk profile, thus allowing a prompt and adequate therapeutic intervention, as the limitation of myocardial injury during SARS-CoV-2 infection is of paramount importance for both short and long-term prognosis [134,187].

4. Novel Therapeutic Strategies: The Frontline against Inflammation

Studies investigating the efficacy of IL-1 and IL-6 inhibition in lowering mortality rates in patients with SARS-CoV-2 infection have controversial results at the moment, but several trials are currently underway [188]. Biologic response modifiers, also known as immunomodulators, are being used as targeted drug therapy in autoimmune diseases and cancers [189]. The protective myocardial role of immunomodulatory therapies is reported for Tocilizumab and Sarilumab monoclonal antibodies, being agents that block both the soluble and the membrane IL-6 receptors. Additionally, these molecules have been shown to play a significant role in reducing systemic inflammation. Despite its negative effect on the lipid profile, Tocilizumab administration in patients with high cardiovascular risk has led to outstanding improvement in endothelial function [190]. Elevated levels of proinflammatory biomarkers during COVID-19 increase the risk of acute myocardial infarction, but also have an impact on its size [191]. The effectiveness of Tocilizumab in limiting the infarction area and improving the prognosis was demonstrated in a randomized, double-blind, placebo-controlled trial evaluating the myocardial rescue index. Broch et al. have found that the myocardial rescue index measured by magnetic resonance imaging was significantly higher after Tocilizumab administration. Less extensive microvascular obstruction and a significant reduction in CRP levels have also been observed in patients receiving the IL-6 receptor blocker [56]. Tocilizumab was not effective for significantly reducing levels of troponin and NT-proBNP in patients hospitalized with COVID-19. Moreover, an IL-6 blockade was not notably associated with reduced mortality rates in patients admitted for SARS-CoV-2 infection, complications with ARDS, and exacerbated inflammation [188,192].

Different regimens of Anakinra, a recombinant IL-1 receptor antagonist, administered early in patients with moderate immune hyperactivation during COVID-19 pneumonia were associated with reduced mortality risk and a good safety profile [192–194]. Conversely, in a randomized double-blinded controlled-placebo trial, Canakinumab, a fully human monoclonal antibody neutralizing IL-1β, did not significantly increase survivability [195]. The Three C Study, an ongoing randomized controlled trial (NCT04365153) is investigating the role of Canakinumab in improving outcomes in patients with SARS-CoV2-associated myocardial injury and hyperinflammatory status. The dynamics of cardiac enzymes and cardiac function should be further investigated in patients with acute cardiac injury or even ACS and COVID-19 receiving monoclonal antibodies. Promising evidence regarding the effect of immunomodulatory strategies in the setting of ACS is currently emerging, as Canakinumab demonstrated a reduction in mortality and hospitalization for HF in patients with a personal history of myocardial infarction and elevated CRP [104]. Moreover, the use of Anakinra in patients with STEMI decreased all-cause mortality and incidence of newly diagnosed HF without affecting the left ventricular ejection fraction compared to placebo [10]. These data suggest that drugs targeting cytokines may be effective in limiting myocardial damage in SARS-CoV-2 infection as well.

Taken together, IL-6 inhibition yields no benefit in COVID-19 pneumonia progression, while an IL-1 blockade has shown only moderate benefit. A more robust clinical positive impact exerted by IL-1 might be its upstream position in the inflammatory cascade; compared to IL-6, a successful IL-1 inhibition potentially leads to the downstream suppression of IL-6 and other inflammatory biomarkers [104,192]. A current matter of debate and future investigations is if an IL-6 and IL-1 blockade truly offers advantages over the standard management in COVID-19, particularly if associated with acute cardiac injury. Additional studies regarding the benefit, safety, and regimens of immunotherapy in preventing and treating the cardiovascular complications of COVID-19 are needed [97,180,185,196].

5. Conclusions

Currently, it is generally accepted that the SARS-CoV-2 infection is associated with an increased prevalence of acute cardiac injury, regardless of potential underlying cardiac causes. The abnormal immune response, endothelial dysfunction, and O_2 supply-demand imbalance are the essential pathophysiological mechanisms contributing to the disease severity in COVID-19, while also being common features in acute cardiac injury. Direct myocardial injury, along with a plethora of indirect mechanisms, represents the substrate of myocardial damage in SARS-CoV-2-related acute cardiac injury pathogenesis. The occurrence of myocardial injury portends a severe course of the disease and is an independent predictor of mortality, therefore an early diagnosis combined with prompt therapeutic management represents the cornerstones for the short-term prognosis of infected patients. In this context, it is essential to make use of the full array of diagnostic tools, highlighting the growing role of cardio-inflammatory biomarkers. An effective assessment of inflammatory status may act as a bridge toward the identification of new, effective, therapeutic strategies that address both COVID-19 and the eventual cardiovascular complications.

Funding: This research received no external funding.

Conflicts of Interest: The authors declare no conflict of interest.

References

1. Clerkin, K.J.; Fried, J.A.; Raikhelkar, J.; Sayer, G.; Griffin, J.M.; Masoumi, A.; Burkhoff, D.; Kumaraiah, D.; Rabbani, L.; Schwartz, A.; et al. Coronavirus disease 2019 (COVID-19) and cardiovascular disease. *Circulation* **2020**, *141*, 1648–1655. [CrossRef] [PubMed]
2. Paludan, S.R.; Mogensen, T.H. Innate immunological pathways in COVID-19 pathogenesis. *Sci. Immunol.* **2022**, *7*, eabm5505. [CrossRef] [PubMed]
3. Shaobo, S.; Mu, Q.; Yuli, C.; Tao, L.; Bo, S.; Fan, Y.; Sheng, C.; Xu, L.; Yaozu, X.; Qinyan, Z.; et al. Characteristics and clinical significance of myocardial injury in patients with severe coronavirus disease 2019. *Eur. Heart J.* **2020**, *41*, 2070–2079. [CrossRef]
4. Izquierdo, A.; Mojón, D.; Bardají, A.; Carrasquer, A.; Calvo-Fernández, A.; Carreras-Mora, J.; Giralt, T.; Pérez-Fernández, S.; Farré, N.; Soler, C.; et al. Myocardial Injury as a Prognostic Factor in Mid- and Long-Term Follow-Up of COVID-19 Survivors. *J. Clin. Med.* **2021**, *10*, 5900. [CrossRef] [PubMed]
5. Chen, T.; Wu, D.; Chen, H. Clinical characteristics of 113 deceased patients with coronavirus disease 2019: Retrospective study. *BMJ* **2020**, *368*, m1091. [CrossRef] [PubMed]
6. Lu, Y.F.; Pan, L.Y.; Zhang, W.W.; Cheng, F.; Hu, S.S.; Zhang, X.; Jiang, H.Y. A meta-analysis of the incidence of venous thromboembolic events and impact of anticoagulation on mortality in patients with COVID-19. *Int. J. Infect. Dis.* **2020**, *100*, 34–41. [CrossRef] [PubMed]
7. Wang, D.; Hu, B.; Hu, C.; Zhu, F.; Liu, X.; Zhang, J.; Wang, B.; Xiang, H.; Cheng, Z.; Xiong, Y.; et al. Clinical Characteristics of 138 Hospitalized Patients With 2019 Novel Coronavirus-Infected Pneumonia in Wuhan, China. *JAMA* **2020**, *323*, 1061–1069. [CrossRef] [PubMed]
8. Xie, Y.; Xu, E.; Bowe, B. Long-term cardiovascular outcomes of COVID-19. *Nat. Med.* **2022**, *28*, 583–590. [CrossRef] [PubMed]
9. Deng, F.; Zhao, Q.; Deng, Y.; Wu, Y.; Zhou, D.; Liu, W.; Yuan, Z.; Zhou, J. Prognostic significance and dynamic change of plasma macrophage migration inhibitory factor in patients with acute ST-elevation myocardial infarction. *Medicine* **2018**, *97*, e12991. [CrossRef]
10. Abate, S.M.; Mantefardo, B.; Nega, S.; Chekole, Y.A.; Basu, B.; Ali, S.A.; Taddesse, M. Global burden of acute myocardial injury associated with COVID-19: A systematic review, meta-analysis, and meta-regression. *Ann. Med. Surg.* **2012**, *68*, 102594. [CrossRef] [PubMed]
11. Li, X.; Guan, B.; Su, T.; Liu, W.; Chen, M.; Bin-Waleed, K.; Guan, X.; Gary, T.; Zhu, Z. Impact of cardiovascular disease and cardiac injury on in-hospital mortality in patients with COVID-19: A systematic review and meta-analysis. *Heart* **2020**, *106*, 1142–1147. [CrossRef] [PubMed]

12. Lala, A.; Johnson, K.W.; Januzzi, J.L.; Russak, A.J.; Paranjpe, I.; Richter, F.; Zhao, S.; Somani, S.; Van Vleck, T.; Vaid, A.; et al. Mount Sinai COVID Informatics Center. Prevalence and Impact of Myocardial Injury in Patients Hospitalized with COVID-19 Infection. *J. Am. Coll. Cardiol.* **2020**, *76*, 533–546. [CrossRef] [PubMed]
13. Lasica, R.; Djukanovic, L.; Mrdovic, I.; Savic, L.; Ristic, A.; Zdravkovic, M.; Simic, D.; Krljanac, G.; Popovic, D.; Simeunovic, D.; et al. Acute Coronary Syndrome in the COVID-19 Era—Differences and Dilemmas Compared to the Pre-COVID-19 Era. *J. Clin. Med.* **2022**, *11*, 3024. [CrossRef] [PubMed]
14. Schiavone, M.; Gobbi, C.; Biondi-Zoccai, G.; D'Ascenzo, F.; Palazzuoli, A.; Gasperetti, A.; Mitacchione, G.; Viecca, M.; Galli, M.; Fedele, F.; et al. Acute coronary syndromes and COVID-19: Exploring the uncertainties. *J. Clin. Med.* **2020**, *9*, 1683. [CrossRef] [PubMed]
15. De Rosa, S.; Spaccarotella, C.; Basso, C.; Calabrò, M.P.; Curcio, A.; Filardi, P.P.; Mancone, M.; Mercuro, G.; Muscoli, S.; Nodari, S.; et al. Reduction of hospitalizations for myocardial infarction in Italy in the COVID-19 era. *Eur. Heart J.* **2020**, *41*, 2083–2088. [CrossRef] [PubMed]
16. De Filippo, O.; D'Ascenzo, F.; Angelini, F.; Bocchino, P.P.; Conrotto, F.; Saglietto, A.; Secco, G.G.; Campo, G.; Gallone, G.; Verardi, R.; et al. Reduced Rate of Hospital Admissions for ACS during COVID-19 Outbreak in Northern Italy. *N. Engl. J. Med.* **2020**, *383*, 88–89. [CrossRef] [PubMed]
17. Hamadeh, A.; Aldujeli, A.; Briedis, K.; Tecson, K.M.; Sanz-Sánchez, J.; Al Dujeili, M.; Al-Obeidi, A.; Diez, J.L.; Žaliūnas, R.; Stoler, R.C.; et al. Characteristics and Outcomes in Patients Presenting With COVID-19 and ST-Segment Elevation Myocardial Infarction. *Am. J. Cardiol.* **2020**, *131*, 1–6. [CrossRef]
18. Xiang, D.; Xiang, X.; Zhang, W.; Yi, S.; Zhang, J.; Gu, X.; Xu, Y. Management and Outcomes of Patients with STEMI During the COVID-19 Pandemic in China. *J. Am. Coll. Cardiol.* **2020**, *76*, 1318–1324. [CrossRef] [PubMed]
19. Basu-Ray, I.; Almaddah, N.K.; Adeboye, A.; Soos, M.P. *Cardiac Manifestations of Coronavirus (COVID-19)*; StatPearls: Treasure Island, FL, USA, 2022.
20. Hendren, N.S.; Drazner, M.H.; Bozkurt, B.; Cooper, L.T., Jr. Description and Proposed Management of the Acute COVID-19 Cardiovascular Syndrome. *Circulation* **2020**, *141*, 1903–1914. [CrossRef]
21. Jackson, C.B.; Farzan, M.; Chen, B.; Choe, H. Mechanisms of SARS-CoV-2 entry into cells. *Nat. Rev. Mol. Cell. Biol.* **2022**, *23*, 3–20. [CrossRef] [PubMed]
22. Guzik, T.J.; Mohiddin, S.A.; Dimarco, A.; Patel, V.; Savvatis, K.; Marelli-Berg, F.; Madhur, M.S.; Tomaszewski, M.; Maffia, P.; D'Acquisto, F.; et al. COVID-19 and the cardiovascular system: Implications for risk assessment, diagnosis, and treatment options. *Cardiovasc. Res.* **2020**, *116*, 1666–1687. [CrossRef] [PubMed]
23. Zheng, Y.Y.; Ma, Y.T.; Zhang, J.Y.; Xie, X. COVID-19 and the cardiovascular system. *Nat. Rev. Cardiol.* **2020**, *17*, 259–260. [CrossRef]
24. Zhosbøl, E.L.; Butt, J.H.; Østergaard, L.; Andersson, C.; Selmer, C.; Kragholm, K.; Schou, M.; Phelps, M.; Gislason, G.H.; Gerds, T.A.; et al. Association of Angiotensin-Converting Enzyme Inhibitor or Angiotensin Receptor Blocker Use With COVID-19 Diagnosis and Mortality. *JAMA* **2020**, *324*, 168–177. [CrossRef]
25. Zhang, P.; Zhu, L.; Cai, J.; Lei, F.; Qin, J.J.; Xie, J.; Liu, Y.M.; Zhao, Y.C.; Huang, X.; Lin, L.; et al. Association of Inpatient Use of Angiotensin-Converting Enzyme Inhibitors and Angiotensin II Receptor Blockers with Mortality Among Patients with Hypertension Hospitalized With COVID-19. *Circ. Res.* **2020**, *126*, 1671–1681. [CrossRef]
26. Guo, T.; Fan, Y.; Chen, M.; Wu, X.; Zhang, L.; He, T.; Wang, H.; Wan, J.; Wang, X.; Lu, Z. Cardiovascular Implications of Fatal Outcomes of Patients with Coronavirus Disease 2019 (COVID-19). *JAMA Cardiol.* **2020**, *5*, 811–818. [CrossRef] [PubMed]
27. Imai, Y.; Kuba, K.; Rao, S.; Huan, Y.; Guo, F.; Guan, B.; Yang, P.; Sarao, R.; Wada, T.; Leong-Poi, H.; et al. Angiotensin-converting enzyme 2 protects from severe acute lung failure. *Nature* **2005**, *436*, 112–116. [CrossRef] [PubMed]
28. Liu, K.; Fang, Y.Y.; Deng, Y.; Liu, W.; Wang, M.F.; Ma, J.P.; Xiao, W.; Wang, Y.N.; Zhong, M.H.; Li, C.H.; et al. Clinical characteristics of novel coronavirus cases in tertiary hospitals in Hubei Province. *Chin. Med. J.* **2020**, *133*, 1025–1031. [CrossRef] [PubMed]
29. Kilic, T.; Ural, D.; Ural, E.; Yumuk, Z.; Agacdiken, A.; Sahin, T.; Kahraman, G.; Kozdag, G.; Vural, A.; Komsuoglu, B. Relation between proinflammatory to anti-inflammatory cytokine ratios and long-term prognosis in patients with non-ST elevation acute coronary syndrome. *Heart* **2006**, *92*, 1041–1046. [CrossRef] [PubMed]
30. Metkus, T.S.; Sokoll, L.J.; Barth, A.S.; Czarny, M.J.; Hays, A.G.; Lowenstein, C.J. Myocardial Injury in Severe COVID-19 Compared with Non-COVID-19 Acute Respiratory Distress Syndrome. *Circulation* **2021**, *143*, 553–565. [CrossRef] [PubMed]
31. Galani, I.E.; Rovina, N.; Lampropoulou, V.; Triantafyllia, V.; Manioudaki, M.; Pavlos, E. Untuned antiviral immunity inCOVID-19 revealed by temporal type I/III interferon patterns and flu comparison. *Nat. Immunol.* **2021**, *22*, 32–40. [CrossRef]
32. Sette, A.; Crotty, S. Adaptive immunity to SARS-CoV-2 and COVID-19. *Cell* **2021**, *184*, 861–880. [CrossRef]
33. Fajgenbaum, D.C.; June, C.H. Cytokine Storm. *N. Engl. J. Med.* **2020**, *383*, 2255–2273. [CrossRef] [PubMed]
34. Wu, C.; Hu, X.; Song, J.; Du, C.; Xu, J.; Yang, D.; Chen, D.; Zhong, M.; Jiang, J.; Xiong, W.; et al. Heart injury signs are associated with higher and earlier mortality in coronavirus disease 2019 (COVID-19). *medRxiv* 2002. [CrossRef]
35. Huertas, A.; Montani, D.; Savale, L.; Pichon, J.; Tu, L.; Parent, F.; Guignabert, C.; Humbert, M. Endothelial cell dysfunction: A major player in SARS-CoV-2 infection (COVID-19)? *Eur. Respir. J.* **2020**, *56*, 2001634. [CrossRef] [PubMed]
36. Koupenova, M.; Clancy, L.; Corkrey, H.A.; Freedman, J.E. Circulating platelets as mediators of immunity, inflammation, and thrombosis. *Circ. Res.* **2018**, *122*, 337–351. [CrossRef]
37. Varga, Z.; Flammer, A.J.; Steiger, P.; Haberecker, M.; Andermatt, R.; Zinkernagel, A.S.; Mehra, M.R.; Schuepbach, R.A.; Ruschitzka, F.; Moch, H. Endothelial cell infection and endotheliitis in COVID-19. *Lancet* **2020**, *395*, 1417–1418. [CrossRef]

38. Koupenova, M.; Kehrel, B.E.; Corkrey, H.A.; Freedman, J.E. Thrombosis and platelets: An update. *Eur. Heart J.* **2017**, *38*, 785–791. [CrossRef]
39. Gómez-Mesa, J.E.; Galindo-Coral, S.; Montes, M.C.; Muñoz Martin, A.J. Thrombosis and Coagulopathy in COVID-19. *Curr. Probl. Cardiol.* **2021**, *46*, 100742. [CrossRef]
40. Kipshidze, N.; Dangas, G.; White, C.J.; Kipshidze, N.; Siddiqui, F.; Lattimer, C.R.; Carter, C.A.; Fareed, J. Viral Coagulopathy in Patients with COVID-19: Treatment and Care. *Clin. Appl. Thromb. Hemost.* **2020**, *26*, 1076029620936776. [CrossRef] [PubMed]
41. Wolf, D.; Ley, K. Immunity and Inflammation in Atherosclerosis. *Circ. Res.* **2019**, *124*, 315–327. [CrossRef]
42. Cohen, M.; Visveswaran, G. Defining and managing patients with non-ST-elevation myocardial infarction: Sorting through type 1 vs other types. *Clin. Cardiol.* **2020**, *43*, 242–250. [CrossRef] [PubMed]
43. Eposito, L.; Cancro, F.P.; Silverio, A.; Di Maio, M.; Iannece, P.; Damato, A.; Alfano, C.; De Luca, G.; Vecchione, C.; Galasso, G. COVID-19 and Acute Coronary Syndromes: From Pathophysiology to Clinical Perspectives. *Oxid. Med. Cell. Longev.* **2021**, *2021*, 4936571. [CrossRef]
44. Katsoularis, I.; Fonseca-Rodríguez, O.; Farrington, P.; Lindmark, K.; Connolly, A.-M.F. Risk of acute myocardial infarction and ischaemic stroke following COVID-19 in Sweden: A self-controlled case series and matched cohort study. *Lancet* **2021**, *398*, 599–607. [CrossRef]
45. Shaw, P.; Senguttuvan, N.B.; Raymond, G.; Sankar, S.; Mukherjee, A.G.; Kunale, M.; Kodiveri Muthukaliannan, G.; Baxi, S.; Mani, R.R.; Rajagopal, M.; et al. COVID-19 Outcomes in Patients Hospitalised with Acute Myocardial Infarction (AMI): A Protocol for Systematic Review and Meta-Analysis. *COVID* **2022**, *2*, 138–147. [CrossRef]
46. Modin, D.; Claggett, B.; Sindet-Pedersen, C.; Lassen, M.C.H.; Skaarup, K.G.; Jensen, J.U.S.; Fralick, M.; Schou, M.; Lamberts, M.; Gerds, T.; et al. Acute COVID-19 and the Incidence of Ischemic Stroke and Acute Myocardial Infarction. *Circulation* **2020**, *142*, 2080–2082. [CrossRef] [PubMed]
47. Min, C.K.; Cheon, S.; Ha, N.Y.; Sohn, K.M.; Kim, Y.; Aigerim, A.; Kim, Y.S.; Shin, H.M.; Choi, J.Y.; Inn, K.S.; et al. Comparative and kinetic analysis of viral shedding and immunological responses in MERS patients representing a broad spectrum of disease severity. *Sci. Rep.* **2016**, *6*, 25359. [CrossRef]
48. Sagris, M.; Theofilis, P.; Antonopoulos, A.S.; Tsioufis, C.; Oikonomou, E.; Antoniades, C.; Crea, F.; Kaski, J.C.; Tousoulis, D. Inflammatory Mechanisms in COVID-19 and Atherosclerosis: Current Pharmaceutical Perspectives. *Int. J. Mol. Sci.* **2021**, *22*, 6607. [CrossRef]
49. Guizani, I.; Fourti, N.; Zidi, W.; Feki, M.; Allal-Elasmi, M. SARS-CoV-2 and pathological matrix remodeling mediators. *Inflamm. Res.* **2021**, *70*, 847–858. [CrossRef]
50. Kattoor, A.J.; Pothineni, N.V.K.; Palagiri, D.; Mehta, J.L. Oxidative Stress in Atherosclerosis. *Curr. Atheroscler. Rep.* **2017**, *19*, 42. [CrossRef]
51. Ridker, P.M.; Danielson, E.; Fonseca, F.A.; Genest, J.; Gotto, A.M.; Kastelein, J.J.; Koenig, W.; Libby, P.; Lorenzatti, A.J.; MacFadyen, J.G.; et al. Rosuvastatin to prevent vascular events in men and women with elevated C-reactive protein. *N. Engl. J. Med.* **2008**, *359*, 2195–2207. [CrossRef]
52. Bergqvist, R.; Ahlqvist, V.H.; Lundberg, M.; Hergens, M.P.; Sundström, J.; Bell, M.; Magnusson, C. HMG-CoA reductase inhibitors and COVID-19 mortality in Stockholm, Sweden: A registry-based cohort study. *PLoS Med.* **2021**, *18*, e1003820. [CrossRef] [PubMed]
53. Tang, Y.; Hu, L.; Liu, Y.; Zhou, B.; Qin, X.; Ye, J.; Shen, M.; Wu, Z.; Zhang, P. Possible mechanisms of cholesterol elevation aggravating COVID-19. *Int. J. Med. Sci.* **2021**, *18*, 3533–3543. [CrossRef] [PubMed]
54. Theofilis, P.; Sagris, M.; Antonopoulos, A.S.; Oikonomou, E.; Tsioufis, C.; Tousoulis, D. Inflammatory Mediators of Platelet Activation: Focus on Atherosclerosis and COVID-19. *Int. J. Mol. Sci.* **2021**, *22*, 11170. [CrossRef] [PubMed]
55. Keeley, E.C.; Boura, J.A.; Grines, C.L. Primary angioplasty versus intravenous thrombolytic therapy for acute myocardial infarction: A quantitative review of 23 randomised trials. *Lancet* **2003**, *361*, 13–20. [CrossRef]
56. Broch, K.; Anstensrud, A.K.; Woxholt, S.; Sharma, K.; Tøllefsen, I.M.; Bendz, B.; Aakhus, S.; Ueland, T.; Amundsen, B.H.; Damås, J.K.; et al. Randomized Trial of Interleukin-6 Receptor Inhibition in Patients with Acute ST-Segment Elevation Myocardial Infarction. *J. Am. Coll. Cardiol.* **2021**, *77*, 1845–1855. [CrossRef]
57. Ezekowitz, J.A.; Kaul, P.; Bakal, J.A.; Armstrong, P.W.; Welsh, R.C.; McAlister, F.A. Declining in-hospital mortality and increasing heart failure incidence in elderly patients with first myocardial infarction. *J. Am. Coll. Cardiol.* **2009**, *53*, 13–20. [CrossRef]
58. Halade, G.V.; Lee, D.H. Inflamation and resolution signaling in cardiac repair and heart failure. *eBioMedicine* **2022**, *79*, 103992. [CrossRef]
59. Giustino, G.; Pinney, S.P.; Lala, A.; Reddy, V.Y.; Johnston-Cox, H.A.; Mechanick, J.I.; Halperin, J.L.; Fuster, V. Coronavirus and cardiovascular disease, myocardial injury, and arrhythmia: JACC focus seminar. *J. Am. Coll. Cardiol.* **2020**, *76*, 2011–2023. [CrossRef]
60. Manolis, A.S.; Manolis, A.A.; Manolis, T.A.; Melita, H. COVID-19 and Acute Myocardial Injury and Infarction: Related Mechanisms and Emerging Challenges. *J. Cardiovasc. Pharmacol. Ther.* **2021**, *26*, 399–414. [CrossRef]
61. Pergola, V.; Cabrelle, G.; Previtero, M.; Fiorencis, A.; Lorenzoni, G.; Dellino, C.M.; Montonati, C.; Continisio, S.; Masetto, E.; Mele, D.; et al. Impact of the "atherosclerotic pabulum" on in-hospital mortality for SARS-CoV-2 infection. Is calcium score able to identify at-risk patients? *Clin. Cardiol.* **2022**, *45*, 629–640. [CrossRef]
62. Greer, J.R. Pathophysiology of cardiovascular dysfunction in sepsis. *BJA Educ.* **2015**, *15*, 316–321. [CrossRef]

63. Basso, C.; Leone, O.; Rizzo, S.; De Gaspari, M.; van der Wal, A.C.; Aubry, M.C.; Bois, M.C.; Lin, P.T.; Maleszewski, J.J.; Stone, J.R. Pathological features of COVID-19 associated myocardial injury: A multicentre cardiovascular pathology study. *Eur. Heart J.* **2020**, *41*, 3827–3835. [CrossRef] [PubMed]
64. Shamsi, F.; Hasan, K.Y.; Hashmani, S.; Jamal, S.F.; Ellaham, S. Review Article—Clinical Overview of Myocardial Infarction Without Obstructive Coronary Artey Disease (MINOCA). *J. Saudi. Heart. Assoc.* **2021**, *33*, 9–15. [CrossRef] [PubMed]
65. Sheikh, A.B.; Ijaz, Z.; Javed, N.; Upadyay, S.; Shekhar, R. COVID-19 with non-obstructive coronary artery disease in a young adult. *J. Community Hosp. Int. Med. Perspect.* **2021**, *11*, 111–114. [CrossRef] [PubMed]
66. Italia, L.; Tomasoni, D.; Bisegna, S.; Pancaldi, E.; Stretti, L.; Adamo, M.; Metra, M. COVID-19 and Heart Failure: From Epidemiology During the Pandemic to Myocardial Injury, Myocarditis, and Heart Failure Sequelae. *Front. Cardiovasc. Med.* **2021**, *8*, 713560. [CrossRef]
67. Nguyen, N.; Nguyen, H.; Ukoha, C.; Hoang, L.; Patel, C.; Ikram, F.G.; Acharya, P.; Dhillon, A.; Sidhu, M. Relation of interleukin-6 levels in COVID-19 patients with major adverse cardiac events. *Bayl. Univ. Med. Cent. Proc.* **2021**, *3*, 6–9. [CrossRef]
68. Rad, F.; Dabbagh, A.; Dorgalaleh, A.; Biswas, A. The Relationship between Inflammatory Cytokines and Coagulopathy in Patients with COVID-19. *J. Clin. Med.* **2021**, *10*, 2020. [CrossRef]
69. Song, Y.; Gao, P.; Ran, T.; Qian, H.; Guo, F.; Chang, L.; Wu, W.; Zhang, S. High Inflammatory Burden: A Potential Cause of Myocardial Injury in Critically Ill Patients With COVID-19. *Front. Cardiovasc. Med.* **2020**, *7*, 128. [CrossRef]
70. Timpau, A.S.; Miftode, R.; Petris, A.O.; Costache, I.I.; Miftode, I.L.; Rosu, F.M.; Anton-Paduraru, D.T.; Leca, D.; Miftode, E.G. Mortality Predictors in Severe COVID-19 Patients from an East European Tertiary Center: A Never-Ending Challenge for a No Happy Ending Pandemic. *J. Clin. Med.* **2021**, *11*, 58. [CrossRef]
71. Siripanthong, B.; Nazarian, S.; Muser, D.; Deo, R.; Santangeli, P.; Khanji, M.Y.; Cooper, L.T., Jr.; Chahal, C.A.A. Recognizing COVID-19-related myocarditis: The possible pathophysiology and proposed guideline for diagnosis and management. *Heart Rhythm* **2020**, *17*, 1463–1471. [CrossRef]
72. Dabbagh, M.F.; Aurora, L.; D'Souza, P.; Weinmann, A.J.; Bhargava, P.; Basir, M.B. Cardiac tamponade secondary to COVID-19. *J. Am. Coll. Cardiol.* **2020**, *2*, 1326–1330. [CrossRef]
73. Fernandes, F.; Ramires, F.J.A.; Fernandes, F.D.; Simões, M.V.; Mesquita, E.T.; Mady, C. Pericardial Affections in Patients with COVID-19: A Possible Cause of Hemodynamic Deterioration. *Arq. Bras. Cardiol.* **2020**, *115*, 569–573. [CrossRef]
74. Imazio, M.; Spodick, D.H.; Brucato, A.; Trinchero, R.; Adler, Y. Controversial issues in the management of pericardial diseases. *Circulation* **2010**, *121*, 916–928. [CrossRef]
75. Priyadarshni, S.; Westra, J.; Kuo, Y.F.; Baillargeon, J.G.; Khalife, W.; Raji, M. COVID-19 Infection and Incidence of Myocarditis: A Multi-Site Population-Based Propensity Score-Matched Analysis. *Cureus* **2022**, *14*, e21879. [CrossRef]
76. Ammirati, E.; Lupi, L.; Palazzini, M.; Hendren, N.S.; Grodin, J.L.; Cannistraci, C.V.; Schmidt, M.; Hekimian, G.; Peretto, G.; Bochaton, T.; et al. Prevalence, Characteristics, and Outcomes of COVID-19-Associated Acute Myocarditis. *Circulation* **2022**, *145*, 1123–1139. [CrossRef]
77. Singer, M.E.; Taub, I.B.; Kaelber, D.C. Risk of Myocarditis from COVID-19 Infection in People Under Age 20: A Population-Based Analysis. *medRxiv* 2022. [CrossRef]
78. Imazio, M.; Gaita, F. Diagnosis and treatment of pericarditis. *Heart* **2015**, *101*, 1159–1168. [CrossRef]
79. Lindner, D.; Fitzek, A.; Bräuninger, H.; Aleshcheva, G.; Edler, C.; Meissner, K.; Scherschel, K.; Kirchhof, P.; Escher, F.; Schultheiss, H.P.; et al. Association of Cardiac Infection With SARS-CoV-2 in Confirmed COVID-19 Autopsy Cases. *JAMA Cardiol.* **2020**, *5*, 1281–1285. [CrossRef]
80. Kažukauskienė, I.; Baltrūnienė, V.; Jakubauskas, A.; Žurauskas, E.; Maneikienė, V.V.; Daunoravičius, D.; Čelutkienė, J.; Ručinskas, K.; Grabauskienė, V. Prevalence and prognostic relevance of myocardial inflammation and cardiotropic viruses in non-ischemic dilated cardiomyopathy. *Cardiol. J.* **2022**, *29*, 441–453. [CrossRef]
81. Natanson, C.; Eichenholz, P.W.; Danner, R.L. Endotoxin and tumor necrosis factor challenges in dogs simulate the cardiovascular profile of human septic shock. *J. Exp. Med.* **1989**, *169*, 823–832. [CrossRef]
82. L'Heureux, M.; Sternberg, M.; Brath, L.; Turlington, J.; Kashiouris, M.G. Sepsis-Induced Cardiomyopathy: A Comprehensive Review. *Curr. Cardiol. Rep.* **2020**, *22*, 35. [CrossRef]
83. Ehrman, R.R.; Sullivan, A.N.; Favot, M.J.; Sherwin, R.L.; Reynolds, C.A.; Abidov, A.; Levy, P.D. Pathophysiology, echocardiographic evaluation, biomarker findings, and prognostic implications of septic cardiomyopathy: A review of the literature. *Crit. Care* **2018**, *22*, 112. [CrossRef]
84. Vasques-Nóvoa, F.; Laundos, T.L.; Madureira, A.; Bettencourt, N.; Nunes, J.P.L.; Carneiro, F.; Paiva, J.A.; Pinto-do-Ó, P.; Nascimento, D.S.; Leite-Moreira, A.F.; et al. Myocardial Edema: An Overlooked Mechanism of Septic Cardiomyopathy? *Shock* **2020**, *53*, 616–619. [CrossRef]
85. Salah, H.M.; Mehta, J.L. Takotsubo cardiomyopathy and COVID-19 infection. *Eur. Heart J. Cardiovasc. Imaging* **2020**, *21*, 1299–1300. [CrossRef]
86. Sisti, N.; Valente, S.; Mandoli, G.E.; Santoro, C.; Sciaccaluga, C.; Franchi, F.; Cameli, P.; Mondillo, S.; Cameli, M. COVID-19 in patients with heart failure: The new and the old epidemic. *Postgad. Med. J.* **2021**, *97*, 175–179. [CrossRef]
87. Park, J.F.; Banerjee, S.; Umar, S. In the eye of the storm: The right ventricle in COVID-19. *Pulm. Circ.* **2020**, *10*, 2045894020936660. [CrossRef]

88. Miftode, R.S.; Petriș, A.O.; Onofrei Aursulesei, V.; Cianga, C.; Costache, I.I.; Mitu, O.; Miftode, I.L.; Șerban, I.L. The Novel Perspectives Opened by ST2 in the Pandemic: A Review of Its Role in the Diagnosis and Prognosis of Patients with Heart Failure and COVID-19. *Diagnostics* **2021**, *11*, 175. [CrossRef]
89. Alserawan, L.; Peñacoba, P.; Orozco Echevarría, S.E.; Castillo, D.; Ortiz, E.; Martínez-Martínez, L.; Moga Naranjo, E.; Domingo, P.; Castellví, I.; Juárez, C.; et al. Growth Differentiation Factor 15 (GDF-15): A Novel Biomarker Associated with Poorer Respiratory Function in COVID-19. *Diagnostics* **2021**, *11*, 1998. [CrossRef]
90. Miftode, R.S.; Constantinescu, D.; Cianga, C.M.; Petris, A.O.; Timpau, A.-S.; Crisan, A.; Costache, I.I.; Mitu, O.; Anton-Paduraru, D.T.; Miftode, I.L.; et al. A Novel Paradigm Based on ST2 and Its Contribution towards a Multimarker Approach in the Diagnosis and Prognosis of Heart Failure: A Prospective Study during the Pandemic Storm. *Life* **2021**, *11*, 1080. [CrossRef]
91. Kaufmann, C.C.; Ahmed, A.; Burger, A.L.; Muthspiel, M.; Jäger, B.; Wojta, J.; Huber, K. Biomarkers Associated with Cardiovascular Disease in COVID-19. *Cells* **2022**, *11*, 922. [CrossRef]
92. Zethelius, B.; Johnston, N.; Venge, P. Troponin I as a predictor of coronary heart disease and mortality in 70-year-old men: A community-based cohort study. *Circulation* **2006**, *113*, 1071–1078. [CrossRef]
93. Gaze, D.C. Clinical utility of cardiac troponin measurement in COVID-19 infection. *Ann. Clin. Bioch.* **2020**, *57*, 202–205. [CrossRef]
94. Wibowo, A.; Pranata, R.; Akbar, M.R.; Purnomowati, A.; Martha, J.W. Prognostic performance of troponin in COVID-19: A diagnostic meta-analysis and meta-regression. *Int. J. Infect. Dis.* **2021**, *105*, 312–318. [CrossRef] [PubMed]
95. Wereski, R.; Kimenai, D.M.; Taggart, C.; Doudesis, D.; Lee, K.K.; Lowry, M.T.H.; Bularga, A.; Lowe, D.J.; Fujisawa, T.; Apple, F.S.; et al. Cardiac Troponin Thresholds and Kinetics to Differentiate Myocardial Injury and Myocardial Infarction. *Circulation* **2021**, *144*, 528–538. [CrossRef] [PubMed]
96. Zhou, F.; Yu, T.; Du, R.; Fan, G.; Liu, Y.; Liu, Z.; Xiang, J.; Wang, Y.; Song, B.; Gu, X.; et al. Clinical course and risk factors for mortality of adult inpatients with COVID-19 in Wuhan, China: A retrospective cohort study. *Lancet* **2020**, *395*, 1054–1062. [CrossRef]
97. Shi, S.; Qin, M.; Shen, B.; Cai, Y.; Liu, T.; Yang, F.; Gong, W.; Liu, X.; Liang, J.; Zhao, Q.; et al. Association of Cardiac Injury with Mortality in Hospitalized Patients With COVID-19 in Wuhan, China. *JAMA Cardiol.* **2020**, *5*, 802–810. [CrossRef]
98. Akwe, J.; Halford, B.; Kim, E.; Miller, A. A Review of Cardiac and Non-Cardiac Causes of Troponin Elevation and Clinical Relevance Part II Non Cardiac Causes. *J. Cardiol. Curr. Res.* **2018**, *11*, 00364. [CrossRef]
99. McCarthy, C.P.; Raber, I.; Chapman, A.R.; Sandoval, Y.; Apple, F.S.; Mills, N.L.; Januzzi, J.L., Jr. Myocardial Injury in the Era of High-Sensitivity Cardiac Troponin Assays: A Practical Approach for Clinicians. *JAMA Cardiol.* **2019**, *4*, 1034–1042. [CrossRef]
100. Nishiga, M.; Wang, D.W.; Han, Y.; Lewis, D.B.; Wu, J.C. COVID-19 and cardiovascular disease: From basic mechanisms to clinical perspectives. *Nat. Rev. Cardiol.* **2020**, *17*, 543–558. [CrossRef]
101. Guo, Y.; Hu, K.; Li, Y.; Lu, C.; Ling, K.; Cai, C.; Wang, W.; Ye, D. Targeting TNF-α for COVID-19: Recent Advanced and Controversies. *Front. Public Health* **2022**, *10*, 833967. [CrossRef]
102. Piccioni, A.; Brigida, M.; Loria, V.; Zanza, C.; Longhitano, Y.; Zaccaria, R.; Racco, S.; Gasbarrini, A.; Ojetti, V.; Franceschi, F.; et al. Role of troponin in COVID-19 pandemic: A review of literature. *Eur. Rev. Med. Pharmacol. Sci.* **2020**, *24*, 10293–10300. [CrossRef] [PubMed]
103. Januzzi, J.L. Troponin and BNP Use in COVID-19. *Cardiol. Mag.* **2020**, *18*. Available online: https://www.acc.org/latest-in-cardiology/articles/2020/03/18/15/25/troponin-and-bnp-use-in-covid19 (accessed on 15 May 2022).
104. Dinarello, C.A. Interleukin-1 in the pathogenesis and treatment of inflammatory diseases. *Blood* **2011**, *117*, 3720–3732. [CrossRef] [PubMed]
105. McGonagle, D.; Sharif, K.; O'Regan, A.; Bridgewood, C. The Role of Cytokines including Interleukin-6 in COVID-19 induced Pneumonia and Macrophage Activation Syndrome-Like Disease. *Autoimmun. Rev.* **2020**, *19*, 102537. [CrossRef] [PubMed]
106. Yang, J.; Savvatis, K.; Kang, J.S.; Fan, P.; Zhong, H.; Schwartz, K.; Barry, V.; Mikels-Vidgal, A.; Karpinski, S.; Komyeyev, D.; et al. Targeting LOXL2 for cardiac interstitial fibrosis and heart failure treatment. *Nat. Commun.* **2016**, *7*, 13710. [CrossRef]
107. Ridker, P.M. From C-reactive protein to interleukin-6 to interleukin-1: Moving upstream to identify novel targets for atheroprotection. *Circ. Res.* **2016**, *118*, 145–156. [CrossRef]
108. Bergsbaken, T.; Fink, S.; Cookson, B. Pyroptosis: Host cell death and inflammation. *Nat. Rev. Microbiol.* **2009**, *7*, 99–109. [CrossRef]
109. Frangogiannis, N.G. Interleukin-1 in cardiac injury, repair, and remodeling: Pathophysiologic and translational concepts. *Discoveries* **2015**, *3*, e41. [CrossRef]
110. Saxena, A.; Chen, W.; Su, Y.; Rai, V.; Uche, O.U.; Li, N.; Frangogiannis, N.G. IL-1 Induces Proinflammatory Leukocyte Infiltration and Regulates Fibroblast Phenotype in the Infarcted Myocardium. *J. Immunol.* **2013**, *191*, 4838–4848. [CrossRef]
111. Fahey, E.; Doyle, S.L. IL-1 Family Cytokine Regulation of Vascular Permeability and Angiogenesis. *Front. Immunol.* **2019**, *10*, 1426. [CrossRef]
112. Everett, B.M.; Cornel, J.H.; Lainscak, M.; Anker, S.D.; Abbate, A.; Thuren, T.; Libby, P.; Glynn, R.J.; Ridker, P.M. Anti-Inflammatory Therapy with Canakinumab for the Prevention of Hospitalization for Heart Failure. *Circulation* **2019**, *139*, 1289–1299. [CrossRef] [PubMed]
113. Orn, S.; Ueland, T.; Manhenke, C.; Sandanger, O.; Godang, K.; Yndestad, A.; Mollnes, T.E.; Dickstein, K.; Aukrust, P. Increased interleukin-1beta levels are associated with left ventricular hypertrophy and remodelling following acute ST segment elevation myocardial infarction treated by primary percutaneous coronary intervention. *J. Intern. Med.* **2012**, *272*, 267–276. [CrossRef]

114. Yang, C.; Deng, Z.; Li, J.; Ren, Z.; Liu, F. Meta-analysis of the relationship between interleukin-6 levels and the prognosis and severity of acute coronary syndrome. *Clinics* **2021**, *76*, e2690. [CrossRef] [PubMed]
115. Feng, Y.; Ye, D.; Wang, Z.; Pan, H.; Lu, X.; Wang, M.; Xu, Y.; Yu, J.; Zhang, J.; Zhao, M.; et al. The Role of Interleukin-6 Family Members in Cardiovascular Diseases. *Front. Cardiovasc. Med.* **2022**, *9*, 818890. [CrossRef] [PubMed]
116. Sawa, Y.; Ichikawa, H.; Kagisaki, K.; Ohata, T.; Matsuda, H. Interleukin-6 derived from hypoxic myocytes promotes neutrophil-mediated reperfusion injury in myocardium. *J. Thorac. Cardiovasc. Surg.* **1998**, *116*, 511–515. [CrossRef]
117. Rusu, I.; Turlacu, M.; Micheu, M.M. Acute myocardial injury in patients with COVID-19: Possible mechanisms and clinical implications. *World J. Clin. Cases* **2022**, *10*, 762–776. [CrossRef]
118. Zhang, C.; Wu, Z.; Li, J.W.; Zhao, H.; Wang, G.Q. Cytokine release syndrome in severe COVID-19: Interleukin-6 receptor antagonist tocilizumab may be the key to reduce mortality. *Int. J. Antimicrob. Agents* **2020**, *55*, 105954. [CrossRef]
119. Tanaka, T.; Narazaki, M.; Kishimoto, T. IL-6 in inflammation, immunity, and disease. *Cold Spring Harb. Perspect. Biol.* **2014**, *6*, a016295. [CrossRef]
120. Chin, B.S.; Conway, D.S.; Chung, N.A.; Blann, A.D.; Gibbs, C.R.; Lip, G.Y. Interleukin-6, tissue factor and von Willebrand factor in acute decompensated heart failure: Relationship to treatment and prognosis. *Blood Coagul. Fibrinolysis* **2003**, *14*, 515–521. [CrossRef]
121. Streetz, K.L.; Luedde, T.; Manns, M.P.; Trautwein, C. Interleukin 6 and liver regeneration. *Gut* **2000**, *47*, 309–312. [CrossRef]
122. Lin, Z.Q.; Kondo, T.; Ishida, Y.; Takayasu, T.; Mukaida, N. Essential involvement of IL-6 in the skin wound-healing process as evidenced by delayed wound healing in IL-6-deficient mice. *J. Leukoc. Biol.* **2003**, *73*, 713–721. [CrossRef] [PubMed]
123. Erta, M.; Quintana, A.; Hidalgo, J. Interleukin-6, a major cytokine in the central nervous system. *Int. J. Biol. Sci.* **2012**, *8*, 1254–1266. [CrossRef] [PubMed]
124. Fontes, J.A.; Rose, N.R.; Čiháková, D. The varying faces of IL-6: From cardiac protection to cardiac failure. *Cytokine* **2015**, *74*, 62–68. [CrossRef]
125. Niculet, E.; Chioncel, V.; Elisei, A.M.; Miulescu, M.; Buzia, O.D.; Nwabudike, L.C.; Craescu, M.; Draganescu, M.; Bujoreanu, F.; Marinescu, E.; et al. Multifactorial expression of IL-6 with update on COVID-19 and the therapeutic strategies of its blockade (Review). *Exp. Ther. Med.* **2021**, *21*, 263. [CrossRef] [PubMed]
126. Gabriel, A.S.; Martinsson, A.; Wretlind, B.; Ahnve, S. IL-6 levels in acute and post myocardial infarction: Their relation to CRP levels, infarction size, left ventricular systolic function, and heart failure. *Eur. J. Intern. Med.* **2004**, *15*, 523–528. [CrossRef] [PubMed]
127. Jong, W.M.; Ten, C.H.; Linnenbank, A.C.; de Boer, O.J.; Reitsma, P.H.; de Winter, R.J.; Zuurbier, C.J. Reduced acute myocardial ischemia-reperfusion injury in IL-6-deficient mice employing a closed-chest model. *Inflamm. Res.* **2016**, *65*, 489–499. [CrossRef]
128. Yang, L.; Xie, X.; Tu, Z.; Fu, J.; Xu, D.; Zhou, Y. The signal pathways and treatment of cytokine storm in COVID-19. *Sig. Transduct. Target. Ther.* **2021**, *6*, 255. [CrossRef]
129. Groot, H.E.; Al Ali, L.; van der Horst, I.C.C.; Schurer, R.A.J.; van der Werf, H.W.; Lipsic, E.; van Veldhuisen, D.J.; Karper, J.C.; van der Harst, P. Plasma interleukin 6 levels are associated with cardiac function after ST-elevation myocardial infarction. *Clin. Res. Cardiol.* **2019**, *108*, 612–621. [CrossRef]
130. Gager, G.M.; Biesinger, B.; Hofer, F.; Winter, M.P.; Hengstenberg, C.; Jilma, B.; Eyileten, C.; Postula, M.; Lang, I.M.; Siller-Matula, J.M. Interleukin-6 level is a powerful predictor of long-term cardiovascular mortality in patients with acute coronary syndrome. *Vascul. Pharmacol.* **2020**, *135*, 106806. [CrossRef]
131. Hayama, N.; Ide, S.; Kitami, Y.; Hara, H.; Kutsuna, S.; Hiroi, Y. Interleukin-6 is upregulated and may be associated with myocardial injury in some patients who have recovered from COVID-19. *Glob. Health Med.* **2022**, *4*, 61–63. [CrossRef]
132. Albini, A.; Calabrone, L.; Carlini, V.; Benedetto, N.; Lombardo, M.; Bruno, A.; Noonan, D.M. Preliminary Evidence for IL-10-Induced ACE2 mRNA Expression in Lung-Derived and Endothelial Cells: Implications for SARS-Cov-2 ARDS Pathogenesis. *Front. Immunol.* **2021**, *12*, 718136. [CrossRef] [PubMed]
133. Peng, X.; Wang, Y.; Xi, X.; Jia, Y.; Tian, J.; Yu, B.; Tian, J. Promising Therapy for Heart Failure in Patients with Severe COVID-19: Calming the Cytokine Storm. *Cardiovasc. Drugs. Ther.* **2021**, *35*, 231–247. [CrossRef] [PubMed]
134. Melillo, F.; Napolano, A.; Loffi, M.; Regazzoni, V.; Boccellino, A.; Danzi, G.B.; Cappelletti, A.M.; Rovere-Querini, P.; Landoni, G.; Ingallina, G.; et al. Myocardial injury in patients with SARS-CoV-2 pneumonia: Pivotal role of inflammation in COVID-19. *Eur. J. Clin. Investig.* **2022**, *52*, e13743. [CrossRef] [PubMed]
135. Arévalos, V.; Ortega-Paz, L.; Rodríguez-Arias, J.J.; Calvo, M.; Castrillo, L.; Salazar, A.; Roque, M.; Dantas, A.P.; Sabaté, M.; Brugaletta, S. Myocardial Injury in COVID-19 Patients: Association with Inflammation, Coagulopathy and In-Hospital Prognosis. *J. Clin. Med.* **2021**, *10*, 2096. [CrossRef] [PubMed]
136. de Falco, R.; Vargas, M.; Palma, D.; Savoia, M.; Miscioscia, A.; Pinchera, B.; Vano, M.; Servillo, G.; Gentile, I.; Fortunato, G. B-Type Natriuretic Peptides and High-Sensitive Troponin I as COVID-19 Survival Factors: Which One Is the Best Performer? *J. Clin. Med.* **2021**, *10*, 2726. [CrossRef]
137. Villacorta, H.; Maisel, A.S. Soluble ST2 testing: A promising biomarker in the management of heart failure. *Arq. Bras. Cardiol.* **2016**, *106*, 145–152. [CrossRef]
138. Saraiva, M.; Vieira, P.; O'Garra, A. Biology and therapeutic potential of interleukin-10. *J. Exp. Med.* **2020**, *217*, e20190418. [CrossRef]

139. Han, H.; Ma, Q.; Li, C.; Liu, R.; Zhao, L.; Wang, W.; Zhang, P.; Liu, X.; Gao, G.; Liu, F.; et al. Profiling Serum Cytokines in COVID-19 Patients Reveals IL-6 and IL-10 Are Disease Severity Predictors. *Emerg. Microbes Infect.* **2020**, *9*, 1123–1130. [CrossRef]
140. Islam, H.; Chamberlain, T.C.; Mui, A.L.; Little, J.P. Elevated Interleukin-10 Levels in COVID-19: Potentiation of Pro-Inflammatory Responses or Impaired Anti-Inflammatory Action? *Front. Immunol.* **2021**, *12*, 677008. [CrossRef]
141. Lu, L.; Zhang, H.; Dauphars, D.J.; He, Y.W. A Potential Role of Interleukin 10 in COVID-19 Pathogenesis. *Trends Immunol.* **2021**, *42*, 3–5. [CrossRef]
142. Antoniv, T.T.; Ivashkiv, L.B. Dysregulation of Interleukin-10-Dependent Gene Expression in Rheumatoid Arthritis Synovial Macrophages. *Arthritis. Rheum.* **2006**, *54*, 2711–2721. [CrossRef] [PubMed]
143. Zheng, M.; Gao, Y.; Wang, G.; Song, G.; Liu, S.; Sun, D.; Xu, Y.; Tian, Z. Functional Exhaustion of Antiviral Lymphocytes in COVID-19 Patients. *Cell. Mol. Immunol.* **2020**, *17*, 533–535. [CrossRef] [PubMed]
144. Potteaux, S.; Esposito, B.; van Oostrom, O.; Brun, V.; Ardouin, P.; Groux, H.; Tedgui, A.; Mallat, Z. Leukocyte-derived interleukin 10 is required for protection against atherosclerosis in low-density lipoprotein receptor knockout mice. *Arterioscler. Thromb. Vasc. Biol.* **2004**, *24*, 1474–1478. [CrossRef]
145. Nijm, J.; Wikby, A.; Tompa, A.; Olsson, A.G.; Jonasson, L. Circulating levels of proinflammatory cytokines and neutrophil-platelet aggregates in patients with coronary artery disease. *Am. J. Cardiol.* **2005**, *95*, 452–456. [CrossRef]
146. Rajappa, M.; Sen, S.K.; Sharma, A. Role of pro-/anti-inflammatory cytokines and their correlation with established risk factors in South Indians with coronary artery disease. *Angiology* **2009**, *60*, 419–426. [CrossRef]
147. Yamashita, H.; Shimada, K.; Seki, E.; Mokuno, H.; Daida, H. Concentrations of interleukins, interferon, and C-reactive protein in stable and unstable angina pectoris. *Am. J. Cardiol.* **2003**, *91*, 133–134. [CrossRef]
148. Heeschen, C.; Dimmeler, S.; Hamm, C.W.; Fichtlscherer, S.; Boersma, E.; Simoons, M.L.; Zeiher, A.M. Serum level of the anti-inflammatory cytokine interleukin-10 is an important prognostic determinant in patients with acute coronary syndromes. *Circulation* **2003**, *107*, 2109–2114. [CrossRef]
149. Malarstig, A.; Eriksson, P.; Hamsten, A.; Lindahl, B.; Wallentin, L.; Siegbahn, A. Raised interleukin-10 is an indicator of poor outcome and enhanced systemic inflammation in patients with acute coronary syndrome. *Heart* **2008**, *94*, 724–729. [CrossRef]
150. Mueller, C.; Giannitsis, E.; Jaffe, A.S.; Huber, K.; Mair, J.; Cullen, L.; Hammarsten, O.; Möckel, M.; Krychtiuk, K.; Thygesen, K.; et al. ESC Study Group on Biomarkers in Cardiology of the Acute Cardiovascular Care Association. Cardiovascular biomarkers in patients with COVID-19. *Eur. Heart. J. Acute Cardiovasc. Care* **2021**, *10*, 310–319. [CrossRef]
151. Guler, N.; Siddiqui, F.; Fareed, J. Is the Reason of Increased D-Dimer Levels in COVID-19 Because of ACE-2-Induced Apoptosis in Endothelium? *Clin. Appl. Thromb. Hemost.* **2020**, *26*, 1076029620935526. [CrossRef]
152. Trimaille, A.; Thachil, J.; Marchandot, B.; Curtiaud, A.; Leonard-Lorant, I.; Carmona, A.; Matsushita, K.; Sato, C.; Sattler, L.; Grunebaum, L.; et al. D-Dimers Level as a Possible Marker of Extravascular Fibrinolysis in COVID-19 Patients. *J. Clin. Med.* **2021**, *10*, 39. [CrossRef]
153. Qeadan, F.; Tingey, B.; Gu, L.Y.; Packard, A.H.; Erdei, E.; Saeed, A.I. Prognostic Values of Serum Ferritin and D-Dimer Trajectory in Patients with COVID-19. *Viruses* **2021**, *13*, 419. [CrossRef] [PubMed]
154. Poudel, A.; Poudel, Y.; Adhikari, A.; Aryal, B.B.; Dangol, D.; Bajracharya, T.; Maharjan, A.; Gautam, R. D-dimer as a biomarker for assessment of COVID-19 prognosis: D-dimer levels on admission and its role in predicting disease outcome in hospitalized patients with COVID-19. *PLoS ONE* **2021**, *16*, e0256744. [CrossRef] [PubMed]
155. Kudlinski, B.; Zgoła, D.; Stolińska, M.; Murkos, M.; Kania, J.; Nowak, P.; Noga, A.; Wojciech, M.; Zaborniak, G.; Zembron-Lacny, A. Systemic Inflammatory Predictors of In-Hospital Mortality in COVID-19 Patients: A Retrospective Study. *Diagnostics* **2022**, *12*, 859. [CrossRef] [PubMed]
156. He, L.-P.; Tang, X.-Y.; Ling, W.-H.; Chen, W.-Q.; Chen, Y.-M. Early C-reactive protein in the prediction of long-term outcomes after acute coronary syndromes: A meta-analysis of longitudinal studies. *Heart* **2010**, *96*, 339–346. [CrossRef]
157. Kim, H.-L.; Lim, W.-H.; Seo, J.-B.; Kim, S.-H.; Zo, J.-H.; Kim, M.-A. Improved Prognostic Value in Predicting Long-Term Cardiovascular Events by a Combination of High-Sensitivity C-Reactive Protein and Brachial–Ankle Pulse Wave Velocity. *J. Clin. Med.* **2021**, *10*, 3291. [CrossRef] [PubMed]
158. Sadeghi-Haddad-Zavareh, M.; Bayani, M.; Shokri, M.; Ebrahimpour, S.; Babazadeh, A.; Mehraeen, R.; Moudi, E.; Rostami, A.; Barary, M.; Hosseini, A.; et al. C-Reactive Protein as a Prognostic Indicator in COVID-19 Patients. *Interdiscip. Perspect. Infect. Dis.* **2021**, *2021*, 5557582. [CrossRef]
159. Qin, C.; Zhou, L.; Hu, Z.; Zhang, S.; Yang, S.; Tao, Y.; Xie, C.; Ma, K.; Shang, K.; Wang, W.; et al. Dysregulation of immune response in patients with coronavirus 2019 (COVID-19) in Wuhan, China. *Clin. Infect. Dis.* **2020**, *71*, 762–768. [CrossRef]
160. Lionte, C.; Sorodoc, V.; Haliga, R.E.; Bologa, C.; Ceasovschih, A.; Petris, O.R.; Coman, A.E.; Stoica, A.; Sirbu, O.; Puha, G.; et al. Inflammatory and Cardiac Biomarkers in Relation with Post-Acute COVID-19 and Mortality: What We Know after Successive Pandemic Waves. *Diagnostics* **2022**, *12*, 1373. [CrossRef]
161. Holzknecht, M.; Tiller, C.; Reindl, M.; Lechner, I.; Fink, P.; Lunger, P.; Mayr, A.; Henninger, B.; Brenner, C.; Klug, G.; et al. Association of C-Reactive Protein Velocity with Early Left Ventricular Dysfunction in Patients with First ST-Elevation Myocardial Infarction. *J. Clin. Med.* **2021**, *10*, 5494. [CrossRef]
162. Mahat, R.K.; Panda, S.; Rathore, V.; Swain, S.; Yadav, L.; Sah, S.P. The dynamics of inflammatory markers in coronavirus disease-2019 (COVID-19) patients: A systematic review and meta-analysis. *Clin. Epidemiol. Glob. Health* **2021**, *11*, 100727. [CrossRef]

163. Esposito, F.; Matthes, H.; Schad, F. Seven COVID-19 Patients Treated with C-Reactive Protein (CRP) Apheresis. *J. Clin. Med.* **2022**, *11*, 1956. [CrossRef] [PubMed]
164. Liu, F.; Li, L.; Xu, M.; Wu, J.; Luo, D.; Zhu, Y.; Li, B.; Song, X.; Zhou, X. Prognostic value of interleukin-6, C-reactive protein, and procalcitonin in patients with COVID-19. *J. Clin. Virol.* **2020**, *127*, 104370. [CrossRef] [PubMed]
165. Luo, X.; Zhou, W.; Yan, X.; Guo, T.; Wang, B.; Xia, H.; Ye, L.; Xiong, J.; Jiang, Z.; Liu, Y.; et al. Prognostic Value of C-Reactive Protein in Patients with Coronavirus 2019. *Clin. Infect. Dis.* **2020**, *71*, 2174–2179. [CrossRef] [PubMed]
166. Kim, W.S.; Park, S.H. Correlation between N-Terminal Pro-Brain Natriuretic Peptide and Doppler Echocardiographic Parameters of Left Ventricular Filling Pressure in Atrial Fibrillation. *J. Cardiovasc. Ultrasound* **2011**, *19*, 26–31. [CrossRef]
167. Bessière, F.; Khenifer, S.; Dubourg, J.; Durieu, I.; Lega, J.C. Prognostic value of troponins in sepsis: A meta-analysis. *Intensive Care. Med.* **2013**, *39*, 1181–1189. [CrossRef]
168. Dmour, B.A.; Miftode, R.S.; Iliescu Halitchi, D.; Anton-Paduraru, D.T.; Iliescu Halitchi, C.O.; Miftode, I.L.; Mitu, O.; Costache, A.D.; Stafie, C.S.; Costache, I.I. Latest Insights into Mechanisms behind Atrial Cardiomyopathy: It Is Not always about Ventricular Function. *Diagnostics* **2021**, *11*, 449. [CrossRef]
169. Lin, S.C.; Tsai, Y.J.; Huang, C.T.; Kuo, Y.W.; Ruan, S.Y.; Chuang, Y.C.; Yu, C.J. Prognostic value of plasma N-terminal pro B-type natriuretic peptide levels in pneumonia patients requiring intensive care unit admission. *Respirology* **2013**, *18*, 933–934. [CrossRef]
170. Sorrentino, S.; Cacia, M.; Leo, I.; Polimeni, A.; Sabatino, J.; Spaccarotella, C.A.M.; Mongiardo, A.; De Rosa, S.; Indolfi, C. B-Type Natriuretic Peptide as Biomarker of COVID-19 Disease Severity—A Meta-Analysis. *J. Clin. Med.* **2020**, *9*, 2957. [CrossRef]
171. Caro-Codón, J.; Rey, J.R.; Buño, A.; Iniesta, A.M.; Rosillo, S.O.; Castrejon-Castrejon, S.; Rodriguez-Sotelo, L.; Martinez, L.A.; Marco, I.; Merino, C.; et al. Characterization of NT-proBNP in a large cohort of COVID-19 patients. *Eur. J. Heart Fail.* **2021**, *23*, 456–464. [CrossRef]
172. Jirak, P.; Pistulli, R.; Lichtenauer, M.; Wernly, B.; Paar, V.; Motloch, L.J.; Rezar, R.; Jung, C.; Hoppe, U.C.; Schulze, P.C.; et al. Expression of the Novel Cardiac Biomarkers sST2, GDF-15, suPAR, and H-FABP in HFpEF Patients Compared with ICM, DCM, and Controls. *J. Clin. Med.* **2020**, *9*, 1130. [CrossRef]
173. Najjar, E.; Faxén, U.L.; Hage, C.; Donal, E.; Daubert, J.-C.; Linde, C.; Lund, L.H. ST2 in heart failure with preserved and reduced ejection fraction. *Scand. Cardiovasc. J.* **2019**, *53*, 21–27. [CrossRef] [PubMed]
174. Biasucci, L.M.; Maino, A.; Grimaldi, M.C.; Cappannoli, L.; Aspromonte, N. Novel Biomarkers in Heart Failure: New Insight in Pathophysiology and Clinical Perspective. *J. Clin. Med.* **2021**, *10*, 2771. [CrossRef]
175. Zeng, Z.; Hong, X.Y.; Li, Y. Serum-soluble ST2 as a novel biomarker reflecting inflammatory status and illness severity in patients with COVID-19. *Biomark. Med.* **2020**, *14*, 1619–1629. [CrossRef] [PubMed]
176. Wendt, R.; Lingitz, M.-T.; Laggner, M.; Mildner, M.; Traxler, D.; Graf, A.; Krotka, P.; Moser, B.; Hoetzenecker, K.; Kalbitz, S.; et al. Clinical Relevance of Elevated Soluble ST2, HSP27 and 20S Proteasome at Hospital Admission in Patients with COVID-19. *Biology* **2021**, *10*, 1186. [CrossRef] [PubMed]
177. Miftode, R.S.; Costache, I.I.; Cianga, P.; Petris, A.O.; Cianga, C.M.; Maranduca, M.A.; Miftode, I.L.; Constantinescu, D.; Timpau, A.S.; Crisan, A.; et al. The Influence of Socioeconomic Status on the Prognosis and Profile of Patients Admitted for Acute Heart Failure during COVID-19 Pandemic: Overestimated Aspects or a Multifaceted Hydra of Cardiovascular Risk Factors? *Healthcare* **2021**, *9*, 1700. [CrossRef]
178. Ragusa, R.; Basta, G.; Del Turco, S.; Caselli, C. A possible role for ST2 as prognostic biomarker for COVID-19. *Vascul. Pharmacol.* **2021**, *138*, 106857. [CrossRef]
179. Gao, Q.; Li, Y.; Pan, X. Lentivirus expressing soluble ST2 alleviates bleomycin-induced pulmonary fibrosis in mice. *Int. Immunopharmacol.* **2016**, *30*, 188–193. [CrossRef]
180. Xu, J.; Zheng, J.; Song, P. IL33/ST2 pathway in a bleomycin induced pulmonary fibrosis model. *Mol. Med. Rep.* **2016**, *14*, 1704–1708. [CrossRef]
181. Burian, E.; Jungmann, F.; Kaissis, G.A. Intensive care risk estimation in COVID-19 pneumonia based on clinical and imaging parameters: Experiences from the Munich cohort. *J. Clin. Med.* **2020**, *9*, 1514. [CrossRef]
182. Que, Y.; Hu, C.; Wan, K.; Hu, P.; Wang, R.; Luo, J.; Li, T.; Ping, R.; Hu, Q.; Sun, Y.; et al. Cytokine release syndrome in COVID-19: A major mechanism of morbidity and mortality. *Int. Rev. Immunol.* **2022**, *41*, 217–230. [CrossRef]
183. Tanaka, T.; Narazaki, M.; Kishimoto, T. Immunotherapeutic implications of IL-6 blockade for cytokine storm. *Immunotherapy* **2016**, *8*, 959–970. [CrossRef]
184. Pathan, N.; Hemingway, C.A.; Alizadeh, A.A.; Stephens, A.C.; Boldrick, J.C.; Oragui, E.E.; McCabe, C.; Welch, S.B.; Whitney, A.; O'Gara, P.; et al. Role of interleukin 6 in myocardial dysfunction of meningococcal septic shock. *Lancet* **2004**, *363*, 203–209. [CrossRef]
185. Jamilloux, Y.; Henry, T.; Belot, A.; Viel, S.; Fauter, M.; El Jammal, T.; Walzer, T.; François, B.; Sève, P. Should we stimulate or suppress immune responses in COVID-19? Cytokine and anti-cytokine interventions. *Autoimmun. Rev.* **2020**, *19*, 102567. [CrossRef] [PubMed]
186. Mitu, O.; Crisan, A.; Redwood, S.; Cazacu-Davidescu, I.-E.; Mitu, I.; Costache, I.-I.; Onofrei, V.; Miftode, R.-S.; Costache, A.-D.; Haba, C.M.S.; et al. The Relationship between Cardiovascular Risk Scores and Several Markers of Subclinical Atherosclerosis in an Asymptomatic Population. *J. Clin. Med.* **2021**, *10*, 955. [CrossRef]
187. Chapman, A.R.; Bularga, A.; Mills, N.L. High-Sensitivity Cardiac Troponin Can Be an Ally in the Fight Against COVID-19. *Circulation* **2020**, *141*, 1733–1735. [CrossRef]

188. Salvarani, C.; Dolci, G.; Massari, M.; Merlo, D.F.; Cavuto, S.; Savoldi, L.; Bruzzi, P.; Boni, F.; Braglia, L.; Turrà, C.; et al. Effect of Tocilizumab vs Standard Care on Clinical Worsening in Patients Hospitalized With COVID-19 Pneumonia: A Randomized Clinical Trial. *JAMA Intern. Med.* **2021**, *181*, 24–31. [CrossRef] [PubMed]
189. Sapkota, B.; Makandar, S.N.; Acharya, S. *Biologic Response Modifiers (BRMs)*; StatPearls: Treasure Island, FL, USA, 2022.
190. Bacchiega, B.C.; Bacchiega, A.B.; Usnayo, M.J.; Bedirian, R.; Singh, G.; Pinheiro, G.D. Interleukin 6 Inhibition and Coronary Artery Disease in a High-Risk Population: A Prospective Community-Based Clinical Study. *J. Am. Heart. Assoc.* **2017**, *6*, e005038. [CrossRef]
191. Hausenloy, D.J.; Kharbanda, R.; Rahbek Schmidt, M.; Møller, U.K.; Ravkilde, J.; Okkels Jensen, L.; Engstrøm, T.; Garcia Ruiz, J.M.; Radovanovic, N.; Christensen, E.F.S.; et al. Effect of remote ischaemic conditioning on clinical outcomes in patients presenting with an ST-segment elevation myocardial infarction undergoing rimary percutaneous coronary intervention. *Eur. Heart J.* **2015**, *36*, 1846–1848.
192. Cavalli, G.; De Luca, G.; Campochiaro, C.; Della-Torre, E.; Ripa, M.; Canetti, D.; Oltolini, C.; Castiglioni, B.; Tassan Din, C.; Boffini, N.; et al. Interleukin-1 blockade with high-dose anakinra in patients with COVID-19, acute respiratory distress syndrome, and hyperinflammation: A retrospective cohort study. *Lancet Rheumatol.* **2020**, *2*, e325–e331. [CrossRef]
193. Huet, T.; Beaussier, H.; Voisin, O. Anakinra for severe forms of COVID-19: A cohort study. *Lancet Rheumatol.* **2020**, *2*, e393–e400. [CrossRef]
194. Cauchois, R.; Koubi, M.; Delarbre, D. Early IL-1 receptor blockade in severe inflammatory respiratory failure complicating COVID-19. *Proc. Natl. Acad. Sci. USA* **2020**, *117*, 18951–18953. [CrossRef] [PubMed]
195. Caricchio, R.; Abbate, A.; Gordeev, I.; Meng, J.; Hsue, P.Y.; Neogi, T.; Arduino, R.; Fomina, D.; Bogdanov, R.; Stepanenko, T.; et al. Effect of Canakinumab vs Placebo on Survival Without Invasive Mechanical Ventilation in Patients Hospitalized with Severe COVID-19: A Randomized Clinical Trial. *JAMA* **2021**, *326*, 230–239. [CrossRef] [PubMed]
196. Shirazi, L.F.; Bissett, J.; Romeo, F.; Mehta, J.L. Role of inflammation in heart failure. *Curr. Atheroscler. Rep.* **2017**, *19*, 27. [CrossRef] [PubMed]

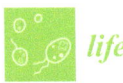

Review

Myocardial Ischemia in Patients with COVID-19 Infection: Between Pathophysiological Mechanisms and Electrocardiographic Findings

Ștefania Teodora Duca [1,2,†], Adriana Chetran [1,2,*], Radu Ștefan Miftode [1,2], Ovidiu Mitu [1,2], Alexandru Dan Costache [1,3,†], Ana Nicolae [1,2], Dan Iliescu-Halițchi [1,4], Codruța-Olimpiada Halițchi-Iliescu [5,6], Florin Mitu [1,3] and Irina Iuliana Costache [1,2]

1. Department of Internal Medicine I, Faculty of Medicine, University of Medicine and Pharmacy "Grigore T. Popa", 700145 Iasi, Romania; stefania-teodora.duca@email.umfiasi.ro (Ș.T.D.); radu-stefan.miftode@umfiasi.ro (R.Ș.M.); ovidiu.mitu@umfiasi.ro (O.M.); dan-alexandru.costache@umfiasi.ro (A.D.C.); ana_nicolae@umfiasi.ro (A.N.); halitchi.iliescu@umfiasi.ro (D.I.-H.); florin.mitu@umfiasi.ro (F.M.); irina.costache@umfiasi.ro (I.I.C.)
2. Department of Cardiology, "St. Spiridon" Emergency County Hospital, 700111 Iasi, Romania
3. Department of Cardiovascular Rehabilitation, Clinical Rehabilitation Hospital, 700661 Iasi, Romania
4. Department of Cardiology, Arcadia Hospital, 700620 Iasi, Romania
5. Department of Mother and Child Medicine-Pediatrics, University of Medicine and Pharmacy "Grigore T. Popa", 700115 Iasi, Romania; olimpiada.iliescu@umfiasi.ro
6. Department of Pediatrics, Arcadia Hospital, 700620 Iasi, Romania
* Correspondence: adriana.ion@umfiasi.ro; Tel.: +40-741089910
† These authors contributed equally to this work.

Abstract: Given the possible pathophysiological links between myocardial ischemia and SARS-CoV-2 infection, several studies have focused attention on acute coronary syndromes in order to improve patients' morbidity and mortality. Understanding the pathophysiological aspects of myocardial ischemia in patients infected with SARS-CoV-2 can open a broad perspective on the proper management for each patient. The electrocardiogram (ECG) remains the easiest assessment of cardiac involvement in COVID-19 patients, due to its non-invasive profile, accessibility, low cost, and lack of radiation. The ECG changes provide insight into the patient's prognosis, indicating either the worsening of an underlying cardiac illnesses or the acute direct injury by the virus. This indicates that the ECG is an important prognostic tool that can affect the outcome of COVID-19 patients, which important to correlate its aspects with the clinical characteristics and patient's medical history. The ECG changes in myocardial ischemia include a broad spectrum in patients with COVID-19 with different cases reported of ST-segment elevation, ST-segment depression, and T wave inversion, which are associated with severe COVID-19 disease.

Keywords: COVID-19; myocardial ischemia; electrocardiography

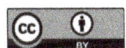

1. Introduction

In the last month of 2019, an outbreak of atypical respiratory disease occurred in China, in the city of Wuhan. Shortly after the first cases, it was discovered that a novel coronavirus was responsible for the next pandemic, as the World Health Organization declared. Since it was structurally related to the virus that caused acute respiratory distress syndrome during 2002–2003, the novel coronavirus was named as the severe acute respiratory syndrome coronavirus-2 (SARS-CoV-2) and the outbreak was called Coronavirus disease 19 (COVID-19) [1,2].

The most common presentation of COVID-19 is pneumonia, but different reports describe different complications, from thromboembolism, myocarditis, and acute coronary syndrome to multiple organ failure [3–5]. Because of the possible pathophysiological links between myocardial ischemia and the SARS-CoV-2 infection, several studies have focused on them in order to improve patients' morbidity and mortality [3,6]. As acute coronary syndromes have been reported to be up to 30%, they may have a significant role in worsening clinical outcomes in patients with COVID-19 [6,7]. Moreover, long COVID-19 syndrome is characterized by persistent tissue damage and inflammation following an acute bout of SARS-CoV-2 infection, mainly manifested through chronic fatigue and dyspnea, but also, among others, with cardiac symptoms. The inflammation of the heart tissues, especially myocardial inflammation which is as prevalent as 78% in post-COVID-19 patients, leads to tachycardia, palpitations, and chest pain in the months post-discharge [8,9].

A series of case reports published have shown that patients following acute COVID-19 infections have developed postural tachycardia syndrome (POTS). This involves an increase in over 30 beats per minute in the heart rate in adults or over 40 beats per minute in patients between the ages of 12–19 in the first 10 min since standing in an orthostatic position, associated with orthostatic intolerance, in the absence of orthostatic hypotension, for a minimum of 3 months [10].

Since the epidemic of COVID-19, multiple studies of hypercoagulability have attracted attention; the pathophysiology aspects of myocardial ischemia have been studied in detail and we focused on electrocardiographic changes in infected individuals [11].

The electrocardiogram (ECG) remains the most facile assessment method for cardiac involvement in COVID-19 patients, due to its non-invasiveness, accessibility, low cost, and radiation-free investigative profile [12–14]. Although the management during a patient's admission is safer when laboratory values and imaging become available, ECG can be quickly performed without exposing a large number of people to SARS-CoV-2 [12,15].

Therefore, we propose a review of different publications regarding the ECG findings in patients with COVID-19 and myocardial ischemia and the pathophysiological pathways behind them. The ECG pattern can predict the severity of the COVID-19 infection and clinical outcomes such as mortality, as several studies have shown [11,16–18]. In the COVID-19 era, patients with chest pain require more attention and high clinical suspicion. ECG interpretation is more challenging, as it can also show chronic abnormalities of an underlying cardiac disease [19,20].

The ECG changes in myocardial ischemia include a broad spectrum in patients with COVID-19, different cases of ST-segment elevation, ST-segment depression, and T-wave inversion being reported, which were associated with a severe form of COVID-19 disease [21,22]. Several authors have described P-wave changes, in the context of atrial infarction, which is supplied in 60% of cases by the right coronary artery and in 40% by the circumflex artery through the superior ramus ostium cava [23].

We searched PubMed and Google Scholar for articles published from December 2019 to March 2022 and compiled a database using the keywords "COVID-19", "SARS-CoV-2", "coronavirus", "ECG", "electrocardiography", "myocardial ischemia", "myocardial infarction", "acute coronary syndrome", "hypercoagulability", "pathophysiology" and all their combinations.

The results included original papers, retrospective studies, prospective studies, reports, systematic reviews, meta-analyses, and case reports, focusing on COVID-19 and ECG changes in myocardial ischemia. We reviewed relevant articles for data to comprehensively discuss and describe the pathophysiological mechanisms and ECG changes in patients with COVID-19 and acute coronary syndrome.

2. Pathophysiology of Myocardial Ischemia in COVID-19 Patients

In the recent COVID-19 pandemic, there were challenges on several levels, from the difficulties of controlling the spread of the disease, to the complexity of diagnosing and treating the multisystemic complications of this infection. Even though it is primarily an infectious disease, the impact of COVID-19 on the cardiovascular system is significant, with complications such as pericarditis, myocarditis, pulmonary embolism, myocardial infarction, and exacerbation of chronic heart failure being described more often as the pandemic progressed [24,25].

Acute and chronic coronary diseases, already some of the most prevalent diseases in the general population, have played a major role in the years of COVID-19 infection as factors of severity and mortality [25]. The problems related to coronary heart disease in the context of COVID-19 infection were multiple: late patient presentation to the hospital, misleading symptoms by the interference of the two diseases, reduced intensive care unit (ICU) capacity, delayed treatment by COVID-19 testing and protocols, hs-troponin values altered by lung infection, and severe prognosis due to coronary heart disease and associated COVID-19 infection. All these issues challenge the diagnostic and therapeutic approach of coronary artery diseases, which reaches beyond guidelines and requires new studies on the particular mechanisms of myocardial ischemia in the context of COVID-19 infection [26–28].

Typical symptoms of coronary disease (chest pain, fatigue, and dyspnea) have lost their specificity and sensitivity as COVID-19 infection often has similar manifestations which delays the diagnosis [29]. Cardiac troponin, a cornerstone biomarker in the diagnosis of myocardial infarction, had elevated values above the 99th percentile in 8–62% of patients with COVID-19 infection, with the highest incidence and mortality recorded in patients with severe infection [30]. In addition to cardiac causes for high troponin values (acute coronary syndrome, myocarditis, and Takotsubo syndrome), several noncardiac conditions, such as sepsis, critical illness, and pulmonary embolism, can lead to increased troponin [30]. Therefore, ECG changes are critical in establishing the diagnosis of coronary diseases. Particular aspects of ECG tracing in patients with COVID-19 have also been described and should be recognized for the proper management of these cases [29,30].

Among coronavirus patients, a substantial number developed myocardial injury or acute coronary syndrome, complications more prevalent if the patient had a previous cardiovascular disease, worsening his prognosis and mortality [31–33].

For a better understanding of the diverse mechanisms involved in the ECG ischemia changes in patients with COVID-19, it is important to make the distinction between two main entities: acute cardiac injury (ACI) and acute coronary syndrome (ACS). ACI is defined as the elevation of high-sensitivity cardiac troponin (hs-cTn) above the 99th percentile of its upper limit of normal, usually with stable and unchanging values, or evidence of new electrocardiographic (ECG) or echocardiographic abnormalities, and may have ischemic or non-ischemic etiology [34].

The causes for ACI may involve an ACS (type I myocardial infarction-due to plaque rupture or thrombosis, type II myocardial infarction-due to oxygen supply/demand mismatch, or myocardial injury due to disseminated intravascular coagulation) or a non-ischemic etiology as: myocarditis, Takotsubo cardiomyopathy (stress-induced cardiomyopathy), acute pulmonary embolism, cytokine release syndrome, and direct viral myocardial invasion. The differential diagnosis between an ischemic and a non-ischemic cause for the ACI may need additional imaging tests (CT Coronary Angiography (CTCA), lung CT scan, or cardiac magnetic resonance (CMR)), guided also by serial hs-cTn testing. It was noted that patients with ACI caused by an ACS have dynamically changing values of hs-cTn, with a rise and fall, as opposed to other types of ACI where troponin had steadily increasing values [34,35].

According to European Society of Cardiology (ESC) guidelines, ACS defines the clinical situations of acute myocardial ischemia or infarction, which can be further classified in three types: unstable angina, Non-ST-elevation myocardial infarction (NSTEMI), and ST-elevation MI (STEMI) [36]. Acute myocardial infarction (AMI) is defined by consistent myocardial ischemia that leads to cardiomyocyte necrosis. The diagnosis involves the detection of dynamic changes in hs-cTn associated with at least one of the following: symptoms of myocardial ischemia, new ischemic ECG changes, development of pathological Q waves on ECG, imaging evidence of viable myocardium loss or new regional wall motion abnormality in a pattern consistent with an ischemic etiology, or intracoronary thrombus detected on angiography or autopsy [36].

The presence of ACS has been reported in a significant number of patients with COVID-19 infection, which has had a negative impact on the prognosis [31,32]. For these patients, some particularities for ACS were noticed such as higher incidence of stent thrombosis, multiple thrombotic culprit lesions, high thrombus burden, and angiographic evidence of non-obstructed coronary arteries, which raised concerns about the diverse mechanisms involved [37,38]. In addition to the usual cardiovascular risk factors, to date, the main mechanisms involved in the development of ACS in COVID-19 patients are: prothrombotic activation of the coagulation cascade, endothelial dysfunction, cytokine-mediated systemic inflammatory response, and hypoxic injury due to oxygen supply/demand imbalance [39].

The effects of COVID-19 infection on the coagulation cascade are not yet fully understood, involving either direct viral aggression or an exacerbated cytokine-mediated inflammatory response [40]. The presence of hemostatic abnormalities was suggested in these patients by higher D-dimer values, decreased platelets count, prolonged prothrombin time, and increased levels of fibrinogen degradation products [41,42]. These abnormalities have been reported in severe cases of COVID-19 pneumonia and are associated with a negative prognosis [41–44]. The prothrombotic state is maintained by the overexpression of ultra-large von Willebrand factor multimers and tissue factor, induced by the cytokines produced during the systemic inflammatory response, which triggers the activation of the coagulation cascade [45]. Another possible mechanism for SARS-CoV-2-related coagulopathy is the presence of lupus anticoagulant antibodies, that may be induced in any infectious or inflammatory disease. The exposed phospholipids of the endothelium to the immune system leads to thrombus formation [46].

Endothelial cells have the ability to respond to many humoral and hemodynamic stimuli by producing regulatory molecules that are part of the defense mechanism of vascular homeostasis. The endothelium plays a significant role in controlling the immune response by promoting leukocyte migration into extravascular spaces, which helps fight infections and promotes tissue repair [47]. In response to inflammatory cytokines such as interleukin IL-1, IL-6, and tumor necrosis factor-α (TNF-α), endothelial cells exhibit adhesion molecules on their surface (e.g., E-selectin, P-selectin, intercellular adhesion molecule-1, vascular cell adhesion molecule-1 (VCAM-1), and integrins), which increases leukocyte binding [48]. Accumulation of inflammatory cells causes endothelial dysfunction through reduced NO bioavailability and increased oxidative stress via activation of NADPH oxidase [49]. The studies confirm the role of adhesion molecules in COVID-19 complications, indicating that high circulating levels of VCAM-1 and E-selectin are associated with increased COVID-19 severity, as a meta-analysis from 2021 showed [50]. Furthermore, in critically ill patients with COVID-19 a high expression of inflammatory cytokines, supporting the role of the cytokine release storm in severe cases has been identified [51].

Endothelial dysfunction is the main cause for coronary artery disease in patients with traditional cardiovascular risk factors (diabetes, smoking, hypertension, and older age) [52]. As the thrombotic complications in patients with COVID-19 increase, endothelial injury is incriminated, either by a direct viral effect or by the action of inflammatory cytokines [53,54]. A direct effect of SARS-CoV-2 on the vascular endothelial glycocalyx (VEGLX) is suspected [55]. Glycocalyx damage usually is associated with pathological situations as inflammatory response, hyperglycemia, hypoxia, and ischemia/reperfusion injury, which may also be present in COVID-19 pneumonia [55–58]. The theory is supported by the measurements of circulating levels of VEGLX components in COVID-19 patients, where higher concentrations were detected for VEGLX injury biomarkers such as syndecan-1, hyaluronic acid, and sTie-2 [27,59]. In the presence of an inflammatory state, the endothelium loses its antithrombotic, anticoagulant, and profibrinolytic capacity as a result of tissue factor expression, von Willebrand factor release, thromboxane production, and plasminogen activator inhibitor-1 (PAI-1) production [60]. Moreover, the inflammatory cytokines act on the endothelial cells to generate superoxide anions, with enhanced local oxidative stress [61]. Overproduction of endothelin-1 contributes, as well, to the endothelial imbalance, acting as a prothrombotic agent and vasoconstrictor [62].

Atherosclerotic disease progression is enhanced by the presence of inflammatory response, which maintains a prothrombotic state and promotes vasoconstriction through sympathetic activity [63,64]. The disturbed balance between prothrombotic and antithrombotic factors promotes erosion or rupture of the atherosclerotic plaque, resulting in coronary thrombosis and ACS [65]. In COVID-19 infection, an exaggerated immune response and a cytokine chain reaction, known as cytokine storm (CS), has been observed [40]. The CS starts with the production of interleukin-1 (IL-1), which has some particularities: it may induce its own gene expression, but also promotes the production of other inflammatory factors such as tumor necrosis factor-alpha (TNFα), interleukin-6 (IL-6), and chemoattractant molecules [66]. All these factors create a prothrombotic and antifibrinolytic imbalance, generating thrombosis and local tissue injury [67]. In SARS-CoV-2 patients, increased levels of inflammatory mediators, part of the CS, such as IL-1, IL-6, IL-10, IFN, granulocyte colony stimulating factor (G-CSF), monocyte chemoattractant protein (MCP1), macrophage inflammatory protein 1 alpha (MIP1A), platelet-derived growth factor (PDGF), TNFα, and vascular endothelial growth factor (VEGF) were detected, which supports the contribution of CS to the development of ACS (Figure 1) [44,68,69].

Prothrombotic activation of the coagulation cascade, endothelial dysfunction, and cytokine-mediated systemic inflammatory response are mechanisms that involve the presence and progression of atherosclerotic lesions, that become unstable and clinically manifest as a type I myocardial infarction (MI). However, a significant number of COVID-19 patients showed ECG signs of ischemia in the absence of atherothrombotic lesions [70–72]. In these patients a type II MI is suspected, due to a mismatch between oxygen supply and demand. The severe hypoxic state, tachyarrhythmias, anemia, sepsis, hypotension, and shock may induce myocardial damage and have often been described in critically ill patients with COVID-19 [73]. Due to the severe situations that induce type II MI, the prognosis is worse, with a higher rate of in-hospital mortality compared with type I MI [74].

Cases of myocardial infarction with nonobstructive coronary arteries (MINOCA) were reported in some case series of STEMI and COVID-19 patients [75,76]. The possible mechanisms involved include coronary vasospasm, microthrombi, and plaque erosion, triggered by the exaggerated inflammatory response, oxidative stress and endothelial dysfunction [76–78]. The limited access to more advanced techniques as intravascular imaging, pharmacological provocation test, and cardiac magnetic resonance, in COVID-19 patients, constitutes an obstacle to a complete understanding of the underlying mechanisms [78,79].

Troponin is the gold standard biomarker used for detection of myocardial ischemia, as reflects the presence of cardiomyocyte damage. In ACS, either STEMI or NSTEMI, the dynamic of circulating troponin levels is similar, regardless of the ECG pattern (ST-elevation, ST-depression, or inverted T wave), the main factor influencing its value is the moment of detection after symptom onset [80]. Typically, troponin cannot be detected in the first 1–2 h of myocardial necrosis, but only approximately 2–4 h after the onset of myocardial injury. Thereby, in cases where patients seek early medical advice, the troponin levels may be normal or slightly increased, which is an indication for repeating the troponin measurements. Serum levels can persist being elevated for up to 4–7 days for troponin I, and 10–14 days for troponin T [81]. We did not find studies indicating correlations between troponin levels and particular ECG aspects of myocardial ischemia or infarction. However, a certain type of ACS that should be mentioned is Wellens syndrome which, despite its great severity and high risk, manifests frequently with troponin within normal limits, which can be falsely reassuring [82]. In COVID-19 patients, troponin levels have often been elevated as a result of cardiac injury, with or without AMI, which highlights the important role of ECG in establishing the diagnosis [83]. However, troponin proved to be valuable in anticipating the prognosis of COVID-19 patients, as Santoso et al. presented in a meta-analysis, which concluded that troponin levels were associated with higher mortality, need for care in the intensive care unit (ICU) and a more severe form of COVID-19 infection [84]. The hypothesis is also confirmed by a study that investigated the risk of mortality in patients with COVID-19, new T-wave inversions (TWI) and troponin levels. Jorge Romero et al.

showed in their study that patients with elevated troponin and TWI had an 80% mortality risk, compared with a 35% mortality risk when isolated TWI with normal values of troponin were present [85].

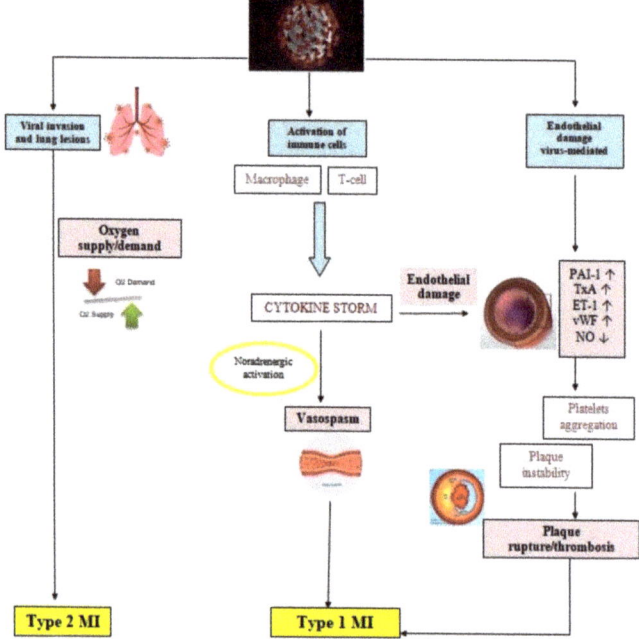

Figure 1. Pathophysiology of myocardial ischemia in COVID-19 patients. COVID-19 infection acts by biding to the ACE2 receptors present on the surface of the host cell, which may be pneumocytes, macrophages, or endothelial cells. Pulmonary infection may range from mild disease to pneumonia and ARDS in severe forms, which in cases of severe respiratory impairment causes hypoxia and due to an oxygen supply/demand mismatch, a type 2 MI. An aberrant inflammatory response is typically described in COVID-19 infection, with the release of cytokines and molecules involved in inflammation, such as IL-1, IL-6, IL-7, TNFα, and IFNγ. The negative effects of cytokines manifest by increasing the production of oxidative stress agents and prothrombotic factors, which damage the endothelial function. Furthermore, SARS-CoV-2 may interact directly with the molecules expressed on the surface of the endothelial cells. The inflammatory environment promotes platelets activation and aggregation, upregulates the sympathetic nervous system, increasing the risk of instability of preexisting atheromatous plaques and coronary spasm. All these mechanisms predispose to plaque rupture and thrombosis, leading to type 1 MI. ACS: acute coronary syndrome; ACE2: angiotensin-converting enzyme 2; COVID-19: coronavirus disease 2019; IFNγ: interferon γ; IL-1: interleukin 1; IL-6: interleukin 6; IL-7: interleukin 7; MI: myocardial infarction; SARS-CoV-2: severe acute respiratory syndrome coronavirus 2; TNFα: tumor necrosis factor α.

3. Electrocardiographic Changes in Myocardial Ischemia in COVID-19 Patients

3.1. ST-T Abnormalities

ST-T abnormalities are well-known and described in patients with myocardial ischemia and they include ST-elevation or depression, T-wave inversion, and nonspecific ST-T-wave changes. While acute subendocardial ischemia causes ST-segment depression, acute transmural ischemia causes ST-segment elevation, due to the electrical repolarization currents responsible for the ST-segment, which are deviated towards the inner layer of the heart in the first case and towards the outer layer of the heart in the latter. Even though the

ECG signs of an acute ST-elevation are more accurate than an acute non-ST-elevation, the repolarization abnormalities of a myocardial infarction can persist indefinitely [86,87].

Patients infected with SARS-CoV-2 who associate myocardial injury may show ST-segment elevation, ST-segment depression, or T-wave inversion on ECG [18,19]. Howbeit, the ST-segment elevation in COVID-19 patients requires differential diagnosis with pericarditis and myocarditis, while myocardial ischemia may be due to both obstructive coronary artery diseases and a mismatch between oxygen supply and demand [88]; these findings have been observed more frequently in severe patients [13,22]. Among the critically ill patients, an abnormal ECG with ST-T changes reaches a frequency of 48.5%, while in patients with a severe type of COVID-19, 25.7% have this abnormality according to Wang et al. [89]. Most studies found that ST-T abnormalities were the most common changes, occurring in up to 40% of patients from different hospitals, including Wuhan Asia General Hospital [15,19,88,90]. T-wave inversion was the most common repolarization change in several studies, including the one of Galidevara et al., who reported that 27.7% of ECG changes were due to this abnormality [7,22]. However, while Rosen et al. reported in his study that 21% patients had an ECG with ST-T modification, Poterucha et al. reported that 10% of the presentations had this abnormality, T-wave inversion was observed in up to 29% of this group, which is similar to other studies. This may be due to the number of patients included in the studies, the second one having a number of patients seven times higher [14,91].

Regarding the localization of the repolarization abnormality, lateral and antero-lateral changes on the ECG were the most frequently described, being also associated with worse clinical outcomes [92–94].

The ST-T modifications on the ECG can be used as an indicator for poor prognosis, including more frequent need for mechanical ventilatory support, increased need for ICU admission, and finally increased mortality [13,19,89]. Patients with ST-T changes on the admission ECG are more likely to show progression towards a severe form, being associated with the severity of the COVID-19 infection and a worse prognosis [13,22,95]. Therefore, the COVID-19 patients detected with myocardial ischemia on the ECG should be monitored for sudden cardiac death [13].

Patients with ST-T abnormalities had elevated cardiac biomarkers, such as troponin, and more frequent requirement for vasoactive treatment [14,96,97]. Although mild troponin elevation was a frequent finding in the study of Chorin et al., which is often associated with non-vascular etiologies, biomarkers of cardiac damage should alert clinicians of a poor prognosis [97].

3.1.1. STEMI Pattern

The ST-segment elevation is sometimes associated with a fatal evolution or a worse prognosis in patients, especially in those with COVID-19 infection. Several studies attest the presence of an ST-segment elevation, characteristic for myocardial infarction, in patients with SARS-CoV-2 infection. Therefore, it is important, especially in patients with COVID-19, to differentiate the ischemic ST-elevation from the one in a possible myopericarditis [11,76,98].

The ST-segment elevation myocardial infarction (STEMI) is defined as new ST-elevation at the J point in two or more contiguous leads, ≥ 0.25 mV in men below the age of 40 years, ≥ 0.2 mV in men over the age of 40 years, or ≥ 0.15 mV in women in leads V2–V3, and/or ≥ 0.1 mV in other leads [86,99,100].

A multicenter case series study from six hospitals in New York, which included patients with ST-segment elevation and COVID-19, showed that in 44% of patients a diagnosis of myocardial infarction was established, whereas 56% had a non-coronary myocardial injury. Half of the patients underwent invasive intervention with angiography, but only two-thirds of them had obstructive disease. This finding suggests that a more prevalent COVID-19 was associated with a non-obstructive type of MI, probably determined by type 2 myocardial infarction [11,76,98]. However, univariate analyses showed that ST-segment elevation had a strong correlation with patients' mortality, being an independent prognostic factor. Sonzor et al. demonstrated in their article in American Journal of The Medical Science that ST-segment elevation can be associated with clinical outcomes in hospitalized patients with COVID-19 [101]. Moreover, the occurrence of ST-segment elevation during hospitalization is also an alarm sign for a poor prognosis, this manifestation being due to the side effects of therapeutic agents, the direct attack of the virus on myocardial tissue, or an indicator of myocardial ischemia [102].

Mccullough et al. reported that only 0.7% of the presentations had localized ST-segment elevation on the ECG, their data suggesting that this was not a common finding in the New York Presbyterian Hospital in the first months of the pandemic [15]. These data were sustained by another study which showed that localized ST-segment elevation was observed in only 0.5% of the presentations during the same months [97].

There was no specific localization of the myocardial infarction in COVID-19 patients as several studies have shown, some concluding that inferior myocardial infarction was the most frequent, while others showing that anterior myocardial injury was the most common type [75,94,100]. An important aspect to mention is that STEMI represented the first clinical manifestation of COVID-19 for most patients with myocardial infarction and only a few developed ST-segment elevation during hospitalization for COVID-19 [75]. Even though we need to be aware of the atypical clinical presentation of COVID-19 with cardiovascular manifestations, physicians should not misdiagnose STEMI even after admission, especially if the patient has chest pain [3,103]. We researched almost all published cases of STEMI and we found an approximately equal localization of the myocardial infarction, with no statistical significance between the affected walls: inferior myocardial infarction-5 cases, inferolateral myocardial infarction-4 cases, anterior myocardial infarction-5 cases, or anterolateral myocardial infarction-3 cases. Interestingly, patients who had a subacute myocardial infarction, with ST-segment elevation and Q waves, had an anterior STEMI with late presentation [3,11,103–111]. Patients with COVID-19 and STEMI who were admitted to the hospital had several cardiovascular risk factors with a past medical history of type 2 diabetes mellitus, hypertension, hyperlipidemia, or overweight body mass index (BMI) [98,104]. This suggests that cardiovascular risk factors in patients with COVID-19 infection play an important role, as this association leads to a more prevalent occurrence of a myocardial infarction. The mean age of the total cases of STEMI associated with COVID-19 infection found in literature was 54.4 years of age, and the majority of patients were male, only four being female with acute STEMI [3,11,103–111]. However, it was observed that the youngest patients with ST-segment elevation myocardial infarction and COVID-19 were female [109,110]. Different authors published articles which included patients with STEMI, but without COVID-19 and concluded that the prognostic for those patients was better, not only because they did not have SARS-CoV-2 infection, but also because the angiography was performed faster [104].

We also found studies with cases of transient ST-segment elevation on the ECG, the possible explanations being a type 2 myocardial infarction due to inflammatory activation, respiratory failure, and severe hypoxia [97,112]. MINOCA due to type 2 acute myocardial infarction causes the appearance of deep Q waves on the subsequent electrocardiograms [113]. Stefanini et al. showed in their study that in approximately 40% of patients with COVID-19 and STEMI, a culprit lesion was not identifiable in the angiography [75]. Therefore, it is not necessary to perform an angiography in all patients with STEMI and COVID-19, but we need to place in balance the risks and benefits and to understand the pathophysiological mechanisms behind de ECG aspects [104,108].

3.1.2. ST-Depression Pattern

ST-segment depression is defined as a new horizontal or down-sloping ST-depression of at least 0.05 mV in two contiguous leads [87,99]. The non-ST-elevation myocardial infarction (NSTEMI) is seen on ECG as ST-segment depression, T-wave inversion or nonspecific ST-segment, and T-wave changes [86]. The variety of ECG findings requires a detailed analysis and raises differential diagnosis problems, as ST-T abnormalities were the most reported ECG findings in patients with COVID-19 infection [88–90].

Although various studies have not shown any cases of ST-segment elevation, they have found ST-segment depression, reported in approximately 5.3% of cases, this manifestation also being associated with a high mortality [6,20,114]. As we described above, MINOCA can be challenging due to the atypical clinical presentation, especially in patients with NSTEMI [6]. Moreover, ST-segment depression related to MINOCA was associated with high levels of cardiac biomarkers [101]. Antwi-Amoabeng et al. showed an incidence of 8.6% of ST-segment depression, with a significant association between this ECG finding and troponin levels [115]. Due to the more frequent cases of ST-segment depression compared with ST-segment elevation, we did not find in literature specific cases of NSTEMI, but only studies on large cohorts [6,114,116].

3.1.3. T-Wave Inversion and Other Patterns of ST-Abnormalities

T waves are normally inverted in leads III, aVR, and V1. T-wave inversions (TWI) produced by myocardial ischemia are classically narrow, symmetric, and have variable depth. Moreover, they have mirror patterns, start in the second part of the repolarization, and may be accompanied by a positive or negative U wave [99,115].

Heberto et al. showed that ischemic T-wave inversion was the most frequent electrocardiographic finding in COVID-19 patients and observed a relationship with mortality in these patients [117]. Other studies demonstrated that T-wave abnormalities were present in up to 49% of the COVID-19 patients [118,119]. Almost all studies showed that T-wave inversion appeared more frequently in the cardiac injury group and in patients over 74 years of age [111,120]. However, Capaccione et al. reported a case of a 36-year-old patient with myocardial ischemia and inferior T-wave inversion, confirming the hypothesis of various studies showing that patients with COVID-19 infection have an increased risk of developing severe cardiovascular disease at a younger age [121]. The number of leads with T-wave inversion pattern was significantly correlated with the elevation of cardiac injury biomarkers, such as troponin [119]. Both of these findings were associated with increased mortality and the need for intubation. Romero et al. conducted a study on 3225 patients with COVID-19 infection, where T-wave inversion was observed in 6% of patients, with the most frequent localization (71%) in the lateral leads (DI, aVL, V5–V6) [18]. Therefore, T-wave inversion remains the most frequent repolarization abnormality and is associated with poor outcomes and death, especially in those with elevated troponin levels [14,121]. The issue for patients with T-wave inversions due to NSTEMI is that during the COVID-19 era, even if the patients were classified as high-risk NSTEMI, angiography was not performed, and conservative treatment during isolation was preferred due to the high risk of infection. However, this strategy may contribute to increasing mortality, as Suryawan et al. reported in their case presentation [122,123].

3.2. Q Waves

Pathological Q waves are defined as the occurrence of Q waves in at least two contiguous leads as follows: any Q wave in leads V2–V3 of at least 0.02 s or QS complex in leads V2 and V3; Q wave of at least 0.03 s and at least 0.1 mV deep or QS complex in leads I, II, aVL, aVF, or V4–V6; R wave of at least 0.04 s in V1–V2 and R/S of at least one with a concordant positive [86,99].

We found in literature some cases of subacute myocardial infarction in COVID-19 patients, with Q wave being observed on ECG in approximately 4% of cases. The location was in both the anterior and inferior territories, and the patients maintained the ST-segment elevation on ECG [20,92]. Because the Q wave remains the only sign of myocardial infarction on ECG, a remote myocardial infarction is more difficult to recognize. Moroni et al. presented three cases of myocardial infarction with late presentation, due to the patients' fear of being infected with COVID-19 in the hospital, who treated themselves at home and were hospitalized long after a good therapeutical procedure could have been performed (Table 1) [105]. This is an alarm signal for patient educational programs, as the SARS-CoV-2 infection alone does not have a poor prognosis, but it can exacerbate preexisting conditions [92,105].

Table 1. Patients with subacute myocardial infarction (adapted after Moroni et al., 2020).

Age	Sex	Symptoms	Time to in-Hospital Presentation	Treatment at Home	ECG Aspect
64	M [1]	Chest pressure Shortness of breath	10 days	Homemade natural remedies	Q waves and ST-segment elevation on the anterior leads
65	F [1]	Epigastric tightness Dyspnea Orthopnea	5 days	Antiacids	Q waves and ST-segment elevation on the anterior leads
60	M [1]	Hypotension Diaphoresis Respiratory distress	4 days	None	Q waves and ST-segment elevation on the anterior leads

[1] M: male; F: female.

3.3. Specific Electrocardiographic Patterns

Cases of COVID-19 patients who had specific electrocardiographic patterns were described in literature.

3.3.1. Takotsubo Pattern

Takotsubo syndrome (TTS) was first described in the 1990s, as an acute myocardial infarction, but with normal angiography and patients recovering within days or weeks. Even though it was initially considered a benign disease, subsequent studies have demonstrated a higher mortality rate than in the normal population. The most common finding on ECG is the ST-segment elevation in the precordial leads, with less common ST-segment depression or abnormal Q waves than for myocardial infarction and with transient changes [124–127].

TTS occurs in 90% of cases in women, often being preceded by emotional stress, therefore the COVID-19 pandemic can be considered a triggering factor [128]. The pathophysiology is associated with high plasma levels of catecholamines, the impact of adrenergic activity on cardiac myocytes causing ascending ST-segment elevation and J point depression. Moreover, high catecholamine levels might increase oxygen demand, inducing vasospasm and myocardial injury, patients with SARS-CoV-2 infection being exposed to a high endogenous secretion as a compensatory intravenous infusion, which are used as a therapeutic method [23,129]. Another determinant mechanism involves the hypothalamic-pituitary-adrenal (HPA) axis, which is activated in COVID-19; several studies have shown that cortisol and adrenocorticotrophic hormones were dysregulated. As the levels of cortisol are significantly higher in COVID-19 patients and the HPA axis induces catecholamine secretion, a relationship between TTS and hypercortisolemia was described. An important aspect to mention is the BNP/troponin ratio used to differentiate TTS from acute myocardial infarction, as TTS is associated with higher brain natriuretic peptide (BNP) and lower troponin levels [129].

Literature presents many cases of TTS in patients with COVID-19, the most specific ECG abnormalities being ST-segment elevation in the anterior leads [11]. Approximately 2–4% of patients with COVID-19 had TTS, with a higher prevalence in critically ill patients, as some studies have reported. Although TTS predominates in women, about 30% of the patients with COVID-19 and TTS are males [129]. The first typical case of TTS with apical ballooning observed on echocardiography in a patient with COVID-19 was reported by Meyer et al. Both emotional and physical stress by the pandemic were considered trigger factors [130].

ST-segment elevation in leads I and aVL and diffuse ST-T-wave changes were found in two female patients with COVID-19, who were subsequently diagnosed with TTS because the cardiac catheterization revealed normal coronary arteries. One of them even admitted to feeling anxious by the reports and images of the COVID-19 pandemic, TTS being an indirect outcome of quarantine-induced stress [128–130].

Although it was considered a benign disease, TTS patients with COVID-19 have a higher mortality rate than patients who have only TTS [131,132]. Furthermore, Barbieri et al. showed that in a hospital from Lombardy, during the COVID-19 pandemic, more patients with TTS have been diagnosed with TTS than in the same months of the previous years. This is an additional argument for the impact of COVID-19 on stress-induced cardiomyopathy [133].

3.3.2. Wellens Pattern

Wellens syndrome is a specific disease for critical stenosis of the proximal left anterior descending coronary artery. The ECG shows deeply inverted or biphasic T waves in leads V2–V3, often in leads V1 and V4 and occasionally in leads V5–V6 (Figure 2). Patients with Wellens syndrome are at risk of a large anterior wall myocardial infarction, even though they are pain-free and the cardiac enzymes are normal [82,134,135].

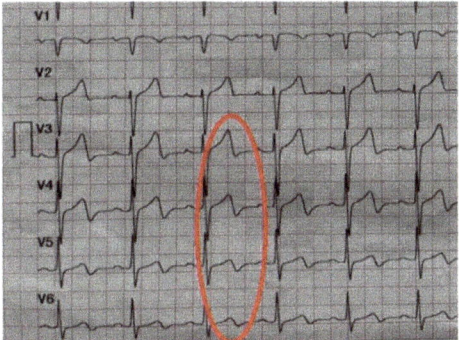

Figure 2. Wellens pattern: deeply biphasic T waves in leads V3–V6 (The collection of the "St. Spiridon" Hospital's Cardiology Clinic, Iasi, Romania).

We found in literature four cases of Wellens syndrome in patients with SARS-CoV-2 infection, three of them were male and one female (Table 2). The mean age was 73 years old, significatively higher than the group with ST-segment elevation. On the ECG, all patients had biphasic T waves in V2–V3, three of them with additionally negative T waves in leads V4–V6. Only one patient had typical chest pain, three patients had only dyspnea. The female patient did not have an angiography performed, in one patient an emergency angiography was performed and the other two patients had a coronary angiography after a few days of medical treatment. All patients were treated with drugs for NSTEMI, with a high-intensity statin, dual antiplatelet aspirin, P2Y12 inhibitors, and anticoagulant [135,136]. Regarding the therapeutic approach, we observed a difference during the pandemic. If the first published case of Wellens syndrome did not receive an angiography because of the COVID-19 status and the risk of infection, Caiati et al., the authors who published the latest case of Wellens syndrome during the COVID-19 pandemic, chose another therapeutic approach and the patient underwent an angiography [136–139]. This may be due to the fact that at the beginning of the pandemic, information about COVID-19 was scarce, a conservatory treatment was preferred in order to keep as little physical contact as possible. Even though for the diagnosis of Wellens syndrome physicians need to perform an angiography, during the pandemic, the European Society of Cardiology and the American College of Cardiology recommended medical management during the acute phase [136].

Table 2. Patients with Wellens syndrome and COVID-19 infection.

Article	Age	Sex	Symptoms	ECG Findings	Treatment	Angiography
Prousi et al.	75	F [1]	Fatigue Dyspnea	Diffuse T-wave inversions in precordial leads Biphasic T waves in V1–V2	Statin Aspirin P2Y12 inhibitors Heparin	Not performed
Elkholy et al.	86	M [1]	Dyspnea	Biphasic T wave in V2–V3 T-wave inversion in V4–V6	Statin Aspirin P2Y12 inhibitors Enoxaparin	Chronic total occlusion of the right coronary artery. Severe disease of the first diagonal. Severe stenosis of the distal obtuse marginal 1
Di Spigno et al.	62	M [1]	Atypical chest pain Dyspnea	Biphasic T waves in V2	-	Subocclusion of the proximal left anterior descending artery
Caiati et al.	69	M [1]	Typical chest pain Dyspnea	T-waves inversion in V2–V3 T-wave flattening in V4–V6	Statin Aspirin P2Y12 inhibitors Heparin	Subocclusive stenosis of the proximal LAD

[1] M: male; F: female.

In addition to the ECG aspect, patients should be investigated for cardiovascular risk factors, as well as a structural evaluation with echocardiography, coronary angiography being the investigation that assists the ECG findings [136]. However, because the high risk of infection during the COVID-19 pandemic required new diagnostic methods, Caiati et al. proposed a non-invasive way that can assess the obstructive atherosclerosis through transthoracic enhanced Doppler echocardiography (E-Doppler TTE). This allows the identification of the coronary blood flow velocity, even though this investigation has never been tested in a Wellens syndrome. The authors used it for the first time the E-Doppler TTE in an acute syndrome and this can open new perspectives on the management of an acute coronary syndrome [139].

3.3.3. De Winter Pattern

The De Winter ECG pattern shows an upsloping ST-segment depression at the J-point in leads V1–V6, followed by peaked symmetrical T waves, being associated with left anterior descending artery occlusion, with a positive predictive value of 95% [140–142].

Almendro-Delia et al. published the only case of De Winter syndrome associated with COVID-19 infection, which occurred in a 33-year-old male patient. Due to his infectious disease, atypical chest pain suggestive for pericarditis, and the ECG aspect with ST-segment depression in V1–V6 followed by tall T waves, the first diagnosis was acute pericarditis (Figure 3). The laboratory result which revealed high troponin levels and the echocardiographic aspect with apical and antero-lateral hypokinesis with an apical thrombus at this region, led to the reinterpretation of the ECG as a De Winter aspect. The angiography confirmed the thrombotic occlusion of the proximal left anterior descending artery, the outcome being favorable. Therefore, in the COVID-19 era, it is necessary to make a detailed differential diagnosis, even in apparently young healthy patients. The ECG aspects can be misinterpreted as early repolarization or pericarditis, delaying proper reperfusion treatment. Thus, the De Winter pattern is the equivalent of an early STEMI, an aspect which should not be ignored [143].

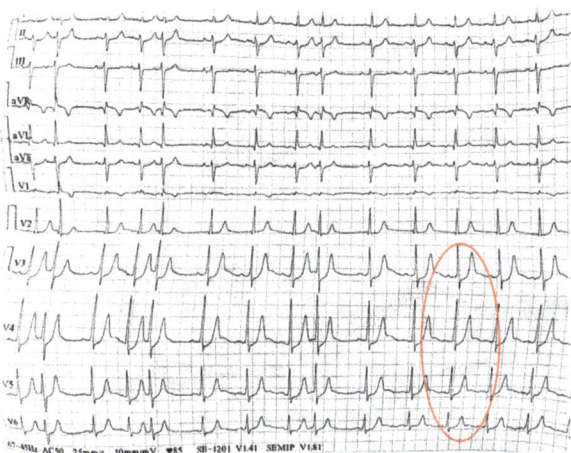

Figure 3. De Winter pattern: upsloping ST-segment depression at the J-point, followed by peaked symmetrical T waves in lead V3, lead V4, lead V5 and lead V6 (The collection of the "St. Spiridon" Hospital's Cardiology Clinic, Iasi, Romania).

3.3.4. Triangular Electrocardiographic Pattern

Another unique ECG presentation of STEMI is represented by the triangular QRS-ST-T waveform, also known as the "shark fin pattern", which is defined as a giant wave resulting from the fusion of the QRS complex, the ST-segment and the T wave [76,144]. This uncommon ECG pattern reflects the left main coronary artery involvement, with a large area of transmural myocardial ischemia and poor in-hospital prognosis [76].

A 32-year-old female patient with COVID-19 infection and shortness of breath, showed a "shark fin pattern" in leads I, II, III, and aVL post-cardiac arrest (Figure 4). Although an angiography was necessary, given her critically ill clinical status and the echocardiographic aspect with mid-wall hypokinesis suggestive for Takotsubo, the intervention was postponed. The "shark fin pattern" is a rare ECG finding, typical for left main coronary artery, but because of the patient's past history of intravenous drug abuse and hepatitis C, over which the COVID-19 infection overlapped, this ECG aspect can be determined by several other factors, such as abnormal laboratory tests [145].

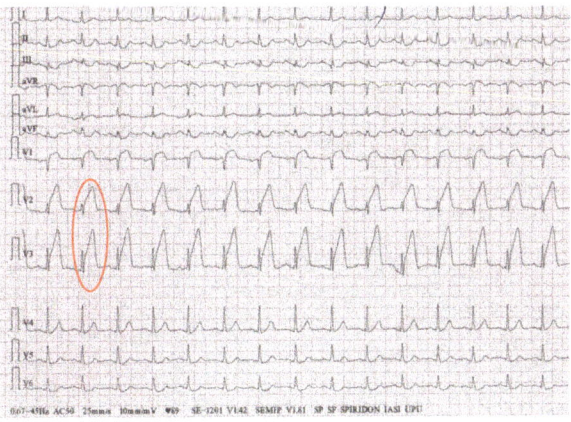

Figure 4. Triangular ECG pattern in leads V2 and V3: fusion of the QRS complex, the ST-segment and the T wave (The collection of the "St. Spiridon" Hospital's Cardiology Clinic, Iasi, Romania).

3.4. Other Electrocardiographic Aspects Associated with Myocardial Ischemia in COVID-19 Patients

Even though new left bundle branch block, right bundle branch block, or poor R-wave progression were described as different changes suggestive for myocardial ischemia, in COVID-19 patients we did not find specific publications or studies regarding only the incidence of these aspects in infected patients [14,93].

4. Why Is It Important to Analyze Myocardial Ischemic-like Electrocardiographic Changes in COVID-19 Patients?

The ECG findings described above are important for differential diagnosis, especially with myopericarditis. In patients with COVID-19 myocarditis, approximately 50% had ST-segment elevation on the ECG, the distinction from myocardial infarction being difficult, although ST-segment elevation in myocarditis is diffuse, not focal as in acute coronary syndrome [18,90]. Moreover, in myopericarditis, ST-segment is characterized by an elevation of the J point with a concave shape, while in STEMI the elevation of the J point has a convex shape. Additional tests are required, troponin being mildly elevated in myopericarditis and the cardiac ultrasound showing increased wall thickness, decreased ejection fraction, or global hypokinesis [18,124]. Finally, late gadolinium enhancement on MRI can reveal the final diagnosis of myocarditis [18]. We found in literature some cases of patients with COVID-19 infection and ST-T abnormalities seen on ECG being interpreted as an acute coronary syndrome with an MRI performed after the angiography showing normal coronary arteries, and thus establishing the diagnosis myopericarditis [11].

Another differential diagnosis to consider is a fever-induced Brugada pattern, as COVID-19 is frequently associated with fever [75].

The management of patients with myocardial infarction suspicion has also suffered changes in the COVID-19 era. Given the difficult differential diagnosis with myocarditis, it is important for the reperfusion therapy not to be postponed in the emergency department. Moreover, in COVID-19 patients with a strong suspicion for NSTEMI, initial medical therapy is the optimal option. Finally, SARS-CoV-2 rapid testing remains mandatory even in the emergency setting and protocols are continuously being adapted [146].

5. Conclusions

Understanding the pathophysiological aspects of myocardial ischemia in patients infected with SARS-CoV-2 can open a broad perspective on the proper management of each patient. The ECG changes provide insight into the patient's prognosis. Although we found the same ECG aspects for myocardial ischemia as before the pandemic, these are much more severe, occur in younger and healthier patients, and the stress-induced cardiomyopathy is much more common in COVID-19 patients. Further studies are needed to elucidate the particular mechanisms of myocardial ischemia in patients infected with COVID-19 in order to promote more specific treatments and to prevent these complications.

Author Contributions: Conceptualization—Ș.T.D.; validation—I.I.C., D.I.-H., C.-O.H.-I., F.M. and A.C.; writing—original draft preparation—Ș.T.D., A.C. and A.D.C.; writing—review and editing—O.M., R.Ș.M. and A.N.; supervision—I.I.C. and A.C. All authors have read and agreed to the published version of the manuscript.

Funding: This research received no external funding.

Conflicts of Interest: The authors declare no conflict of interest.

References

1. Yuki, K.; Fujiogi, M.; Koutsogiannaki, S. COVID-19 pathophysiology: A review. *Clin. Immunol.* **2020**, *215*, 108427. [CrossRef] [PubMed]
2. Fauci, A.S.; Lane, H.C.; Redfield, R.R. COVID-19—Navigating the Uncharted. *N. Engl. J. Med.* **2020**, *382*, 1268–1269. [CrossRef]
3. Genovese, L.; Ruiz, D.; Tehrani, B.; Sinha, S. Acute coronary thrombosis as a complication of COVID-19. *BMJ Case Rep.* **2021**, *14*, e238218. [CrossRef] [PubMed]

4. Yang, L.; Liu, S.; Liu, J.; Zhang, Z.; Wan, X.; Huang, B.; Chen, Y.; Zhang, Y. COVID-19: Immunopathogenesis and Immunotherapeutics. *Signal. Transduct. Target Ther.* **2020**, *5*, 128. [CrossRef] [PubMed]
5. Velavan, T.P.; Meyer, C.G. The COVID-19 epidemic. *Trop. Med. Int. Health* **2020**, *25*, 278–280. [CrossRef]
6. Schiavone, M.; Gobbi, C.; Biondi-Zoccai, G.; D'Ascenzo, F.; Palazzuoli, A.; Gasperetti, A.; Mitacchione, G.; Viecca, M.; Galli, M.; Fedele, F.; et al. Acute Coronary Syndromes and COVID-19: Exploring the Uncertainties. *J. Clin. Med.* **2020**, *9*, 1683. [CrossRef]
7. Anupama, B.K.; Chaudhuri, D. A Review of Acute Myocardial Injury in Coronavirus Disease 2019. *Cureus* **2020**, *12*, e8426.
8. Yong, S.J. Long COVID or post-COVID-19 syndrome: Putative pathophysiology, risk factors, and treatments. *Infect. Dis.* **2021**, *53*, 737–754. [CrossRef]
9. Sykes, D.L.; Holdsworth, L.; Jawad, N.; Gunasekera, P.; Morice, A.H.; Crooks, M.G. Post-COVID-19 Symptom Burden: What is Long-COVID and How Should We Manage It. *Lung* **2021**, *199*, 113–119. [CrossRef] [PubMed]
10. Raj, S.R.; Arnold, A.C.; Barboi, A.; Claydon, V.E.; Limberg, J.K.; Lucci, V.M.; Numan, M.; Peltier, A.; Snapper, H.; Vernino, S. Long-COVID postural tachycardia syndrome: An American Autonomic Society statement. *Clin. Auton. Res.* **2021**, *31*, 365–368. [CrossRef]
11. Mehraeen, E.; Seyed Alinaghi, S.A.; Nowroozi, A.; Dadras, O.; Alilou, S.; Shobeiri, P.; Behnezhad, F.; Karimi, A. A systematic review of ECG findings in patients with COVID-19. *Indian Heart J.* **2020**, *72*, 500–507. [CrossRef]
12. Elias, P.; Poterucha, T.J.; Jain, S.S.; Sayer, G.; Raikhelkar, J.; Fried, J.; Clerkin, K.; Griffin, J.; DeFilippis, E.M.; Gupta, A.; et al. The Prognostic Value of Electrocardiogram at Presentation to Emergency Department in Patients with COVID-19. *Mayo Clin. Proc.* **2020**, *95*, 2099–2109. [CrossRef] [PubMed]
13. Barman, H.A.; Atici, A.; Alici, G.; Sit, O.; Tugrul, S.; Gungor, B.; Okuyan, E.; Sahin, I. The effect of the severity COVID-19 infection on electrocardiography. *Am. J. Emerg. Med.* **2021**, *46*, 317–322. [CrossRef]
14. Rosén, J.; Noreland, M.; Stattin, K.; Lipcsey, M.; Frithiof, R.; Malinovschi, A.; Hultström, M. Uppsala Intensive Care COVID-19 Research Group. ECG pathology and its association with death in critically ill COVID-19 patients, a cohort study. *PLoS ONE* **2021**, *16*, e0261315.
15. McCullough, S.A.; Goyal, P.; Krishnan, U.; Choi, J.J.; Safford, M.M.; Okin, P.M. Electrocardiographic Findings in Coronavirus Disease-19: Insights on Mortality and Underlying Myocardial Processes. *J. Card. Fail.* **2020**, *26*, 626–632. [CrossRef]
16. Haseeb, S.; Gul, E.E.; Çinier, G.; Bazoukis, G.; Alvarez-Garcia, J.; Garcia-Zamora, S.; Lee, S.; Yeung, C.; Liu, T.; Tse, G.; et al. International Society of Electrocardiology Young Community (ISE-YC). Value of electrocardiography in coronavirus disease 2019 (COVID-19). *J. Electrocardiol.* **2020**, *62*, 39–45. [CrossRef] [PubMed]
17. Nemati, R.; Ganjoo, M.; Jadidi, F.; Tanha, A.; Baghbani, R. Electrocardiography in Early Diagnosis of Cardiovascular Complications of COVID-19; a Systematic Literature Review. *Arch. Acad. Emerg. Med.* **2020**, *9*, e10.
18. Romero, J.; Gabr, M.; Diaz, J.C. Electrocardiographic Features of COVID-19 patients: An Updated Review. *Card. Electrophysiol. Clin.* **2021**, *14*, 63–70. [CrossRef]
19. Long, B.; Brady, W.J.; Bridwell, R.E.; Ramzy, M.; Montrief, T.; Singh, M.; Gottlieb, M. Electrocardiographic manifestations of COVID-19. *Am. J. Emerg. Med.* **2021**, *41*, 96–103. [CrossRef]
20. Lanza, G.A.; De Vita, A.; Ravenna, S.E.; D'Aiello, A.; Covino, M.; Franceschi, F.; Crea, F. Electrocardiographic findings at presentation and clinical outcome in patients with SARS-CoV-2 infection. *Europace* **2021**, *23*, 123–129. [CrossRef]
21. Denegri, A.; Pezzuto, G.; D'Arienzo, M.; Morelli, M.; Savorani, F.; Cappello, C.G.; Luciani, A.; Boriani, G. Clinical and electrocardiographic characteristics at admission of COVID-19/SARS-CoV-2 pneumonia infection. *Intern. Emerg. Med.* **2021**, *16*, 1451–1456. [CrossRef] [PubMed]
22. Galidevara, J.; Veeramani Kartheek, A.S. Electrocardiographic findings in COVID-19 patients. *Int. J. Res. Med. Sci.* **2021**, *9*, 378–385. [CrossRef]
23. Predabon, B.; Souza, A.Z.M.; Sumnienski Bertoldi, G.H.; Sales, R.L.; Luciano, K.S.; de March Ronsoni, R. The electrocardiogram in the differential diagnosis of cardiologic conditions related to the covid-19 pandemic. *J. Cardiac. Arrhythmias* **2020**, *33*, 133–141.
24. Boukhris, M.; Hillani, A.; Moroni, F.; Annabi, M.S.; Addad, F.; Ribeiro, M.H.; Mansour, S.; Zhao, X.; Ybarra, L.F.; Abbate, A.; et al. Cardiovascular Implications of the COVID-19 Pandemic: A Global Perspective. *Can. J. Cardiol.* **2020**, *36*, 1068–1080. [CrossRef] [PubMed]
25. Manolis, A.S.; Manolis, T.A. Cardiovascular complications of the coronavirus (COVID-19) infection. *Rhythmos* **2020**, *15*, 23–28.
26. Garcia, S.; Stanberry, L.; Schmidt, C.; Sharkey, S.; Megaly, M.; Albaghdadi, M.S.; Meraj, P.M.; Garberich, R.; Jaffer, F.A.; Stefanescu Schmidt, A.C.; et al. Impact of COVID-19 pandemic on STEMI care: An expanded analysis from the United States. *Catheter. Cardiovasc. Interv.* **2021**, *98*, 217–222. [CrossRef]
27. Xiang, D.; Xiang, X.; Zhang, W.; Yi, S.; Zhang, J.; Gu, X.; Xu, Y.; Huang, K.; Su, X.; Yu, B.; et al. Management and Outcomes of Patients with STEMI during the COVID-19 Pandemic in China. *J. Am. Coll. Cardiol.* **2020**, *76*, 1318–1324. [CrossRef]
28. Cammalleri, V.; Muscoli, S.; Benedetto, D.; Stifano, G.; Macrini, M.; Di Landro, A.; Di Luozzo, M.; Marchei, M.; Mariano, E.G.; Cota, L.; et al. Who Has Seen Patients with ST-Segment-Elevation Myocardial Infarction? First Results from Italian Real-World Coronavirus Disease 2019. *Am. Heart J.* **2020**, *9*, e017526. [CrossRef]
29. Struyf, T.; Deeks, J.J.; Dinnes, J.; Takwoingi, Y.; Davenport, C.; Leeflang, M.M.; Spijker, R.; Hooft, L.; Emperador, D.; Dittrich, S.; et al. Cochrane COVID-19 Diagnostic Test Accuracy Group. Signs and symptoms to determine if a patient presenting in primary care or hospital outpatient settings has COVID-19 disease. *Cochrane Database Syst. Rev.* **2020**, *7*, CD013665.

30. Sandoval, Y.; Januzzi, J.L., Jr.; Jaffe, A.S. Cardiac troponin for the diagnosis and risk-stratification of myocardial injury in COVID-19: JACC review topic of the week. *J. Am. Coll. Cardiol.* **2020**, *76*, 1244–1258. [CrossRef]
31. Giustino, G.; Croft, L.B.; Stefanini, G.G.; Bragato, R.; Silbiger, J.J.; Vicenzi, M.; Danilov, T.; Kukar, N.; Shaban, N.; Kini, A.; et al. Characterization of Myocardial Injury in Patients with COVID-19. *J. Am. Coll. Cardiol.* **2020**, *76*, 2043–2055. [CrossRef] [PubMed]
32. Piazza, G.; Campia, U.; Hurwitz, S.; Snyder, J.E.; Rizzo, S.M.; Pfeferman, M.B.; Morrison, R.B.; Leiva, O.; Fanikos, J.; Nauffal, V.; et al. Registry of Arterial and Venous Thromboembolic Complications in Patients with COVID-19. *J. Am. Coll. Cardiol.* **2020**, *76*, 2060–2072. [CrossRef] [PubMed]
33. Lala, A.; Johnson, K.W.; Januzzi, J.L.; Russak, A.J.; Paranjpe, I.; Richter, F.; Zhao, S.; Somani, S.; Van Vleck, T.; Vaid, A.; et al. Prevalence and Impact of Myocardial Injury in Patients Hospitalized with COVID-19 Infection. *J. Am. Coll. Cardiol.* **2020**, *76*, 533–546. [CrossRef] [PubMed]
34. Manolis, A.S.; Manolis, A.A.; Manolis, T.A.; Melita, H. COVID-19 and Acute Myocardial Injury and Infarction: Related Mechanisms and Emerging Challenges. *J. Cardiovasc. Pharmacol. Ther.* **2021**, *26*, 399–414. [CrossRef] [PubMed]
35. Gaze, D.C. Clinical utility of cardiac troponin measurement in COVID-19 infection. *Ann. Clin. Biochem.* **2020**, *57*, 202–205. [CrossRef]
36. Collet, J.P.; Thiele, H.; Barbato, E.; Barthélémy, O.; Bauersachs, J.; Bhatt, D.L.; Dendale, P.; Dorobantu, M.; Edvardsen, T.; Folliguet, T.; et al. 2020 ESC Guidelines for the management of acute coronary syndromes in patients presenting without persistent ST-segment elevation. *Eur. Heart J.* **2021**, *42*, 1289–1367. [CrossRef] [PubMed]
37. Choudry, F.A.; Hamshere, S.M.; Rathod, K.S.; Akhtar, M.M.; Archbold, R.A.; Guttmann, O.P.; Woldman, S.; Jain, A.K.; Knight, C.J.; Baumbach, A.; et al. High Thrombus Burden in Patients with COVID-19 Presenting With ST-Segment Elevation Myocardial Infarction. *J. Am. Coll. Cardiol.* **2020**, *76*, 1168–1176. [CrossRef]
38. Hamadeh, A.; Aldujeli, A.; Briedis, K.; Tecson, K.M.; Sanz-Sánchez, J.; Al Dujeili, M.; Al-Obeidi, A.; Diez, J.L.; Žaliūnas, R.; Stoler, R.C.; et al. Characteristics and Outcomes in Patients Presenting with COVID-19 and ST-Segment Elevation Myocardial and ST-Segment Elevation Myocardial Infarction. *Am. J. Cariol.* **2020**, *131*, 1–6. [CrossRef]
39. Esposito, L.; Cancro, F.P.; Silverio, A.; Di Maio, M.; Iannece, P.; Damato, A.; Alfano, C.; De Luca, G.; Vecchione, C.; Galasso, G. COVID-19 and Acute Coronary Syndromes: From Pathophysiology to Clinical Perspectives. *Oxid. Med. Cell. Longev.* **2021**, *2021*, 4936571. [CrossRef]
40. Mehta, P.; McAuley, D.F.; Brown, M.; Sanchez, E.; Tattersall, R.S.; Manson, J.J.; HLH Across Speciality Collaboration, UK. COVID-19: Consider cytokine storm syndromes and immunosuppression. *Lancet* **2020**, *395*, 1033–1034. [CrossRef]
41. Lippi, G.; Favaloro, E.J. D-dimer is associated with severity of coronavirus disease 2019: A pooled analysis. *Thromb. Haemost.* **2020**, *120*, 876–878. [CrossRef]
42. Lippi, G.; Plebani, M.; Henry, B.M. Thrombocytopenia is associated with severe coronavirus disease 2019 (COVID-19) infections: A meta-analysis. *Clin. Chim. Acta* **2020**, *506*, 145–148. [CrossRef] [PubMed]
43. Tang, N.; Li, D.; Wang, X.; Sun, Z. Abnormal coagulation parameters are associated with poor prognosis in patients with novel coronavirus pneumonia. *J. Thromb. Haemost.* **2020**, *18*, 844–847. [CrossRef]
44. Huang, C.; Wang, Y.; Li, X.; Ren, L.; Zhao, J.; Hu, Y.; Zhang, L.; Fan, G.; Xu, J.; Gu, X.; et al. Clinical features of patients infected with 2019 novel coronavirus in Wuhan, China. *Lancet* **2020**, *395*, 497–506. [CrossRef]
45. Panigada, M.; Bottino, N.; Tagliabue, P.; Grasselli, G.; Novembrino, C.; Chantarangkul, V.; Pesenti, A.; Peyvandi, F.; Tripodi, A. Hypercoagulability of COVID-19 patients in intensive care unit: A report of thromboelastography findings and other parameters of hemostasis. *J. Thromb. Haemost.* **2020**, *18*, 1738–1742. [CrossRef]
46. Giannakopoulos, B.; Krilis, S.A. The pathogenesis of the antiphospholipid syndrome. *N. Engl. J. Med.* **2013**, *268*, 1033–1044. [CrossRef] [PubMed]
47. Mestas, J.; Ley, K. Monocyte-endothelial cell interactions in the development of atherosclerosis. *Trends Cardiovasc. Med.* **2008**, *18*, 228–232. [CrossRef]
48. Noels, H.; Weber, C.; Koenen, R.R. Chemokines as Therapeutic Targets in Cardiovascular Disease. *Arterioscler. Thromb. Vasc. Biol.* **2019**, *39*, 583–592. [CrossRef]
49. Pober, J.S.; Sessa, W.C. Evolving functions of endothelial cells in inflammation. *Nat. Rev. Immunol.* **2007**, *7*, 803–815. [CrossRef]
50. Lampsas, S.; Tsaplaris, P.; Pantelidis, P.; Oikonomou, E.; Marinos, G.; Charalambous, G.; Souvaliotis, N.; Mystakidi, V.C.; Goliopoulou, A.; Katsianos, E.; et al. The Role of Endothelial Related Circulating Biomarkers in COVID-19. A Systematic Review and Meta-analysis. *Curr. Med. Chem.* **2022**, *29*, 3790–3805. [CrossRef]
51. Del Valle, D.M.; Kim-Schulze, S.; Huang, H.H.; Beckmann, N.D.; Nirenberg, S.; Wang, B.; Lavin, Y.; Swartz, T.H.; Madduri, D.; Stock, A.; et al. An inflammatory cytokine signature predicts COVID-19 severity and survival. *Nat. Med.* **2020**, *26*, 1636–1643. [CrossRef] [PubMed]
52. Gutiérrez, E.; Flammer, A.J.; Lerman, L.O.; Elízaga, J.; Lerman, A.; Fernández-Avilés, F. Endothelial dysfunction over the course of coronary artery disease. *Eur. Heart J.* **2013**, *34*, 3175–3181. [CrossRef]
53. Varga, Z.; Flammer, A.J.; Steiger, P.; Haberecker, M.; Andermatt, R.; Zinkernagel, A.S.; Mehra, M.R.; Schuepbach, R.A.; Ruschitzka, F.; Moch, H. Endothelial cell infection and endotheliitis in COVID-19. *Lancet* **2020**, *395*, 1417–1418. [CrossRef]
54. Klok, F.A.; Kruip, M.J.H.A.; van der Meer, N.J.M.; Arbous, M.S.; Gommers, D.A.M.P.J.; Kant, K.M.; Kaptein, F.H.J.; van Paassen, J.; Stals, M.A.M.; Huisman, M.V.; et al. Incidence of thrombotic complications in critically ill ICU patients with COVID-19. *Thromb. Res.* **2020**, *191*, 145–147. [CrossRef] [PubMed]

55. Stahl, K.; Gronski, P.A.; Kiyan, Y.; Seeliger, B.; Bertram, A.; Pape, T.; Welte, T.; Hoeper, M.M.; Haller, H.; David, S. Injury to the Endothelial Glycocalyx in Critically Ill Patients with COVID-19. *Am. J. Respir. Crit. Care Med.* **2020**, *202*, 1178–1181. [CrossRef]
56. Rubio-Gayosso, I.; Platts, S.H.; Duling, B.R. Reactive oxygen species mediate modification of glycocalyx during ischemia-reperfusion injury. *Am. J. Physiol. Heart Circ. Physiol.* **2006**, *290*, H2247–H2256. [CrossRef]
57. Alphonsus, C.S.; Rodseth, R.N. The endothelial glycocalyx: A review of the vascular barrier. *Anaesthesia* **2014**, *69*, 777–784. [CrossRef]
58. Uchimido, R.; Schmidt, E.P.; Shapiro, N.I. The glycocalyx: A novel diagnostic and therapeutic target in sepsis. *Crit. Care* **2019**, *23*, 6. [CrossRef]
59. Buijsers, B.; Yanginlar, C.; de Nooijer, A.; Grondman, I.; Maciej-Hulme, M.L.; Jonkman, I.; Janssen, N.A.F.; Rother, N.; de Graaf, M.; Pickkers, P.; et al. Increased Plasma Heparanase Activity in COVID-19 Patients. *Front. Immunol.* **2020**, *11*, 575047. [CrossRef]
60. Croce, K.; Libby, P. Intertwining of thrombosis and inflammation in atherosclerosis. *Curr. Opin. Hematol.* **2007**, *14*, 55–61. [CrossRef]
61. Pennathur, S.; Heinecke, J.W. Oxidative stress and endothelial dysfunction in vascular disease. *Curr. Diabetes Rep.* **2007**, *7*, 257–264. [CrossRef] [PubMed]
62. Rafnsson, A.; Matic, L.P.; Lengquist, M.; Mahdi, A.; Shemyakin, A.; Paulsson-Berne, G.; Hansson, G.K.; Gabrielsen, A.; Hedin, U.; Yang, J.; et al. Endothelin-1 increases expression and activity of arginase 2 via ETB receptors and is co-expressed with arginase 2 in human atherosclerotic plaques. *Atherosclerosis* **2020**, *292*, 215–223. [CrossRef] [PubMed]
63. Libby, P.; Ridker, P.M.; Hansson, G.K. Inflammation in atherosclerosis: From pathophysiology to practice. *J. Am. Coll. Cardiol.* **1985**, *54*, 2129–2138. [CrossRef]
64. Ardlie, N.G.; McGuiness, J.A.; Garrett, J.J. Effect on human platelets of catecholamines at levels achieved in the circulation. *Atherosclerosis* **1985**, *58*, 251–259. [CrossRef]
65. Katritsis, D.G.; Pantos, J.; Efstathopoulos, E. Hemodynamic factors and atheromatic plaque rupture in the coronary arteries: From vulnerable plaque to vulnerable coronary segment. *Coron Artery Dis.* **2007**, *18*, 229–237. [CrossRef] [PubMed]
66. Warner, S.J.; Auger, K.R.; Libby, P. Human interleukin 1 induces interleukin 1 gene expression in human vascular smooth muscle cells. *J. Exp. Med.* **1987**, *165*, 1316–1331. [CrossRef]
67. Pons, S.; Arnaud, M.; Loiselle, M.; Arrii, E.; Azoulay, E.; Zafrani, L. Immune Consequences of Endothelial Cells' Activation and Dysfunction During Sepsis. *Crit. Care Clin.* **2020**, *36*, 401–413. [CrossRef]
68. Helms, J.; Tacquard, C.; Severac, F.; Leonard-Lorant, I.; Ohana, M.; Delabranche, X.; Merdji, H.; Clere-Jehl, R.; Schenck, M.; Fagot Gandet, F.; et al. High risk of thrombosis in patients with severe SARS-CoV-2 infection: A multicenter prospective cohort study. *Intensive Care Med.* **2020**, *46*, 1089–1098. [CrossRef]
69. Chen, N.; Zhou, M.; Dong, X.; Qu, J.; Gong, F.; Han, Y.; Qiu, Y.; Wang, J.; Liu, Y.; Wei, Y.; et al. Epidemiological and clinical characteristics of 99 cases of 2019 novel coronavirus pneumonia in Wuhan, China: A descriptive study. *Lancet* **2020**, *395*, 507–513. [CrossRef]
70. Rodriguez-Leor, O.; Cid Alvarez, A.B.; Pérez de Prado, A.; Rossello, X.; Ojeda, S.; Serrador, A.; López-Palop, R.; Martin-Moreiras, J.; Rumoroso, J.R.; Cequier, A.; et al. In-hospital outcomes of COVID-19 ST-elevation myocardial infarction patients. *EuroIntervention* **2021**, *16*, 1426–1433. [CrossRef]
71. Popovic, B.; Varlot, J.; Metzdorf, P.A.; Jeulin, H.; Goehringer, F.; Camenzind, E. Changes in characteristics and management among patients with ST-elevation myocardial infarction due to COVID-19 infection. *Catheter. Cardiovasc. Interv.* **2021**, *97*, E319–E326. [CrossRef] [PubMed]
72. Basso, C.; Leone, O.; Rizzo, S.; De Gaspari, M.; van der Wal, A.C.; Aubry, M.C.; Bois, M.C.; Lin, P.T.; Maleszewski, J.J.; Stone, J.R. Pathological features of COVID-19-associated myocardial injury: A multicentre cardiovascular pathology study. *Eur. Heart J.* **2020**, *41*, 3827–3835. [CrossRef] [PubMed]
73. Shi, S.; Qin, M.; Shen, B.; Cai, Y.; Liu, T.; Yang, F.; Gong, W.; Liu, X.; Liang, J.; Zhao, Q.; et al. Association of Cardiac Injury with Mortality in Hospitalized Patients with COVID-19 in Wuhan, China. *JAMA Cardiol.* **2020**, *5*, 802–810. [CrossRef] [PubMed]
74. Chapman, A.R.; Shah, A.S.V.; Lee, K.K.; Anand, A.; Francis, O.; Adamson, P.; McAllister, D.A.; Strachan, F.E.; Newby, D.E.; Mills, N.L. Long-Term Outcomes in Patients with Type 2 Myocardial Infarction and Myocardial Injury. *Circulation* **2018**, *137*, 1236–1245. [CrossRef]
75. Stefanini, G.G.; Montorfano, M.; Trabattoni, D.; Andreini, D.; Ferrante, G.; Ancona, M.; Metra, M.; Curello, S.; Maffeo, D.; Pero, G.; et al. ST-Elevation Myocardial Infarction in Patients with COVID-19: Clinical and Angiographic Outcomes. *Circulation* **2020**, *141*, 2113–2116. [CrossRef]
76. Bangalore, S.; Sharma, A.; Slotwiner, A.; Yatskar, L.; Harari, R.; Shah, B.; Ibrahim, H.; Friedman, G.H.; Thompson, C.; Alviar, C.L.; et al. ST-Segment Elevation in Patients with COVID-19—A Case Series. *N. Engl. J. Med.* **2020**, *382*, 2478–2480. [CrossRef] [PubMed]
77. Rivero, F.; Antuña, P.; Cuesta, J.; Alfonso, F. Severe coronary spasm in a COVID-19 patient. *Catheter. Cardiovasc. Interv.* **2021**, *97*, E670–E672. [CrossRef] [PubMed]
78. Reynolds, H.R.; Maehara, A.; Kwong, R.Y.; Sedlak, T.; Saw, J.; Smilowitz, N.R.; Mahmud, E.; Wei, J.; Marzo, K.; Matsumura, M.; et al. Coronary Optical Coherence Tomography and Cardiac Magnetic Resonance Imaging to Determine Underlying Causes of Myocardial Infarction with Nonobstructive Coronary Arteries in Women. *Circulation* **2021**, *143*, 624–640. [CrossRef]

79. Dastidar, A.G.; Baritussio, A.; De Garate, E.; Drobni, Z.; Biglino, G.; Singhal, P.; Milano, E.G.; Angelini, G.D.; Dorman, S.; Strange, J.; et al. Prognostic Role of CMR and Conventional Risk Factors in Myocardial Infarction with Nonobstructed Coronary Arteries. *JACC Cardiovasc. Imaging* 2019, 12, 1973–1982. [CrossRef]
80. Daubert, M.A.; Jeremias, A. The utility of troponin measurement to detect myocardial infarction: Review of the current findings. *Vasc. Health Risk Manag.* 2010, 6, 691–699.
81. Adams, J.E.; Abendschein, D.R.; Jaffe, A.S. Biochemical markers of myocardial injury. Is MB creatine kinase the choice for the 1990s. *Circulation* 1993, 88, 750–763. [CrossRef] [PubMed]
82. Rhinehardt, J.; Brady, W.J.; Perron, A.D.; Mattu, A. Electrocardiographic manifestations of Wellens' syndrome. *Am. J. Emerg. Med.* 2002, 20, 638–643. [CrossRef] [PubMed]
83. García de Guadiana-Romualdo, L.; Morell-García, D.; Rodríguez-Fraga, O.; Morales-Indiano, C.; María Lourdes Padilla Jiménez, A.; Gutiérrez Revilla, J.I.; Urrechaga, E.; Álamo, J.M.; Hernando Holgado, A.M.; Lorenzo-Lozano, M.D.C.; et al. Cardiac troponin and COVID-19 severity: Results from BIOCOVID study. *Eur. J. Clin. Investig.* 2021, 51, e13532. [CrossRef] [PubMed]
84. Santoso, A.; Pranata, R.; Wibowo, A.; Al-Farabi, M.J.; Huang, I.; Antariksa, B. Cardiac injury is associated with mortality and critically ill pneumonia in COVID-19: A meta-analysis. *Am. J. Emerg. Med.* 2021, 44, 352–357. [CrossRef] [PubMed]
85. Romero, J.; Alviz, I.; Parides, M.; Diaz, J.C.; Briceno, D.; Gabr, M.; Gamero, M.; Patel, K.; Braunstein, E.D.; Purkayastha, S.; et al. T-wave inversion as a manifestation of COVID-19 infection: A case series. *J. Interv. Card. Electrophysiol.* 2020, 59, 485–493. [CrossRef]
86. Michael, M.A.; El Masry, H.; Khan, B.R.; Das, M.K. Electrocardiographic signs of remote myocardial infarction. *Prog. Cardiovasc. Dis.* 2007, 50, 198–208. [CrossRef]
87. Landesberg, G. Monitoring for myocardial ischemia. *Best Pract. Res. Clin. Anaesthesiol.* 2005, 19, 77–95. [CrossRef]
88. Li, Y.; Liu, T.; Tse, G.; Wu, M.; Jiang, J.; Liu, M.; Tao, L. Electrocardiograhic characteristics in patients with coronavirus infection: A single-center observational study. *Ann. Noninvasive Electrocardiol.* 2020, 25, e12805. [CrossRef]
89. Wang, Y.; Chen, L.; Wang, J.; He, X.; Huang, F.; Chen, J.; Yang, X. Electrocardiogram analysis of patients with different types of COVID-19. *Ann. Noninvasive Electrocardiol.* 2020, 25, e12806. [CrossRef]
90. Angeli, F.; Reboldi, G.; Spanevello, A.; De Ponti, R.; Visca, D.; Marazzato, J.; Zappa, M.; Trapasso, M.; Masnaghetti, S.; Fabbri, L.M.; et al. Electrocardiographic features of patients with COVID-19: One year of unexpected manifestations. *Eur. J. Intern. Med.* 2022, 95, 7–12. [CrossRef]
91. Poterucha, T.J.; Elias, P.; Jain, S.S.; Sayer, G.; Redfors, B.; Burkhoff, D.; Rosenblum, H.; DeFilippis, E.M.; Gupta, A.; Lawlor, M.; et al. Admission Cardiac Diagnostic Testing with Electrocardiography and Troponin Measurement Prognosticates Increased 30-Day Mortality in COVID-19. *J. Am. Heart Assoc.* 2021, 10, e018476. [CrossRef]
92. Sonsoz, M.R.; Oncul, A.; Cevik, E.; Orta, H.; Yilmaz, M.; Ayduk Govdeli, E.; Nalbant, A.; Demirtakan, Z.G.; Tonyali, M.; Durmus, D.; et al. Wide QRS Complex and Lateral ST-T Segment Abnormality Are Associated with Worse Clinical Outcomes in COVID-19 Patients. *Am. J. Med. Sci.* 2021, 361, 591–597. [CrossRef] [PubMed]
93. Li, L.; Zhang, S.; He, B.; Chen, X.; Wang, S.; Zhao, Q. Risk factors and electrocardiogram characteristics for mortality in critical inpatients with COVID-19. *Clin. Cardiol.* 2020, 43, 1624–1630. [CrossRef] [PubMed]
94. Marzieh, M.; Rezvanjeh, S.; Maryam, C. A novel electrocardiogram characteristic in patients with myocardial injury due to COVID-19. *Res. Cardiovasc. Med.* 2021, 10, 83–87.
95. Bergamaschi, L.; D'Angelo, E.C.; Paolisso, P.; Toniolo, S.; Fabrizio, M.; Angeli, F.; Donati, F.; Magnani, I.; Rinaldi, A.; Bartoli, L.; et al. The value of ECG changes in risk stratification of COVID-19 patients. *Ann. Noninvasive Electrocardiol.* 2021, 26, e12815. [CrossRef] [PubMed]
96. Ogungbe, O.; Kumbe, B.; Fadodun, O.; Latha, T.; Meyer, D.; Asala, A.; Davidson, P.M.; Dennison Himmelfarb, C.R.; Post, W.S.; Commodore-Mensah, Y. Subclinical myocardial injury, coagulopathy, and inflammation in COVID-19: A meta-analysis of 41,013 hospitalized patients. *Int. J. Cardiol. Heart Vasc.* 2022, 40, 100950. [CrossRef]
97. Chorin, E.; Dai, M.; Kogan, E.; Wadhwani, L.; Shulman, E.; Nadeau-Routhier, C.; Knotts, R.; Bar-Cohen, R.; Barbhaiya, C.; Aizer, A.; et al. Electrocardiographic Risk Stratification in COVID-19 Patients. *Front Cardiovasc Med.* 2021, 8, 636073. [CrossRef]
98. Bae, J.Y.; Hussein, K.I.; Howes, C.J.; Setaro, F.S. The Challenges of ST-Elevation Myocardial Infarction in COVID-19 Patients. *Case Rep. Cardiol.* 2021, 2021, 9915650. [CrossRef] [PubMed]
99. Thygesen, K.; Alpert, J.S.; Jaffe, A.S.; White, H.D. Diagnostic application of the universal definition of myocardial infarction in the intensive care unit. *Curr. Opin. Crit. Care* 2008, 14, 543–548. [CrossRef]
100. Cipriani, A.; D'Amico, G.; Brunetti, G.; Vescovo, G.M.; Donato, F.; Gambato, M.; Dall'Aglio, P.B.; Cardaioli, F.; Previato, M.; Martini, N.; et al. Electrocardiographic Predictors of Primary Ventricular Fibrillation and 30-Day Mortality in Patients Presenting with ST-Segment Elevation Myocardial Infarction. *J. Clin. Med.* 2021, 10, 5933. [CrossRef]
101. Centurión, O.A. Wide QRS Complex and Left Ventricular Lateral Repolarization Abnormality: The Importance of ECG Markers on Outcome Prediction in Patients with COVID-19. *Am. J. Med. Sci.* 2021, 362, 1–2. [CrossRef] [PubMed]
102. Haji Aghajani, M.; Toloui, A.; Aghamohammadi, M.; Pourhoseingholi, A.; Taherpour, N.; Sistanizad, M.; Madani Neishaboori, A.; Asadpoordezaki, Z.; Miri, R. Electrocardiographic Findings and In-Hospital Mortality of COVID-19 Patients; a Retrospective Cohort Study. *Arch. Acad. Emerg. Med.* 2021, 9, e45. [PubMed]
103. Siddamreddy, S.; Thotakura, R.; Dandu, V.; Kanuru, S.; Meegada, S. Corona Virus Disease 2019 (COVID-19) Presenting as Acute ST Elevation Myocardial Infarction. *Cureus* 2020, 12, e7782. [CrossRef] [PubMed]

104. Xiao, Z.; Xu, C.; Wang, D.; Zeng, H. The experience of treating patients with acute myocardial infarction under the COVID-19 epidemic. *Catheter. Cardiovasc. Interv.* **2021**, *97*, E244–E248. [CrossRef]
105. Moroni, F.; Gramegna, M.; Ajello, S.; Beneduce, A.; Baldetti, L.; Vilca, L.M.; Cappelletti, A.; Scandroglio, A.M.; Azzalini, L. Collateral Damage: Medical Care Avoidance Behavior among Patients with Myocardial Infarction during the COVID-19 Pandemic. *JACC Case Rep.* **2020**, *2*, 1620–1624. [CrossRef]
106. Eid, M.M.; Zubaidi, A.A. ST-elevation myocardial infarction in a patient with COVID-19. *Vis. J. Emerg. Med.* **2021**, *25*, 101151. [CrossRef]
107. Ehrman, R.R.; Brennan, E.E.; Creighton, T.; Ottenhoff, J.; Favot, M.J. ST Elevation in the COVID-19 Era: A Diagnostic Challenge. *J. Emerg. Med.* **2021**, *60*, 103–106. [CrossRef]
108. Yolcu, M.; Gunesdogdu, F.; Bektas, M.; Bayirli, D.T.; Serefhanoglu, K. Coronavirus disease 2019 (COVID-19) and simultaneous acute anteroseptal and inferior ST-segment elevation myocardial infarction. *Cardiovasc. J. Afr.* **2020**, *31*, 335–338. [CrossRef]
109. Hulkoti, V.; Acharya, S.; Talwar, D.; Khanna, S. Medical Science l Case Report Myocardial infarction in a young female: A rare case report. *Med. Sci.* **2021**, *25*, 1281–1285.
110. Harari, R.; Bangalore, S.; Chang, E.; Shah, B. COVID-19 complicated by acute myocardial infarction with extensive thrombus burden and cardiogenic shock. *Catheter. Cardiovasc. Interv.* **2021**, *97*, E661–E666. [CrossRef]
111. Bertini, M.; Ferrari, R.; Guardigli, G.; Malagù, M.; Vitali, F.; Zucchetti, O.; D'Aniello, E.; Volta, C.A.; Cimaglia, P.; Piovaccari, G.; et al. Electrocardiographic features of 431 consecutive, critically ill COVID-19 patients: An insight into the mechanisms of cardiac involvement. *Europace* **2020**, *22*, 1848–1854. [CrossRef] [PubMed]
112. Asif, T.; Ali, Z. Transient ST Segment Elevation in Two Patients with COVID-19 and a Normal Transthoracic Echocardiogram. *Eur. J. Case Rep. Intern. Med.* **2020**, *7*, 001672. [PubMed]
113. Meizinger, C.; Klugherz, B. Focal ST-segment elevation without coronary occlusion: Myocardial infarction with no obstructive coronary atherosclerosis associated with COVID-19—A case report. *Eur. Heart J. Case Rep.* **2021**, *5*, ytaa532. [CrossRef]
114. Angeli, F.; Spanevello, A.; De Ponti, R.; Visca, D.; Marazzato, J.; Palmiotto, G.; Feci, D.; Reboldi, G.; Fabbri, L.M.; Verdecchia, P. Electrocardiographic features of patients with COVID-19 pneumonia. *Eur. J. Intern. Med.* **2020**, *78*, 101–106. [CrossRef]
115. Channer, K.; Morris, F. ABC of clinical electrocardiography: Myocardial ischaemia. *BMJ* **2002**, *324*, 1023–1026. [CrossRef] [PubMed]
116. Antwi-Amoabeng, D.; Beutler, B.D.; Singh, S.; Taha, M.; Ghuman, J.; Hanfy, A.; Manasewitsch, N.T.; Ulanja, M.B.; Ghuman, J.; Awad, M.; et al. Association between electrocardiographic features and mortality in COVID-19 patients. *Ann. Noninvasive Electrocardiol.* **2021**, *26*, e12833. [CrossRef]
117. Heberto, A.B.; Carlos, P.C.J.; Antonio, C.R.J.; Patricia, P.P.; Enrique, T.R.; Danira, M.P.J.; Benito, G.Á.E.; Alfredo, M.R.J. Implications of myocardial injury in Mexican hospitalized patients with coronavirus disease 2019 (COVID-19). *Int. J. Cardiol. Heart Vasc.* **2020**, *30*, 100638. [CrossRef]
118. Abrams, M.P.; Wan, E.Y.; Waase, M.P.; Morrow, J.P.; Dizon, J.M.; Yarmohammadi, H.; Berman, J.P.; Rubin, G.A.; Kushnir, A.; Poterucha, T.J.; et al. Clinical and cardiac characteristics of COVID-19 mortalities in a diverse New York City Cohort. *J. Cardiovasc. Electrophysiol.* **2020**, *31*, 3086–3096. [CrossRef]
119. Chen, L.; Feng, Y.; Tang, J.; Hu, W.; Zhao, P.; Guo, X.; Huang, N.; Gu, Y.; Hu, L.; Duru, F.; et al. Surface electrocardiographic characteristics in coronavirus disease 2019: Repolarization abnormalities associated with cardiac involvement. *ESC Heart Fail.* **2020**, *7*, 4408–4415. [CrossRef]
120. Maeda, T.; Obata, R.; Rizk, D.; Kuno, T. Cardiac Injury and Outcomes of Patients with COVID-19 in New York City. *Heart Lung Circ.* **2021**, *30*, 848–853. [CrossRef]
121. Capaccione, K.M.; Leb, J.S.; D'souza, B.; Utukuri, P.; Salvatore, M.M. Acute myocardial infarction secondary to COVID-19 infection: A case report and review of the literature. *Clin. Imaging* **2021**, *72*, 178–182. [CrossRef] [PubMed]
122. De Carvalho, H.; Leonard-Pons, L.; Segard, J.; Goffinet, N.; Javaudin, F.; Martinage, A.; Cattin, G.; Tiberghien, S.; Therasse, D.; Trotignon, M.; et al. Electrocardiographic abnormalities in COVID-19 patients visiting the emergency department: A multicenter retrospective study. *BMC Emerg. Med.* **2021**, *21*, 141. [CrossRef] [PubMed]
123. Suryawan, I.G.R.; Bakhriansyah, J.; Puspitasari, M.; Gandi, P.; Intan, R.E.; Alkaff, F.F. To reperfuse or not to reperfuse: A case report of Wellens' syndrome with suspected COVID-19 infection. *Egypt. Heart J.* **2020**, *72*, 58. [CrossRef] [PubMed]
124. Mansoor, A.; Chang, D.; Mitra, R. Rhythm, conduction, and ST elevation with COVID-19: Myocarditis or myocardial infarction? *HeartRhythm Case Rep.* **2020**, *6*, 671–675. [CrossRef] [PubMed]
125. Pelliccia, F.; Kaski, J.C.; Crea, F.; Camici, P.G. Pathophysiology of Takotsubo Syndrome. *Circulation* **2017**, *135*, 2426–2441. [CrossRef]
126. Frangieh, A.H.; Obeid, S.; Ghadri, J.R.; Imori, Y.; D'Ascenzo, F.; Kovac, M.; Ruschitzka, F.; Lüscher, T.F.; Duru, F.; Templin, C.; et al. ECG Criteria to Differentiate between Takotsubo (Stress) Cardiomyopathy and Myocardial Infarction. *J. Am. Heart Assoc.* **2016**, *5*, e003418. [CrossRef]
127. Dichtl, W.; Tuovinen, N.; Barbieri, F.; Adukauskaite, A.; Senoner, T.; Rubatscher, A.; Hintringer, F.; Siedentopf, C.; Bauer, A.; Gizewski, E.R.; et al. Functional neuroimaging in the acute phase of Takotsubo syndrome: Volumetric and functional changes of the right insular cortex. *Clin. Res. Cardiol.* **2020**, *109*, 1107–1113. [CrossRef]
128. Minhas, A.S.; Scheel, P.; Garibaldi, B.; Liu, G.; Horton, M.; Jennings, M.; Jones, S.R.; Michos, E.D.; Hays, A.G. Takotsubo Syndrome in the Setting of COVID-19. *JACC Case Rep.* **2020**, *2*, 1321–1325. [CrossRef]

129. Moady, G.; Atar, S. Takotsubo Syndrome during the COVID-19 Pandemic: State-of-the-Art Review. *CJC Open* **2021**, *3*, 1249–1256. [CrossRef]
130. Okura, H. Update of takotsubo syndrome in the era of COVID-19. *J. Cardiol.* **2021**, *77*, 361–369. [CrossRef]
131. O'Keefe, E.L.; Torres-Acosta, N.; O'Keefe, J.H.; Sturgess, J.E.; Lavie, C.J.; Bybee, K.A. Takotsubo Syndrome: Cardiotoxic Stress in the COVID Era. *Mayo Clin. Proc. Innov. Qual. Outcomes* **2020**, *4*, 775–785. [CrossRef] [PubMed]
132. Desai, H.D.; Sharma, K.; Jadeja, D.M.; Desai, H.M.; Moliya, P. COVID-19 pandemic induced stress cardiomyopathy: A literature review. *Int. J. Cardiol. Heart Vasc.* **2020**, *31*, 100628. [CrossRef] [PubMed]
133. Barbieri, L.; Galli, F.; Conconi, B.; Gregorini, T.; Lucreziotti, S.; Mafrici, A.; Pravettoni, G.; Sommaruga, M.; Carugo, S. Takotsubo syndrome in COVID-19 era: Is psychological distress the key. *J. Psychosom. Res.* **2021**, *140*, 110297. [CrossRef]
134. Miner, B.; Grigg, W.S.; Hart, E.H. *Wellens Syndrome*; StatPearls Publishing: Treasure Island, FL, USA, 2022.
135. Tandy, T.K.; Bottomy, D.P.; Lewis, J.G. Wellens' syndrome. *Ann. Emerg. Med.* **1999**, *33*, 347–351. [CrossRef]
136. Prousi, G.S.; Giordano, J.; McCann, P.J. A 75-Year-Old Woman with COVID-19 Pneumonia and Wellens Syndrome Diagnosed by Electrocardiography. *Am. J. Case. Rep.* **2021**, *22*, e930125. [CrossRef] [PubMed]
137. Elkholy, K.O.; Mirashi, E.; Malyshev, Y.; Charles, G.; Sahni, S. Wellens' Syndrome in the Setting of the 2019 Novel Coronavirus (COVID-19). *Cureus* **2021**, *13*, e13290. [CrossRef]
138. Di Spigno, F.; Spezzano, T.; Halasz, G.; Piepoli, M. Un caso di sindrome di Wellens durante la pandemia COVID-19 [A case of Wellens syndrome during the COVID-19 pandemic]. *G Ital. Cardiol.* **2021**, *22*, 888–890.
139. Caiati, C.; Desario, P.; Tricarico, G.; Iacovelli, F.; Pollice, P.; Favale, S.; Lepera, M.E. Wellens' Syndrome from COVID-19 Infection Assessed by Enhanced Transthoracic Coronary Echo Doppler: A Case Report. *Diagnostics* **2022**, *12*, 804. [CrossRef]
140. Huang, W.; Mai, L.; Lu, J.; Li, W.; Huang, Y.; Hu, Y. Evolutionary de Winter pattern: From STEMI to de Winter ECG—A case report. *ESC Heart Fail.* **2022**, *9*, 771–774. [CrossRef]
141. Qayyum, H.; Hemaya, S.; Squires, J.; Adam, Z. Recognising the de Winter ECG pattern—A time critical electrocardiographic diagnosis in the Emergency Department. *J. Electrocardiol.* **2018**, *51*, 392–395. [CrossRef]
142. Xu, J.; Wang, A.; Liu, L.; Chen, Z. The de winter electrocardiogram pattern is a transient electrocardiographic phenomenon that presents at the early stage of ST-segment elevation myocardial infarction. *Clin. Cardiol.* **2018**, *41*, 1177–1184. [CrossRef]
143. Almendro-Delia, M.; Ruíz-Salmerón, R.; García-Del Río, M.; Seoane-García, T.; Trujillo-Berraquero, F.; Hidalgo-Urbano, R. The de Winter electrocardiographic pattern as an ST-elevation myocardial infarction equivalent in a young patient with COVID-19. *Emergencias* **2021**, *33*, 484–485.
144. Miranda, J.M.; de Oliveira, W.S.; de Sá, V.P.; de Sá, I.F.; Neto, N.O. Transient triangular QRS-ST-T waveform with good outcome in a patient with left main coronary artery stenosis: A case report. *J. Electrocardiol.* **2019**, *54*, 87–89. [CrossRef] [PubMed]
145. Celli, D.; Byer, M.; Sancassani, R.; Colombo, R. Triangular ECG Pattern in a Young Female with COVID-19. *Am. J. Med.* **2021**, *134*, 751–753. [CrossRef] [PubMed]
146. Mahmud, E.; Dauerman, H.L.; Welt, F.G.P.; Messenger, J.C.; Rao, S.V.; Grines, C.; Mattu, A.; Kirtane, A.J.; Jauhar, R.; Meraj, P.; et al. Management of acute myocardial infarction during the COVID-19 pandemic: A Consensus Statement from the Society for Cardiovascular Angiography and Interventions (SCAI), the American College of Cardiology (ACC), and the American College of Emergency Physicians (ACEP). *Catheter. Cardiovasc. Interv.* **2020**, *96*, 336–345. [PubMed]

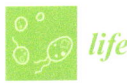

Article

Rare Causes of Acute Coronary Syndrome: Carbon Monoxide Poisoning

Raluca Ecaterina Haliga [1,2], Bianca Codrina Morărașu [1,2,*], Victorița Șorodoc [1,2], Cătălina Lionte [1,2], Oana Sîrbu [1,2], Alexandra Stoica [1,2], Alexandr Ceasovschih [1,2], Mihai Constantin [1,2] and Laurentiu Șorodoc [1,2]

1 Department of Internal Medicine and Toxicology, Saint Spiridon University Regional Emergency Hospital, 700111 Iasi, Romania; raluca.haliga@umfiasi.ro (R.E.H.); victorita.sorodoc@umfiasi.ro (V.Ș.); catalina.lionte@umfiasi.ro (C.L.); oana.sirbu@umfiasi.ro (O.S.); alexandra.rotariu@umfiasi.ro (A.S.); alexandr.ceasovschih@umfiasi.ro (A.C.); mihai.s.constantin@umfiasi.ro (M.C.); laurentiu.sorodoc@umfiasi.ro (L.Ș.)
2 Faculty of Medicine, "Grigore T. Popa" University of Medicine and Pharmacy, 700111 Iasi, Romania
* Correspondence: morarasu.bianca.codrina@gmail.com; Tel.: +40-754-300-395

Abstract: Acute coronary syndrome (ACS) is a spectrum of clinical and paraclinical disorders arising from an imbalance of oxygen demand and supply to the myocardium. The most common cause is atherosclerosis; however, other rare causes such as carbon monoxide (CO) poisoning should be considered. Through tissue hypoxia and direct cell injury, CO poisoning can lead to a broad spectrum of cardiac disorders, especially ACS. **Materials and Methods**. We have conducted a retrospective study in the Toxicology Department of Saint Spiridon Emergency University Hospital, including all patients admitted through the emergency department with CO poisoning. We divided the cohort into event group (myocardial injury) and non-event group (patients without myocardial injury) and performed a subset analysis of the former. **Results**. A total of 65 patients were included, 22 in the event and 43 in the non-event group. The severity of poisoning did not correlate with myocardial injury; however, 50% of the event group had severe poisoning with carboxyhaemoglobin $\geq 20\%$. Cardiac enzyme markers (troponin and creatin-kinase MB) had a statistically significant increase in the event group compared to the non-event group ($p < 0.05$). Most of the patients in the STEMI (50%) and NSTEMI (66.7%) groups had severe CO intoxication. The STEMI group had a mean age of 27.7 years old and no comorbidities. **Conclusions**. Myocardial injury can develop in CO poisoning irrespective of the severity of poisoning, and it can be transient, reversible, or permanent. Our study introduces new information on adverse cardiac events in patients with CO poisoning, focusing on the ACS. We found that the severity of CO poisoning plays an important role in developing myocardial injury, as 50% of patients in the event group were severely intoxicated. While in-hospital mortality in our study was low, further prospective studies should investigate the long-term mortality in these patients.

Keywords: acute coronary syndrome; carbon monoxide poisoning; myocardial injury; severity of poisoning

Citation: Haliga, R.E.; Morărașu, B.C.; Șorodoc, V.; Lionte, C.; Sîrbu, O.; Stoica, A.; Ceasovschih, A.; Constantin, M.; Șorodoc, L. Rare Causes of Acute Coronary Syndrome: Carbon Monoxide Poisoning. *Life* 2022, *12*, 1158. https://doi.org/10.3390/life12081158

Academic Editor: Gopal J. Babu

Received: 14 June 2022
Accepted: 27 July 2022
Published: 29 July 2022

Publisher's Note: MDPI stays neutral with regard to jurisdictional claims in published maps and institutional affiliations.

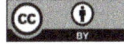

Copyright: © 2022 by the authors. Licensee MDPI, Basel, Switzerland. This article is an open access article distributed under the terms and conditions of the Creative Commons Attribution (CC BY) license (https://creativecommons.org/licenses/by/4.0/).

1. Introduction

Acute coronary syndrome (ACS) is a consequence of a sudden imbalance between oxygen demand and supply to the myocardium. It is represented by a spectrum of clinical and paraclinical presentations, ranging from ST-segment elevation myocardial infarction (STEMI) to non–ST-segment elevation myocardial infarction (NSTEMI) or unstable angina [1]. The most common cause of ACS is atherosclerosis (90%), which is frequently complicated, leading to partial or complete thrombosis of infarct-related coronary artery [2]. There are other rare causes of ACS, such as endocrine or haematological. Spasm, obstruction, inflammation, or trauma of the coronary arteries can cause myocardial injury. Carbon monoxide (CO) poisoning, through different mechanisms, can be the cause of ACS.

CO poisoning is a major public health problem, being one of the leading causes of death and injury worldwide [3]. Cumulative worldwide incidence and mortality of CO poisoning are currently estimated at 137 cases and 4.6 deaths per million, respectively [4]. In Europe, national data provided by 28 European member states on CO poisoning reported an annual rate of 2.2/100,000 CO-related deaths [5].

CO has a specific effect on highly sensitive tissues to hypoxia, such as brain or heart [6]. Its toxicity is the result of hypoxia, increased carboxyhaemoglobin (CoHgb) formation and direct CO-mediated cell damage. Furthermore, CO can induce coronary spasm and intracoronary thrombosis and increase vascular permeability and platelet aggregation [7], which can lead to ACS both on healthy and non-critical atherosclerotic plaque [8].

In this retrospective study, we aim to analyse and describe our experience regarding cardiovascular events in the context of acute CO poisoning, focusing on ACS in relation to the severity of CO intoxication, comorbidities, clinical and biological characteristics, and outcome of patients.

2. Materials and Methods

2.1. Study Design and Selection of Patients

We carried out a retrospective study in "Saint Spiridon" Regional Emergency Hospital, Toxicology Department, a tertiary regional centre for clinical toxicology in northeast Romania. We included all patients aged over 18 with a diagnosis of CO poisoning between 1 January 2013 and 31 December 2021.

Inclusion criteria consisted of patients admitted through the emergency department (ED) with at least one of the following: history of CO exposure, increased COHgb levels, and symptoms consistent with CO poisoning.

The electronic hospital records were searched based on the patient's diagnosis at discharge. We extracted the following data: patient's demographics (gender, age, residential area, smoking status), body mass index (BMI—using the following cut-off: normal—18.5–24.9 kg/m^2, overweight—25–29.9 kg/m^2, obesity $\geq$ 30 kg/m^2) [9], comorbidities (arterial hypertension, ischaemic heart disease, previous myocardial infarction (MI), heart failure, diabetes mellitus type 2, presence of angina type pain, level of COHgb on admission, cardiac enzymes (troponin and creatin-kinase MB (CK-MB)), electrocardiogram (ECG) upon presentation and during admission, if performed by attending physician, need for orotracheal intubation upon presentation, clinical outcome and length of admission. ECGs were retrospectively reviewed by 2 Internal Medicine Trainees (1st and 5th year of training). Subsequently, an Internal Medicine Consultant randomly reviewed the ECGs to ensure accuracy.

We used the following definitions for the severity of poisoning: mild poisoning—COHgb > 10% without clinical signs and symptoms or COHgb < 10% with associated signs and symptoms, moderate poisoning—COHgb 10–19% with clinical signs and symptoms, severe poisoning—COHgb $\geq$ 20% with clinical signs and symptoms [3,10]; for clinical outcome: favourable—the patient was discharged when considered clinically improved by treating physician; against medical advice—the patient discharged himself against medical advice from treating physician; death—patient died due to CO poisoning or associated acute illness in this context. Length of admission was divided into 3 main categories: 1–3 days; 4–7 days and >7 days. Whenever the information was missing, it was mentioned as not available (NA).

Patients younger than 18, with acute concomitant illness requiring a specific approach in a different department, except for the Toxicology Intensive Care Unit (ICU) (e.g., burns, trauma, acute stroke etc.), were excluded from our study.

2.2. Outcomes

The primary outcome was to analyse the incidence and types of cardiac ischemic events by dividing the patients into 2 cohorts: event group (myocardial injury) and non-event group (patients without myocardial injury). We further performed a subset analysis of patients in the event group in relation to the severity of acute CO poisoning. Myocardial injury was identified as evidence of STEMI (new ST-segment elevation ≥ 1 mm in 2 consecutive leads), NSTEMI (new ST-segment depression ≥ 0.5 mm in 2 consecutive leads), other features of ischaemia (new T-wave inversion ≥ 2 mm in 2 consecutive leads). Secondary outcomes were the presence of rhythm and conduction disorders, positive cardiac enzymes, need for intubation, length of admission and clinical outcome.

2.3. Blood Analysis

COHgb concentration in venous blood was measured using the ABL90 Series method (Radiometer, Copenhagen, Denmark) in ED. Cardiac enzymes (troponin and CK-MB) were measured using an ARHITECT clinical chemistry analyser (Abbott Laboratories, Abbott Park, IL, USA). This high-sensitivity troponin assay was introduced in 2018. Throughout the years, we have used several assays with different sensitivities and specificities.

2.4. Treatment

All patients underwent initial assessment and treatment in the ED to ensure the stability of vital signs, carboxyhaemoglobin measurement and 100% oxygen therapy, as well as full blood tests (full blood count, biochemistry, coagulation tests) in symptomatic patients (e.g., malaise, nausea, headache, chest pain, reduced consciousness, coma [3]). Cardiac enzymes were taken as indicated by the emergency medicine/internal medicine/toxicology consultant. In the case of severe poisoning associated with the need for intubation (GCS 8, acute respiratory failure not corrected by non-invasive treatment), severe acidosis (pH < 7.2 despite adequate treatment), fluid-resistant hypotension (MAP < 65 mmHg), or other appropriate criteria, as indicated by the ICU Consultant, patients were managed in the Toxicology ICU department. Those clinically stable (e.g., systolic blood pressure > 90 mmHg, GCS > 9, oxygen saturation > 80 correcting with oxygen therapy, absence of new organ failure) but requiring further observation and/or management of CO poisoning and associated comorbidities were admitted to our Toxicology Department.

2.5. Data Analysis

Statistical analyses were performed with SPSS software for Windows (v.22.0; SPSS, Chicago, IL, USA). Nominal variables are presented as frequencies and percentages, and continuous variables are presented as the mean $\pm$ standard deviation (SD). To identify significant parameters associated with a CO poisoning diagnosis, a two-tailed Student's t-test was used to compare normally distributed continuous variables, whereas the chi-squared test and Cochrane's statistic were used for categorical variables. A p-value < 0.05 was considered statistically significant.

3. Results

3.1. Patients' Characteristics

Sixty-five patients with acute CO poisoning were admitted to our Toxicology department between 2013 and 2021, out of a total of 1780 patients with drug/non-pharmaceutical-induced acute poisonings. In all cases, the poisoning was accidental because of either a house fire, incorrectly installed, or faulty gas-powered generators, heating systems or wood stoves. The demographic characteristics of the cohort are presented in Table 1.

A high percentage (40%) of patients were young, aged between 18 and 39 years old. In total, 55.4% of patients were female, 61.5% lived in urban areas, and 35.4% were current smokers.

3.2. Severity of CO Poisoning

Of the 65 acute CO poisoning patients included in the study, 44.6% had mild, while 35.4% had severe poisoning.

Table 1. Characteristics of patients with acute CO poisoning.

Demographic Data	Total (n = 65)	%
Age interval		
18–39 years	26	40.0
40–59 years	12	18.5
60–79 years	19	29.2
over 80 years	8	12.3
Gender		
Male	29	44.6
Female	36	55.4
Residence		
Urban	40	61.5
Rural	25	38.5
Smoking		
Current smoker	23	35.4
Non-smoker	42	64.6
Body mass index		
Normal	21	32.3
Overweight	7	10.8
Obesity	4	6.2
Not available	33	50.8
Patients' comorbidities		
Diabetes mellitus type 2	7	10.8
Arterial hypertension	12	18.5
Ischemic heart disease	9	13.8
Previous MI	1	1.5
Heart failure	9	13.8
Severity of poisoning		
Mild poisoning	29	44.6
Moderate poisoning	13	20.0
Severe poisoning	23	35.4

3.3. Cardiac Ischemic Events

Out of 65 patients, 22 are in the event group and 43 in the non-event group, with a mean age of 57 years old and 48 years old, respectively (Table 2).

Regarding smoking status and comorbidities, there is no statistically significant difference between the two groups. Approximately one-third of the patients were current smokers in both groups. Comorbidities were present in both groups to a certain degree; arterial hypertension was slightly more present in the event group (27.3%) compared to the non-event group (14.0%).

The severity of poisoning does not correlate with cardiac ischaemic events. For each degree of CO toxicity, there is a similar proportion of affected individuals, both in the event and non-event groups. However, 50% of the event group had severe poisoning with COHgb $\geq$ 20%, while the non-event group had mild poisoning in most cases (48.8%).

Cardiac enzyme markers (troponin and CK-MB) had a statistically significant increase in the event group compared to the non-event group ($p < 0.05$). On the other hand, troponin was not available in 58.1% of the non-event group. There was no difference between groups regarding orotracheal intubation.

Patients with cardiac events had a longer admission, 4–7 days (45.5%), compared to the non-event group, admitted for 1–3 days (55.8%). Most of our patients had a favourable outcome, 77.3% in the first and 55.8% in the second group, with 9.1% and 7% mortality rates in the two groups.

Table 2. Characteristics of event and non-event groups.

Parameter	Event (n = 22)	Non-Event (n = 43)	χ^2 Test	T Test	p Value
Mean Age	57.45 ± 24.27	48.65 ± 21.06		2.292	0.135
Smoking status			0.440		0.507
Current smoker	9 (40.9%)	14 (32.6%)			
Non-smoker	13 (59.1%)	29 (67.4%)			
Angina	3 (13.6%)	1 (2.3%)	3.029		0.082
Comorbidities					
Diabetes mellitus type 2	2 (9.1%)	5 (11.6%)	0.100		0.752
Arterial hypertension	6 (27.3%)	6 (14.0%)	1.646		0.200
Ischemic heart disease	4 (18.2%)	5 (11.6%)	0.507		0.477
Previous myocardial infarction	0 (0.0%)	1 (2.3%)	0.834		0.361
Heart failure	4 (18.2%)	5 (11.6%)	0.507		0.477
Severity of poisoning			3.153		0.207
Mild poisoning	8 (36.4%)	21 (48.8%)			
Moderate poisoning	3 (13.6%)	10 (23.3%)			
Severe poisoning	11 (50.0%)	12 (27.9%)			
Troponin			10.396		0.006
Increased	2 (9.1%)	1 (2.3%)			
Normal	16 (72.7%)	17 (39.5%)			
NA	4 (18.2%)	25 (58.1%)			
CK-MB			9.009		0.011
Increased	5 (22.7%)	13 (30.2%)			
Normal	16 (72.7%)	17 (39.5%)			
NA	1 (4.5%)	13 (30.2%)			
Orotracheal intubation	3 (13.6%)	5 (11.6%)	0.054		0.817
Length of admission			4.067		0.131
1–3 days	7 (31.8%)	24 (55.8%)			
4–7 days	10 (45.5%)	15 (34.9%)			
Over 7 days	5 (22.7%)	4 (9.3%)			
Outcome			4.260		0.119
Favourable	17 (77.3%)	24 (55.8%)			
Death	2 (9.1%)	3 (7.0%)			
Discharged against medical advice	3 (13.6%)	16 (37.2%)			

We further characterised the event group depending on the type of ECG changes (other features of ischaemia, STEMI and NSTEMI). There are nine patients with other features of ischaemia, four patients with STEMI and nine with NSTEMI. The STEMI group is relatively younger, with a mean age of 27.7 years old and no comorbidities. Arterial hypertension and ischaemic heart disease are present in 44.4% and 33.3% of the other features of the ischaemia group, compared to 22.2% and 11.1% in the NSTEMI group. Most patients in other features of the ischaemia group (44.4%) had mild poisoning, while 66.7% of the NSTEMI (66.7%) group had severe CO poisoning (Table 3).

Table 3. Characteristics of the event group depending on the type of ECG changes.

Parameter	Other Features of Ischaemia (n = 9)	STEMI (n = 4)	NSTEMI (n = 9)	p Value for T Test	p Value for Cfi Square Test
Mean Age	58.56 ± 24.42	27.75 ± 9.74	69.56 ± 17.53	0.009	
Smoking status					0.308
Current smoker	3 (33.3%)	2 (50.0%)	3 (33.3%)		
Non-smoker	6 (66.7%)	2 (50.0%)	6 (66.7%)		
Comorbidities					
Diabetes mellitus type 2	1 (11.1%)	0 (0.0%)	1 (11.1%)		0.655
Arterial hypertension	4 (44.4%)	0 (0.0%)	2 (22.2%)		0.144
Ischemic heart disease	3 (33.3%)	0 (0.0%)	1 (11.1%)		0.210
Previous myocardial infarction	0 (0.0%)	0 (0.0%)	0 (0.0%)		-
Heart failure	2 (22.2%)	0 (0.0%)	2 (22.2%)		0.408
Severity of poisoning					0.482
Mild poisoning	4 (44.4%)	2 (50.0%)	2 (22.2%)		
Moderate poisoning	2 (22.2%)	0 (0%)	1 (11.1%)		
Severe poisoning	3 (33.3%)	2 (50.0%)	6 (66.7%)		
Troponin					0.855
Increased	1 (11.1%)	0 (0.0%)	1 (11.1%)		
Normal	7 (77.8%)	2 (50.0%)	6 (66.7%)		
NA	1 (11.1%)	2 (50.0%)	2 (22.2%)		
CK-MB					0.095
Increased	0 (0.0%)	2 (50.0%)	3 (33.3%)		
Normal	8 (88.9%)	2 (50.0%)	6 (66.7%)		
NA	1 (11.1%)	0 (0.0%)	0 (0.0%)		
Orotracheal intubation	1 (11.1%)	2 (50.0%)	1 (11.1%)		0.791
Length of admission					0.495
1–3 days	2 (22.2%)	3 (75.0%)	3 (33.3%)		
4–7 days	5 (55.6%)	1 (25.0%)	3 (33.3%)		
Over 7 days	2 (22.2%)	0 (0.0%)	3 (33.3%)		
Outcome					0.604
Favourable	6 (66.7%)	3 (75.0%)	7 (77.8%)		
Death	1 (11.1%)	1 (25.0%)	1 (11.1%)		
Discharged against medical advice	2 (22.2%)	0 (0.0%)	1 (11.1%)		

Troponin was increased in the other features of ischaemia and NSTEMI groups, but the majority of patients had normal levels. In total, 50% of STEMI and 33% of the NSTEMI population had an increase in CK-MB levels. Half of the patients with STEMI were intubated. The length of admission was equally distributed in the NSTEMI group; 4–7 days for most (55.6%) of the other features of the ischaemia group, and 1–3 days for STEMI. The highest mortality was 25% ($n = 1$) in patients with STEMI and lower (11%) in the other two groups (Table 3).

3.4. Arrhythmias

They were described as more frequent (17.2%) in mild CO poisoning, being represented by the new appearance of either sinus tachycardia, atrial or ventricular extrasystoles, or atrial fibrillation (Table 4).

Table 4. ECG arrhythmias and conduction disorders in patients with acute CO poisoning.

		Severity of Poisoning			*p*-Value
		Mild Poisoning (*n* = 29)	Moderate Poisoning (*n* = 13)	Severe Poisoning (*n* = 23)	
ECG	Arrhythmias	5 (17.2%)	1 (7.7%)	2 (8.7%)	0.552
	Conduction disorders	5 (17.2%)	2 (15.4%)	4 (17.4%)	0.986

Furthermore, ECG atrioventricular (AV) conduction disorders (newly diagnosed bundle branch blocks) were more frequently described (17.2%) in mild CO poisoning. Both arrhythmias and conduction disorders did not show statistical significance depending on CO poisoning severity (Table 4).

4. Discussion

Our study comprises a relatively young cohort with no significant comorbidities and mild poisoning. The severity of poisoning does not have a statistically significant correlation with myocardial injury. On the other hand, one-third of the studied population had either STEMI, NSTEMI or other features of ischaemia on the ECG, and half of them had severe poisoning. Most patients had normal troponin levels. Those with mild poisoning developed arrhythmias (17.2%). This highlights the heterogeneity of CO poisoning patients. They may develop myocardial injury in the absence of significant risk factors. Hence, an individualised approach is necessary when treating CO poisoning. Moreover, future research should address the long-term complications and establish the need for follow-up in this special category of patients.

4.1. Cardiovascular Effects of CO Poisoning

There is a high variability of myocardial involvement based on the cardiovascular status of the affected individual. In most cases, a severe degree of CO poisoning can cause acute coronary syndrome, even in individuals with minimal or no coronary atherosclerosis. However, there are cases in the literature reporting that mild CO poisoning can also lead to severe myocardial injury, especially in older patients with cardiovascular risk factors [11]. Patients may develop angina, which can trigger the physician to further investigate as this symptom seems to correlate with the degree of CO poisoning [12]. On the other hand, cardiac chest pain can develop later in the course of the disease [13], or it can be completely absent [14]. Overall, 13% of our event group developed angina compared to 2.3% in the non-event group. Another study showed that of 104 patients referred to the coronary care unit with unstable angina, three patients had chronic CO poisoning, and five had exposure. This suggests that even environmental CO exposure can result in high COHgb concentrations, causing acute coronary syndrome. In most cases, patients are investigated in the context of acute intoxication; otherwise, this may be overlooked by the physician [15].

There were no major differences in comorbidity profiles between the event and non-event groups. Out of arterial hypertension, diabetes mellitus, ischaemic heart disease, previous MI and heart failure, only the former was slightly more frequent in the event group. These patients do not have the common risk factors of patients with cardiovascular disease, as demonstrated by another retrospective study with a 230 CO poisoning cohort where cardiovascular comorbidities were uncommon, with only 7% of patients having previous MI. Interestingly, arterial hypertension was identified as a predictor of myocardial injury [16].

Smoking is a well-known cardiovascular risk factor determining around 30% of coronary artery disease mortality. [17]. Around 40% of our cohort were active smokers, with no significant difference between the event and non-event group. We can argue that different types of smoking expose individuals to CO, and their baseline COHgb may increase to 10%. This chronic exposure can cause symptoms of fatigue or headache that may worsen in the context of acute exposure and accelerate ischaemic events [18].

It is difficult to determine whether a patient will develop myocardial injury and most studies do not report a statistically significant correlation between levels of COHgb and adverse cardiovascular events. Our study is consistent with these previous findings as the severity of poisoning did not correlate with cardiac ischaemic events. On the other hand, ECG changes and insufficient diagnostic performance of cardiac enzymes may be misleading in appreciating the degree of cardiac impairment. Ischaemic changes have been described in several case reports until larger cohorts were studied. Anderson [19] reports ST segment abnormalities (elevation and depression) in a case series with seven patients but apical thrombus and coronary artery thrombosis in one patient. From a total of 250 patients, Cha YS et al. [20] described ischaemic changes in 3.6% of patients (ST elevation in 0.8%, ST depression 1.6% and T wave inversion in 1.2%), a relatively low incidence, but included patients with less severe CO poisoning (mean initial COHgb was 13.55%). We determined that out of all patients in the event group, 50% had severe poisoning with a COHgb $\geq$ 20%. In the subset analysis of our event group, nine patients had other features of ischaemia, nine had NSTEMI and four of them STEMI. The ECG changes were more frequent in those with NSTEMI and severe poisoning (66.7%). Most patients in the other features of the ischaemia group (44.4%) and STEMI group (50%) had mild poisoning. Another study showed that 85 out of 230 patients developed ST and T wave changes consistent with myocardial injury, and 35% had increased cardiac enzymes [16]. Our STEMI group had no increase in troponin levels. Although troponin, especially high sensitivity troponin, is a key marker of myocardial injury, it cannot be used to predict cardiovascular events in the context of moderate to severe CO poisoning [21]. These changes may be transient and determined by direct CO toxicity, as opposed to atherosclerotic mechanisms. This hypothesis is confirmed by a prospective study that evaluated the cardiac function and structure of patients with CO poisoning. Those with elevated cardiac enzymes were explored with coronary angiography, which was normal in all cases. Coronary spasm was excluded by provocation tests. We can, therefore, argue that increased levels of CK-MB and troponin can arise in anatomically intact coronary arteries [22]. On the other side, STEMI due to left anterior descending coronary artery thrombosis [23], total occlusion of a branch of the right coronary artery [24] or myocardial rupture and tamponade secondary to ACS have also been described in CO poisoning [25].

In the subset analysis groups, most of the patients had normal troponin and CK-MB levels. Troponin was slightly increased in the other features of ischaemia and NSTEMI subgroups of the event cohort, and 50% of STEMI and 33% of the NSTEMI population had an increase in CK-MB levels. Cho et al. [26] found increased troponin in 54% of the 359 patients included in the study. A total of 104 patients underwent cardiac MRI, out of which 72 had late gadolinium enhancement with mid-wall myocardial injury. This cohort included patients with no cardiovascular comorbidities, similar to our STEMI group as our patients were relatively young, with a mean age of 27.7 years old, active smokers (50%), and no comorbidities. In addition to cardiac MRI, SPECT scintigraphy has been proved to provide a significant correlation between the imagistic changes and severity of CO poisoning [27].

Regarding the length of admission, patients in the event group had longer admission compared to the non-event group. Most of our patients had a favourable outcome on discharge. On the other hand, when followed up for a longer period of time, patients with myocardial injury due to CO poisoning may have a three times higher mortality compared to those without myocardial injury and CO poisoning [28]. Henry et al. [29] report that out of the patients with increased cardiac markers and ECG changes consistent with myocardial injury, 38% died after a 7.6-year follow-up. Half of our patients with STEMI were intubated. Length of admission was equally distributed in the NSTEMI group, with 4–7 days and for 55.6% of the ECG ischaemic changes group and 1–3 days for STEMI. The highest mortality was 25% ($n = 1$) in patients with STEMI and lower (11%) in the other two groups. Further studies need to investigate the long-term outcome of patients with cardiac events and CO poisoning.

4.2. Arrhythmias, Conduction Disorders

In our study, arrhythmias were represented by newly diagnosed sinus tachycardia, atrial and ventricular extrasystoles, and atrial fibrillation on ECG. These were more frequent in mild forms of acute CO poisoning. ECG intra-ventricular conduction disorders (newly diagnosed bundle branch blocks) were present in 25% of cases in mild forms, and 17.4% were present in severe forms of acute CO intoxication. Sinus tachycardia was reported in 9 out of 40 patients in one investigation by Aslan et al. [30], while in another study by the same author, it was noted in 26.5% of patients ($n = 83$) [31].

Lee et al. [32] showed in a cohort with 8381 CO poisoning patients that the risk of arrhythmia was twice as high in CO poisoning patients compared with those without CO poisoning. The risk remained significantly higher in patients with associated comorbidities and severe CO poisoning after the adjustment of confounders such as sex, age, or comorbidity. Systemic hypoxia in CO poisoning induces compensatory tachyarrhythmia, increases the oxygen demand, and accelerates CO diffusion, which further exacerbates hypoxic injury of the myocardium. A few cases of intra-ventricular conduction disorders associated with CO poisoning were reported. Most of them were reversible and explained by cardiac ischaemia and toxic effects of CO, such as the case of a young female presenting with a transient left bundle branch block and normal coronary angiography in the context of moderate CO poisoning [33].

4.3. Study Limitations

Our study has several limitations. It is a retrospective study with a review of medical records with some information being unavailable or missing. We conducted the study in a single centre, and the cohort had a relatively small number of patients. Cardiac markers were not available in all patients. Moreover, the troponin assay has changed throughout time, currently providing more accurate and earlier detection of cardiac injury. Since 2018, we have introduced high-sensitivity troponin. This might have affected the number of patients diagnosed with cardiac events prior to 2018, hence the number of patients included in our study.

5. Conclusions

Our study introduces new information on cardiac adverse events in patients with CO poisoning, focusing on the ACS. We found that the severity of CO poisoning plays an important role in developing cardiac ischaemic events, as 50% of patients in the event group were severely intoxicated. On the other side, none of the studied parameters correlated the degree of CO poisoning with the risk of developing myocardial injury.

Taking into account the variability found in our study, we can acknowledge that cardiovascular events in CO poisoning are difficult to predict. This is due to myocardial injury, which can be transient, reversible, or permanent and can arise in both intact or atherosclerotic coronary arteries. Routine investigations, such as ECG, cardiac enzymes or echocardiography, may not be sufficient. On the other hand, invasive and expensive investigations (coronary angiography, cardiac MRI) should be carefully sought as patients may exhibit transient changes. Our in-hospital mortality was low, but future prospective studies are needed to investigate the long-term effects of cardiac involvement at the time of poisoning.

Author Contributions: Conceptualisation, R.E.H., B.C.M. and V.Ș.; data curation, O.S., A.S., A.C., and M.C.; formal analysis, O.S. and A.S.; funding acquisition, V.Ș., O.S., A.S., A.C., M.C. and L.Ș.; investigation, R.E.H., B.C.M., V.Ș., C.L., O.S., A.S., A.C., M.C. and L.Ș.; methodology, R.E.H.; project administration, R.E.H., B.C.M., V.Ș., C.L. and L.Ș.; resources, R.E.H. and B.C.M.; software, B.C.M.; supervision, L.Ș.; validation, R.E.H. and C.L.; visualisation, C.L.; writing—original draft, R.E.H. and B.C.M.; writing—review and editing, R.E.H. and B.C.M. All authors have read and agreed to the published version of the manuscript.

Funding: This research received no external funding.

Institutional Review Board Statement: The study was conducted in accordance with the guidelines of the Helsinki Declaration and approved by the University of Medicine and Pharmacy and Hospital's Ethics Committee.

Informed Consent Statement: Patient consent was waived by our Institutions' Ethics Committee as the research did not pose any risks to the patients, and data were anonymised.

Data Availability Statement: Please contact the corresponding author for any supplement data.

Conflicts of Interest: The authors declare no conflict of interest.

References

1. Collet, J.-P.; Thiele, H.; Barbato, E.; Barthélémy, O.; Bauersachs, J.; Bhatt, D.L.; Dendale, P.; Dorobantu, M.; Edvardsen, T.; Folliguet, T.; et al. 2020 ESC Guidelines for the management of acute coronary syndromes in patients presenting without persistent ST-segment elevation. *Eur. Heart J.* **2021**, *42*, 1289–1367. [CrossRef] [PubMed]
2. Thygesen, K.; Alpert, J.S.; Jaffe, A.S.; Simoons, M.L.; Chaitman, B.R.; White, H.D.; Katus, H.A.; Lindahl, B.; Morrow, D.A.; Joint ESC/ACCF/AHA/WHF Task Force for the Universal Definition of Myocardial Infarction; et al. Third universal definition of myocardial infarction. *Circulation* **2012**, *126*, 2020–2035. [CrossRef] [PubMed]
3. Smollin, C.; Olson, K. Carbon monoxide poisoning (acute). *BMJ Clin. Evid.* **2010**, *2010*, 2103. [PubMed]
4. Mattiuzzi, C.; Lippi, G. Worldwide epidemiology of carbon monoxide poisoning. *Hum. Exp. Toxicol.* **2020**, *39*, 387–392. [CrossRef]
5. Braubach, M.; Algoet, A.; Beaton, M.; Lauriou, S.; Héroux, M.E.; Krzyzanowski, M. Mortality associated with exposure to carbon monoxide in WHO European Member States. *Indoor Air* **2013**, *23*, 115–125. [CrossRef]
6. Kaya, H.; Coşkun, A.; Beton, O.; Zorlu, A.; Kurt, R.; Yucel, H.; Gunes, H.; Yilmaz, M.B. COHgb levels predict the long-term development of acute myocardial infarction in CO poisoning. *Am. J. Emerg. Med.* **2016**, *34*, 840–844. [CrossRef] [PubMed]
7. Rose, J.J.; Wang, L.; Xu, Q.; McTiernan, C.F.; Shiva, S.; Tejero, J.; Gladwin, M.T. Carbon Monoxide Poisoning: Pathogenesis, Management, and Future Directions of Therapy. *Am. J. Respir. Crit. Care Med.* **2017**, *195*, 596–606. [CrossRef]
8. Lichtarska, D.; Feldman, R. Troponin positive acute coronary syndromes in the course of acute carbon monoxide poisoning as the factor exposing primary coronary heart disease previously undiagnosed. *Prz. Lek.* **2011**, *68*, 510–514.
9. Zierle-Ghosh, A.; Jan, A. *Physiology, Body Mass Index*; StatPearls Publishing: Treasure Island, FL, USA, 2021.
10. Palmeri, R.; Gupta, V. *Carboxyhemoglobin Toxicity*; StatPearls Publishing: Treasure Island, FL, USA, 2022.
11. Gao, Y.; Yang, J.; Ma, L.; Zhang, Y.; Li, Z.; Wu, L.; Yang, L.; Wang, H. Non-ST elevation myocardial infarction induced by carbon monoxide poisoning: A case report. *Medicine* **2019**, *98*, e15151. [CrossRef]
12. Koskela, R.S.; Mutanen, P.; Sorsa, J.A.; Klockars, M. Factors predictive of ischemic heart disease mortality in foundry workers exposed to carbon monoxide. *Am. J. Epidemiol.* **2000**, *152*, 628–632. [CrossRef] [PubMed]
13. Henz, S.; Maeder, M. Prospective study of accidental carbon monoxide poisoning in 38 Swiss soldiers. *Swiss Med. Wkly.* **2005**, *135*, 398–408. [PubMed]
14. Thiels, H.; Van Durme, J.P.; Vermeire, P.; Pannier, R. Modifications Electrocardiographiques Immédiates et Tardives au Cours de L'intoxication Oxycarbonée Aiguë. *Lille Med.* **1972**, *17*, 191–195. [PubMed]
15. Balzan, M.V.; Cacciottolo, J.M.; Mifsud, S. Unstable angina and exposure to carbon monoxide. *Postgrad. Med. J.* **1994**, *70*, 699–702. [CrossRef] [PubMed]
16. Satran, D.; Henry, C.R.; Adkinson, C.; Nicholson, C.I.; Bracha, Y.; Henry, T.D. Cardiovascular manifestations of moderate to severe carbon monoxide poisoning. *J. Am. Coll. Cardiol.* **2005**, *45*, 1513–1516. [CrossRef] [PubMed]
17. Gallucci, G.; Tartarone, A.; Lerose, R.; Lalinga, A.V.; Capobianco, A.M. Cardiovascular risk of smoking and benefits of smoking cessation. *J. Thorac. Dis.* **2020**, *12*, 3866–3876. [CrossRef] [PubMed]
18. Dorey, A.; Scheerlinck, P.; Nguyen, H.; Albertson, T. Acute and Chronic Carbon Monoxide Toxicity from Tobacco Smoking. *Mil. Med.* **2020**, *185*, e61–e67. [CrossRef] [PubMed]
19. Anderson, R.F.; Allensworth, D.C.; DeGroot, W.J. Myocardial toxicity from carbon monoxide poisoning. *Ann. Intern. Med.* **1967**, *67*, 1172–1182. [CrossRef]
20. Cha, Y.S.; Cha, K.C.; Kim, O.H.; Lee, K.H.; Hwang, S.O.; Kim, H. Features and predictors of myocardial injury in carbon monoxide poisoned patients. *Emerg. Med. J.* **2014**, *31*, 210–215. [CrossRef]

21. Liu, Q.; Gao, X.; Xiao, Q.; Zhu, B.; Liu, Y.; Han, Y.; Wang, W. A combination of NLR and sST2 is associated with adverse cardiovascular events in patients with myocardial injury induced by moderate to severe acute carbon monoxide poisoning. *Clin. Cardiol.* **2021**, *44*, 401–406. [CrossRef]
22. Kalay, N.; Ozdogru, I.; Cetinkaya, Y.; Eryol, N.K.; Dogan, A.; Gul, I.; Inanc, T.; Ikizceli, I.; Oguzhan, A.; Abaci, A. Cardiovascular effects of carbon monoxide poisoning. *Am. J. Cardiol.* **2007**, *99*, 322–324. [CrossRef]
23. Dziewierz, A.; Ciszowski, K.; Gawlikowski, T.; Rakowski, T.; Kleczyński, P.; Surdacki, A.; Dudek, D. Primary angioplasty in patient with ST-segment elevation myocardial infarction in the setting of intentional carbon monoxide poisoning. *J. Emerg. Med.* **2013**, *45*, 831–834. [CrossRef]
24. Kim, S.; Lim, J.H.; Kim, Y.; Oh, S.; Choi, W.G. A Case of Acute Carbon Monoxide Poisoning Resulting in an ST Elevation Myocardial Infarction. *Korean Circ. J.* **2012**, *42*, 133–135. [CrossRef]
25. Dragelytè, G.; Plenta, J.; Chmieliauskas, S.; Jasulaitis, A.; Raudys, R.; Jovaiša, T.; Badaras, R. Myocardial Rupture following Carbon Monoxide Poisoning. *Case Rep. Crit. Care* **2014**, *2014*, 281701. [CrossRef] [PubMed]
26. Cho, D.H.; Ko, S.M.; Son, J.W.; Park, E.J.; Cha, Y.S. Myocardial Injury and Fibrosis From Acute Carbon Monoxide Poisoning: A Prospective Observational Study. *JACC Cardiovasc. Imaging* **2021**, *14*, 1758–1770. [CrossRef] [PubMed]
27. Pach, J.; Hubalewska-Hoła, A.; Pach, D.; Szpak, D. Usefulness of rest and forced perfusion scintigraphy (SPECT) to evaluate cardiotoxicity in acute carbon monoxide poisoning. *Prz. Lek.* **2001**, *58*, 297–300.
28. Henry, T.D.; Satran, D. Acute Carbon Monoxide Poisoning and Cardiac Magnetic Resonance: The Future Is Now. *JACC Cardiovasc. Imaging* **2021**, *14*, 1771–1773. [CrossRef] [PubMed]
29. Henry, C.R.; Satran, D.; Lindgren, B.; Adkinson, C.; Nicholson, C.I.; Henry, T.D. Myocardial injury and long-term mortality following moderate to severe carbon monoxide poisoning. *JAMA* **2006**, *295*, 398–402. [CrossRef]
30. Aslan, S.; Erol, M.K.; Karcioglu, O.; Meral, M.; Cakir, Z.; Katirci, Y. The investigation of ischemic myocardial damage in patients with carbon monoxide poisoning. *Anadolu Kardiyol. Derg.* **2005**, *5*, 189–193. [PubMed]
31. Aslan, S.; Uzkeser, M.; Seven, B.; Gundogdu, F.; Acemoglu, H.; Aksakal, E.; Varoglu, E. The evaluation of myocardial damage in 83 young adults with carbon monoxide poisoning in the East Anatolia region in Turkey. *Hum. Exp. Toxicol.* **2006**, *25*, 439–446. [CrossRef] [PubMed]
32. Lee, F.Y.; Chen, W.K.; Lin, C.L.; Kao, C.H. Carbon monoxide poisoning and subsequent cardiovascular disease risk: A nationwide population-based cohort study. *Medicine* **2015**, *94*, e624. [CrossRef] [PubMed]
33. Atif, B.; Osman, K.A.; Ilker, A.; Alpasla, U. Reversible left bundle-branch block due to carbon monoxide poisoning: A case report. *Am. J. Emerg. Med.* **2016**, *34*, 342.E1–342.E3.

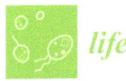

Review

Etiologic Puzzle of Coronary Artery Disease: How Important Is Genetic Component?

Lăcrămioara Ionela Butnariu [1], Laura Florea [2], Minerva Codruta Badescu [3,4,*], Elena Țarcă [5,*], Irina-Iuliana Costache [6] and Eusebiu Vlad Gorduza [1]

1. Department of Medical Genetics, Faculty of Medicine, "Grigore T. Popa" University of Medicine and Pharmacy, 700115 Iași, Romania; ionela.butnariu@umfiasi.ro (L.I.B.); vgord@mail.com (E.V.G.)
2. Department of Nefrology—Internal Medicine, Faculty of Medicine, "Grigore T. Popa" University of Medicine and Pharmacy, 700115 Iași, Romania; laura.florea@umfiasi.ro
3. Department of Internal Medicine, "Grigore T. Popa" University of Medicine and Pharmacy, 16 University Street, 700115 Iași, Romania
4. III Internal Medicine Clinic, "St. Spiridon" County Emergency Clinical Hospital, 1 Independence Boulevard, 700111 Iași, Romania
5. Department of Surgery II—Pediatric Surgery, "Grigore T. Popa" University of Medicine and Pharmacy, 700115 Iași, Romania
6. Department of Internal Medicine (Cardiology), "Grigore T. Popa" University of Medicine and Pharmacy, 16 University Street, 700115 Iași, Romania; irina.costache@umfiasi.ro
* Correspondence: minerva.badescu@umfiasi.ro (M.C.B.); elena.tuluc@umfiasi.ro (E.Ț.)

Abstract: In the modern era, coronary artery disease (CAD) has become the most common form of heart disease and, due to the severity of its clinical manifestations and its acute complications, is a major cause of morbidity and mortality worldwide. The phenotypic variability of CAD is correlated with the complex etiology, multifactorial (caused by the interaction of genetic and environmental factors) but also monogenic. The purpose of this review is to present the genetic factors involved in the etiology of CAD and their relationship to the pathogenic mechanisms of the disease. Method: we analyzed data from the literature, starting with candidate gene-based association studies, then continuing with extensive association studies such as Genome-Wide Association Studies (GWAS) and Whole Exome Sequencing (WES). The results of these studies revealed that the number of genetic factors involved in CAD etiology is impressive. The identification of new genetic factors through GWASs offers new perspectives on understanding the complex pathophysiological mechanisms that determine CAD. In conclusion, deciphering the genetic architecture of CAD by extended genomic analysis (GWAS/WES) will establish new therapeutic targets and lead to the development of new treatments. The identification of individuals at high risk for CAD using polygenic risk scores (PRS) will allow early prophylactic measures and personalized therapy to improve their prognosis.

Keywords: coronary artery disease; ischemic heart disease; atherosclerosis; genetic risk factors; heritability; polymorphism; GWAS; PRS

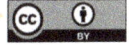

1. Introduction

Despite the remarkable advances made in recent decades in the treatment and prevention of coronary artery disease (CAD), also known as ischemic heart disease (IHD) or coronary heart disease (CHD), it continues to be a major cause of death in industrialized countries. CAD causes more than 3.9 million deaths in Europe, of which 1.8 million in the European Union [1]; in the US, over 18.2 million people have CAD, and annually, more than 805,000 people develope acute coronary syndrome (ACS) (Centers for Disease Control and Prevention, 2019) [2,3]. The risk of CAD and especially acute myocardial infarction (MI) is usually correlated with old age; however, about 5–10% of cases occur before the age of 50. Mortality caused by CAD at a young age has a significant psychological impact on affected families, as well as a substantial negative economic effect. The risk of developing CAD after the age of 40 is about 32% in women and about 49% in men, with women developing CAD a decade later than men due to the protective effect of estrogen hormones, so the onset of the disease follows the onset of menopause [4,5].

The main cause of CAD is the decrease in blood flow in the epicardial coronary arteries caused by obstruction by atherosclerotic plaques (atherosclerotic CAD) [4,6,7].

Some studies have shown that the pathophysiological mechanism of CAD is much more complex and, beyond the presence of epicardial atherosclerotic plaques, coronary microcirculation is crucial in the genesis of CAD [8,9].

Atherosclerotic CAD comprises a wide range of clinical features that include asymptomatic subclinical atherosclerosis and its complications such as angina pectoris (PA), acute myocardial infarction (MI) and sudden cardiac death (SCD) [6]. The etiology of CAD is extremely heterogeneous and, although cases of atherosclerotic CAD with monogenic etiology are described, CAD is considered to have a complex multifactorial etiology, being the consequence of the interaction between genetic factors and many environmental factors (diet, physical activity, smoking, other comorbidities) [9–11].

Numerous epidemiological studies have been conducted in recent years in an attempt to determine which are the risk factors for CAD, in order to develop models that would allow the development of risk scores (CAD risk prediction models) [4,12,13].

The Framingham Heart Study (FHS, 1948) was the first study to attempt to elucidate cardiovascular disease risk factors (CRF), followed by the FINRISK study (Finland, 1972) and other cohort studies conducted at Uppsala University in Sweden (ULSAM, PIVUS, POEM, EpiHealth and SCAPIS), INTERHEART study (a case–control study of acute myocardial infarction in 52 countries) and another study in New Zealand (PREDICT Cardiovascular Disease Cohort). In these studies, CAD risk factors are classified into two categories: modifiable risk factors (hypercholesterolemia, smoking, diabetes mellitus, systolic hypertension, sedentary lifestyle) and non-modifiable risk factors (age, sex, family history for CAD) (Figure 1) [4–8,12–15].

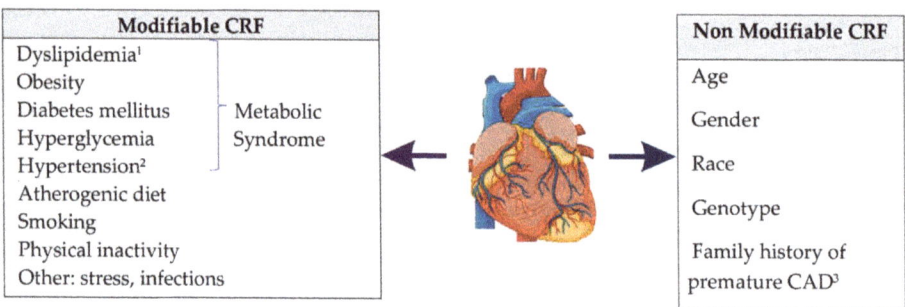

Figure 1. Classification of Cardiovascular Risk Factors (CRF) [4–8,12–15]. [1] Dyslipidemia (total cholesterol > 200 mg/dL; LDL-C > 130 mg/dL; HDL-C < 40 mg/dL; TG > 150 mg/dL) [7]; [2] Hypertension is defined as a blood pressure (BP) $\geq$ 140/90 mm Hg by the European guidelines [8], whereas a lower threshold of BP $\geq$ 130/80 mm Hg is used by the American guidelines [11]; [3] Family history of premature CAD (CAD in male first–degree relative < 55 years, or CAD in female first-degree relative < 65 years) [4–6,12–15].

Currently, the Multi Ethnic Study Group of Atherosclerosis (MESA) is considering the inclusion of coronary artery calcification (CAC) in the category of risk factors for CAD [13]. The European Association for Cardiovascular Prevention and Rehabilitation (EACRP) and the American College of Cardiology/American Heart Association (ACC/AHA) have developed practical guidelines, based on CAD risk prediction models, to reduce the risk of acute coronary syndromes (ACS) [13].

The phenotypic variability in CAD patients is most likely due to complex pathophysiological mechanisms involving numerous interactions between different genetic factors encoding different molecules, as well as their interactions with environmental factors. The identification of risk alleles, which determine an increased susceptibility to CAD, is of great interest. Geneticists point to the need to achieve polygenic risk scores (PRS) that could play an important role in identifying people at high risk for CAD. In their case, the early implementation of prophylactic measures would help to improve the prognosis and life expectancy [6,13].

The aim of our paper is to provide an in-depth analysis of the data available in the literature on the role of genetic factors in the etiology of CAD. We also focused on the complex interaction between genetic and environmental factors. Thus, we performed the most comprehensive analysis of the methods used in the study of genetic factors involved in the etiology of CAD and their results. We highlighted the advantages and limitations of each type of study, as well as the perspectives that these data offer for the implementation of effective prophylactic measures, early diagnosis in order to avoid lethal complications (MI, SCD), personalized therapy, and last but not least, for the development of innovative drugs.

2. Literature Search Strategies and Data Collection

The data synthesized and presented in this review was obtained by examining the literature (Google Scholar, PubMed, MEDLINE, OMIM, MedGen databases) and using the following keywords: ischemic heart disease (IHD), coronary artery disease (CAD), atherosclerosis, genetic risk factors, heritability, monogenic CAD/IHD/CHD, polygenic CAD/IHD/CHD, candidate gene-based association studies (CGS), Linkage-studies (LS), Genetic linkage-analysis (LA), Genome-wide association studies (GWAS) or Whole Exome Sequencing (WES) (Table 1).

Table 1. Genetic etiology of coronary artery disease.

Genetic Transmission Monogenic/Polygenic	Gene(s)	Location/ Chromosome	Disease/CAD-S	Biochemical Changes	Method CGS/GWAS/LA/WES	References
			Monogenic lipid CAD			
	LDLR	19p13.2	FH	↑LDL-C	CGS/GWAS	[4,6,16–18]
	APOB	2p24.1	FHCL2/FDB	↑LDL-C	CGS/GWAS	[4,16,19–22]
	PCSK9	1p34.1-p32	HCHOLA3	↑LDL-C	CGS/GWAS	[16,23–27]
	LDLRAP1	1p34-p35	ARH	↑LDL-C	CGS	[16,28,29]
	APOAI	11q23.3	Apo AI deficiency, Apo-A1 and apo C-III combined deficiency	↓HDL-C	CGS	[4,16,30–34]
	ABCA1	9q31.1	TGD	↓HDL-C	CGS/GWAS	[16,35–37]
	LCAT	16q22.1	LCAT deficiency	↓HDL-C	CGS/GWAS	[10,16,38,39]
	LPL	8p21.3	LPL deficiency/CHLF	↑TG, ↓LDL-C, ↓HDL-C	CGS	[16,40,41]
	APOC2	19q13.2	HL Ib	↑TG	CGS	[16,42]
	ABCG5, ABCG8	2p21	STSL	↑plant sterols	CGS	[6,43,44]
	APOA1/C3/A4/A5	11p14.1-q12.1, 1q21-23, 16q22-24.1	FCHL	↑VLDL, ↑LDL-C, ↑ApoB, ↑TG	LA/GWAS	[6,45–50]
	APOA5	11p14.1-q12.1, 15q11.2-q13.1, 8q11-q13	FHTG	↑TG	LA/GWAS	[4,16,50–53]
	ATHS	19p13.3-p13.2	ATHS/ALP	↑LDL-C, ↑TG, ↓HDL-C	LA	[16,54–58]

Table 1. Cont.

Genetic Transmission Monogenic/Polygenic	Gene(s)	Location/ Chromosome	Disease/CAD-S	Biochemical Changes	Method CGS/GWAS/LA/WES	References
			Other Monogenic CAD			
	MEF2A	15q26	ADCAD1		CGS	[6,59–62]
	ST6GALNAC5	1p31.1			GWAS/WES	[16,63,64]
	CYP27A1	2p35	CTX	↓ LDL, ↓ VLDL, ↑ HDL-C	WES	[16,65–68]
	LRP6	12p13.2		↑ LDL-C, ↑ TG	CGS/GWAS	[16,69,70]
			Polygenic CAD			
	CDKN2A, CDKN2B	9p21	CAD-S		GWAS	[8,10,71–74]
	C6orf105 gene	6p24.1	CAD-S		GWAS	[6,75,76]
	COL4A1/COL4A2, ZC3HC1, CYP17A1	13q34, 7q32.2, 10q24.32	CAD-S		GWAS	[77,78]
	CTSS	1q21	CAD-S		GWAS	[79]
	WDR11-FGFR2	10q26	CAD-S		GWAS	[79]
	RDX-FDX1	11q22	CAD-S		GWAS	[79]
	PSRC1	1p13.3	CAD-S		GWAS	[73,80]
	MIA3	1q41	CAD-S		GWAS	[73,80]
	SMAD3	15q22.3	CAD-S		GWAS	[73,81–83]
Polygenic lipid CAD	APOE, APOB, LPL, OLR1 (LOX1), SORT1, TRIB1,	19q13.32, 2p24.1, 8p21.3, 12p13.2, 1p13.3, 8q24.13	CAD-S		GWAS	[84–91] [6,21,92–94] [80,95–98] [99,100] [101] [80,102,103]
Genes associated with vascular homeostasis	NOS3, TCF21, ADAMTS7, HHIPL1, ACE, AGT, AGT1R, CYP11B2	7q36.1, 6q23.2, 15q25.1, 14q32, 17q23.3, 1q42.2, 3q23, 8q24.3	CAD-S		GWAS	[4,104–106] [80,107,108] [80,109] [110] [80,111–114] [114] [115,116] [117–119]
Genes associated with vascular hemostasis	ITGA2, ITGB2, ITGB3, PAI-1, THBS (1, 2, 4), F5 Leiden (Arg506Gln), F2 gene (Arg 506Gln)	5q11.2, 21q22.3, 17q21.32, 7q22.1, 15q14, 6q27, 5q14.1 1q24.2, 11p11.2	CAD-S		GWAS	[4,120,121] [122,123] [124,125] [126,127] [128] [4,129] [4,129]
HHcy	MTHFR	1p36.22	CAD-S		GWAS	[130–133]
Inflammation	IL-6	7p15.3	CAD-S		GWAS	[4,80,134]
Other genes	POAD CHDS2, CHDS3, AGTR2, IRS1, CAPN10, HDLBPALDH2	1p31 2q21.2-q22, Xq23-q26, Xq23, 2q36-q37.3 12q24	CAD-S		GWAS	[135] [136] [16,136] [136] [5,137,138] [139]

CAD: Coronary artery disease; MI: Acute myocardial infarction; HDL-C: High-density lipoprotein cholesterol; LDL-C: Low-density lipoprotein cholesterol; TG: Triglyceride; CGS: Candidate gene-based association studies; GWAS: Genome-wide association studies; LA: Genetic Linkage analysis; WES: Whole exome sequencing; FH: Familial hypercholesterolemia; FDB: Familial defective apolipoprotein B-100; FHCL2: Hypercholesterolemia, familial, 2; HCHOLA3: Hypercholesterolemia, autosomal dominant, 3; ARH: Autosomal recessive hypercholesterolemia; TGD: Tangier disease; HLIb: Hyperlipoproteinemia type Ib; LPL deficiency: Lipoprotein lipase deficiency; CHLF: Combined hyperlipidemia, familial; STSL: Sitosterolemia; FCHL: Familial combined hyperlipidemia; FHTG: Familial hypertriglyceridemia; CTX: Cerebrotendinous Xanthomatosis; VLDL: Very low-density lipoprotein; APOB: Apolipoprotein B; Atherosclerosis Susceptibility (ATHS)/Atherogenic Lipoprotein Phenotype (ALP); ADCAD1: Coronary artery disease, autosomal dominant, 1; F5 Leiden: Factor V Leiden; F2 gene: prothrombin; CAD-S: CAD Susceptibility; HHcy: Hyperhomocysteinemia.

3. Phenotypic Variability of Coronary Artery Disease

The study of genetic factors involved in the pathogenesis of CAD has proven to be a difficult task due to phenotypic variability which is closely correlated with genetic heterogeneity. However, in recent years, due to the development of molecular technology, significant progress has been made in the genetic and genomic studies of CAD and MI [6].

Coronary atherosclerosis is the main pathogenic mechanism in CAD, regardless of its clinical form, that ranges from subclinical atherosclerosis to chronic and acute coronary sindroms and SCD [6,14]. Some data indicate that about 50% of SCD are due to MI, and about a third of MI cases are silent [6,13]. The average age at which the first MI occurs varies between the two sexes, being 64.9 years for men and 72.3 years for women [1]. In the case of octogenarian patients, a history of atherosclerotic CAD is usually present, often preceded by a long asymptomatic period, but episodes of MI are also present in young adults (<40 years), in the absence of a positive history of coronary atherosclerosis [6].

The formation of atherosclerotic plaque on the wall of the coronary arteries is a chronic process, with an early onset, and is initiated/favored by chronic endothelial lesions. Plaques progress, causing vascular obstruction and tissue ischemia over time. Rupture or ulceration of unstable plaques causes ACS, such as unstable angina, acute myocardial infarction (MI), and sudden cardiac death (SCD). Rupture of a vulnerable atherosclerotic plaque, accumulation and activation of platelets, fibrin deposition, thrombus formation and possible occlusion of vessels are the pathophysiological mechanism of MI [6,9].

The formation and progression of atherosclerotic plaques involves many biochemical processes involving enzymes, receptors and their ligands, molecules that are encoded by various genes that interact with environmental factors. Thus, lipid and apolipoprotein metabolism, inflammatory response, endothelial function, platelet function, thrombosis, homocysteine metabolism, insulin sensitivity and blood pressure regulating mechanism may be disrupted [5,6].

The location of atherosclerotic stenosis in the coronary vessels and may reflect how genetic variability may influence the production of atherosclerosis under certain conditions of dynamic blood flow. Isolated aorto-ostial stenosis (left or right main coronary artery ostium) and bifurcation lesions are more evident in relation to turbulent flow and endothelial response to flow dynamics. In some studies in mice, *PECAM-1* gene polymorphism has been shown to be an important factor in the atherogenic changes seen in ApoE-deficient mice, the effects of which are dependent on the location of atherosclerosis in the coronary arteries. These results suggest that the heterogeneity of atherosclerosis localization could be influenced by certain polymorphisms of genes involved in the process of atherosclerosis, under different dynamic flow conditions [6,140]. On the other hand, diffuse atherosclerosis is more commonly seen in patients with diabetes mellitus (DM) [5–7].

4. Heritability of Atherosclerotic CAD

The importance of genetic factors in the etiology of CAD and MI has been demonstrated by numerous clinical and population studies. Several cohort studies have shown that the family history of CAD is associated with an increased risk of the disease, with family aggregation being reported since the middle of the last century [6,141]. The heritability of CAD is estimated to be between 40–60%, according to family-based association studies, those of twin studies or GWASs [6,140]. Subsequently, a significant association of cases with early-onset CAD was demonstrated in patients who had first-degree relatives with early-onset CAD [142].

The Framingham Heart Study (FHS) later confirmed that a family history of premature CAD (defined as the presence of an affected first-degree relative, male under 55 or female under 65) is an independent risk factor for CAD [143]. The importance of genetic factors is confirmed by the association between the increased number of affected relatives and the lower age of onset. Family-based studies have shown that a positive family history for CAD increases a person's risk of developing the disease two to seven times compared with a person with no family history of the disease. In fact, studies based on the results of coronary angiography have indicated that the etiology of CAD with a positive family history is independent of environmental factors (atherogenic diet, obesity, hypertension, smoking or alcohol consumption) [6,144].

Other population studies (the Western Collaborative Group Study, British Regional Heart Study, German PROCAM study) confirmed the strong independent association between the positive family history for CAD and the risk of CAD and MI in offspring [6].

Twin studies have provided important information on the genetic component of CAD. Thus, in monozygotic (MZ) twins a concordance was observed regarding early-onset CAD and the involvement of the same coronary arteries [4,6]. Data from the Swedish Twin Registry included 20,966 twins, who were followed for 36 years, indicate that if one of the twins died by CAD, the twin brother's risk of developing lethal CAD is 8.1 for monozygotic (MZ) twins and 3.8 for dizygotic (DZ) twin. The estimated heritability of CAD differs between the two sexes, being estimated at 57% in males and 38% in females and the influence of genetic factors was in the age range between 36 and 86 years [145].

A prospective analysis of 8000 pairs of twins included in the Danish Twin Registry showed an increased incidence of CAD deaths in MZ twins compared with DZ twins (44% vs. 14%), with a heritability of mortality due to heart disease (heritability of frailty, liability to death) estimated at 0.53 in men and 0.58 in women [146].

Genetic factors act independently of the environmental factors involved in the etiology of CAD, but the variable phenotype results from their permanent interaction. The study of monogenic mutations that cause atherosclerotic CAD as well as polygenic risk factors (genetic polymorphisms) was performed by two types of studies: linkage analysis (LA) and association studies (CGS, GWAS and WES) [4,7,8].

Genetic Linkage analysis (LA) studies investigate the cosegregation (association with the onset of disease) of polymorphic DNA markers distributed throughout the genome with hereditary transmission of the disease in that family and aims to detect the genomic region where the gene is located, identifying the disease-causing gene variant. It has been used successfully in identifying monogenic mutations that cause disease and, less so in the case of polygenic diseases, given the complexity of their etiology [4–6,9,10].

Association studies are an alternative method of studying polygenic inheritance and usually use the candidate-gene approach (CGA). Starting from the known pathophysiological mechanisms and from the genes that are supposed to intervene in different stages, the hypothesis of the association of these genes with the respective disease is analyzed/tested. In the case of CAD, the genes involved in lipid metabolism, lipopoteins, DM, and hypertension were analyzed. However, this approach is limited by incomplete knowledge of the pathogenic mechanisms of CAD. The advances in the last 20 years in molecular technology have allowed extensive analysis of the whole genome (GWAS) or exome (WES) providing important information on the genetic causes of diseases with complex, multifactorial etiology [4,7,10].

5. Monogenic Etiology of CAD/MI

Candidate gene-based association studies (CGS) and linkage analysis (LA) studies have identified many genes whose mutations cause rare monogenic forms of CAD, most of which are involved in lipid metabolism (atherosclerotic CAD) (Table 1).

5.1. Monogenic Lipid Disorders
5.1.1. Genetic Causes of Elevated Plasma LDL-Cholesterol Level

Atherosclerosis and coronary artery obstruction are the leading causes of CAD, and low-density lipoprotein cholesterol (LDL-C) molecules, in particular, contribute to the development and progression of atherosclerotic plaque. Considering this, mutations of genes involved in lipid metabolism that increase plasma levels of LDL-C have an important contribution to CAD [4–6].

Familial Hypercholesterolemia type 1 (FH)

Mutations of genes encoding the LDL receptor (LDLR), apolipoprotein B-100 (ApoB-100), an LDL-C receptor ligand, and proprotein convertase, subtilisin/kexin-type 9 (PCSK9) cause familial hypercholesterolemia type 1 (FH), (OMIM, 606,945), an autosomal dominant disorder [16].

a. Low-Density Lipoprotein Receptor (LDLR) Gene

The *LDLR* gene (located on chromosome 19p13.2) encodes an 860 amino acid protein (LDLR) that is involved in the absorption and degradation of LDL-C. *LDLR* gene mutations cause about 85–90% of FH cases and are associated with abnormal or dysfunctional LDLR. There are currently 3839 known mutations that are distributed throughout the *LDLR* gene [4–6].

Homozygous mutations in the *LDLR* gene cause early-onset CAD in childhood and are characterized by plasma LDL-C levels approximately 6–10 times higher than normal (600–1200 mg/dL), detected at birth. Extremely high LDL-C levels can cause the first MI to occur before the age of 20, and in the absence of treatment, death occurs before the age of 30. Approximately 5% of people with CAD and MI before the age of 60 have heterozygous mutations of the *LDLR* gene, with 2 times higher plasma levels of LDL-C (300–400 mg/dL) being detected at birth. Among heterozygotes, 75% of men and 45% of women develop CAD by the age of 60, and 50% of men and 15% of women die of MI by this age [17].

In familial cases of CAD, the genetic testing algorithm is based on the initial investigation of the *LDLR* gene, and in case of a negative result the mutations of the *ApoB-100* and *PCSK9* genes are tested [18].

b. APOB Gene

The *APOB* gene (located on chromosome 2p24.1) encodes ApoB-100 apolipoproteins, the main protein component of apolipoproteins synthesized in the liver: chylomicrons (CM), very low-density lipoprotein (VLDL) and low-density lipoprotein (LDL), and ApoB-48 (synthesized exclusively in the intestine). ApoB-100 has an LDLR binding domain, helping to regulate plasma cholesterol levels, removing LDL-C from the body, and binding to heparin and various proteoglycans in arterial walls [4,19].

Two allelic variants of the *APOB* gene: C10580G (p.Arg3527Gln) [20] and C10800T (p.Arg3531Cys) [21] have been associated with decreased affinity for LDLR, leading to familial hypercholesterolemia type 2 (FHCL2) (OMIM 144,010) also called familial defective apolipoprotein B-100 (FDB), an autosomal dominant genetic disorder associated with hyperlipidemia and increased risk of early atherosclerosis [16].

In a study that combined genetic linkage analysis (LA) with WES in a family members with FH (familial hypercholesterolemia type 1, AD), Thomas et al. [22] identified a third mutation (p.Arg50Trp) in exon 3 of the *APOB* gene [22].

Other mutations of the *APOB* gene cause hypobetalipoproteinemia (FHBL) (OMIM, 615,558) and abetalipoproteinemia (ABL) (OMIM, 200,100), two rare, autosomal recessive conditions characterized by hypocholesterolemia and malabsorption of lipid-soluble vitamins, which causes retinal degeneration, neuropathy and coagulopathy [16].

c. PCSK9 Gene

The *PCSK9* gene (proprotein convertase, subtilisin/kexin-type, 9, located on chromosome 1p32.3) encodes neural apoptosis-regulated convertase 1 (NARC 1), a serum protease that reduces both hepatic and extrahepatic LDLR levels, causing increase plasma LDL-C level [23]. Functional mutations in the *PCSK9* gene cause autosomal dominant familial hypercholesterolemia-3 (FHCL3, FH3, HCHOLA3) (OMIM, 603,776) [16].

Initially, nine types of mutations in the *PCSK9* gene were reported in families whose members had a form of autosomal dominant transmitted hypercholesterolemia [24]. These mutations are associated with a decrease in the number of LDLR, the consequence being the increase plasma total cholesterol (TC) levels and LDL-C with the appearance of tendon xanthomas, premature CAD, MI and ischemic stroke. A GWAS study indicated that the single nucleotide polymorphism (SNP) rs11206510 (risk allele T) located on *PCSK9* gene was associated with an increased risk of CAD and MI [25].

The *PCSK9* gene polymorphism is correlated with both plasma lipid levels and the response to lipid-lowering drugs (statins). Studies in patients with hypocholesterolemia (Atherosclerosis Risk in Communities-ARIC and Dallas Heart Study) have found that loss-of-function mutation of *PCSK9* gene have a protective effect against CAD and MI [26].

In a meta-analysis by Chuan et al. [27], the association between the allelic variant rs562556 (c.1420G>A, I474V) located in exon 9 of the *PCSK9* gene and the low plasma total cholesterol (TC) levels and LDL-C was highlighted [27]. These findings have led to the development of *PCSK9* inhibitors as new agents to reduce plasma cholesterol levels [27].

d. *LDLRAP1 Gene*

The loss-of-function mutation in the *LDLRAP1* (LDL receptor adapter protein 1) gene (located on chromosome 1p34-1p35) are extremely rare and lead to the appearance of a truncated or non-functional LDLRAP1 protein (required for internalizing LDLR into hepatocytes). Compound homozygous or heterozygous individuals for pathogenic mutations of *LDLRAP1* show an autosomal recessive form of hypercholesterolemia (ARH/FHCL4) (OMIM, 603813) [16]. ARH can be considered a phenocopy of homozygous familial hypercholesterolemia, which progresses with increased risk for atherosclerotic CAD (with rapid fatal evolution, despite conventional therapies) and, aortic valve stenosis. Lomitapide combined with conventional drugs that reduce plasma LDL-C levels appears to be an effective treatment for ARH [28].

The literature describes 50 cases of ARH, in patients of Mediterranean or Middle Eastern origin. In a study by Arca et al. [29] which included 28 people from 17 unrelated families in Sardinia, two types of mutations of *LDLRAP1* gene were identified: a frameshift mutation C432insA (p.FS170stop) in exon 4 (ARH1) and a nonsense mutation C65G->A (p.Trp22ter) in exon 1 (ARH2). In three of the cases, a compound heterozygous genotype was detected as a result of the ancient recombination of the two mutations ARH1 and ARH2 [29]. Only four of the reported cases had the homozygous genotype ARH1, the patients coming from the Italian mainland [29].

5.1.2. Genetic Causes of Low Plasma HDL-Cholesterol Level

Prospective cohort studies revealed that low high-density lipoprotein-cholesterol (HDL-C) (HDL-C < 35–40 mg/dL according to current guidelines or age-and sex-adjusted plasma HDL-C concentration below the 10th percentile) is a significant, negative risk factor, independent of traditional CAD risk factors [30]. In 40% of CAD cases, low plasma HDL-C levels are detected, and the genetic etiology is incriminated in a proportion of 40–70% [4].

a. *APOA1 Gene*

The *APOA1* gene is located on chromosome 11q23.3 and encodes the apolipoprotein AI (ApoA-I), a component of HDL-C, with a major role in its metabolism. ApoA-I acts as a cofactor for the enzyme LCAT (lecithin-cholesterol acyltransferase), which is responsible for removing cholesterol from tissues and plasma through a cholesterol esterification process. Compound homozygous, heterozygous, and heterozygous mutations in the *APOA1* gene cause familial hypoalphalipoproteinemia (Hypoalphalipoproteinemia, Primary, 2) (OMIM, 618,463), which also includes the Combined Apo-I and apoC-III, both being autosomal recessive diseases [4,16,31].

The *APOA1* gene polymorphism is associated with low plasma HDL-C levels and an increased risk of premature CAD. Homozygous mutations cause complete absence of ApoA-I, with low HDL-C < 5 mg/dL and normal plasma LDL-C and TG levels. Missense mutations in the *APOA1* gene (which are almost always heterozygous) affect the structure of the ApoA-I protein, often causing impairment of its function, associated with low plasma levels of ApoA-I and HDL-C [4,31].

Yamakawa-Kobayashi et al. [32] analyzed the polymorphism of the *APOA1* gene in a group of 67 Japanese children with low plasma HDL-C levels, identifying four different mutations (3 frameshifts mutation and 1 splice site mutation) [32]. In their case, the plasma levels of ApoA-I were reduced by approximately 50% of the normal value (below the first percentile of the general population distribution) (80 mg/dL). The frequency of hypoalphalipoproteinemia due to *APOA1* gene mutations in the Japanese population was estimated at 0.3% in the general population and 6% of individuals with low plasma HDL-C levels [32].

In a Danish study, Haase et al. [33] showed that certain rare allelic variants (eg variant A164S) of the *APOA1* gene are associated with decreased plasma levels of ApoA-I and HDL-C and predispose to amyloidosis, with an increased risk of CAD and MI [33]. The ApoA-I(Milano) and ApoA-I(Paris) variants are rare cysteine variants of ApoA-I which, although they cause decreased plasma HDL-C levels and increased plasma TG levels, have a cardioprotective effect. They can also produce a HDL-C deficiency in the absence of cardiovascular disease (CVD) [34].

b. *ABC1 Gene*

The *ABC1* gene (located on chromosome 9q31.1) encodes ATP-binding cassette transporter 1 (ABCA1) a cellular exporter of cholesterol, which causes the removal of free intracellular cholesterol and phospholipids from extrahepatic cells, having a protective role against CVD. Mutations in the *ABCA1* gene cause loss of transporter protein function and may contribute to the process of atherogenesis present in common inflammatory diseases and metabolic disorders. Compound homozygous or heterozygous mutations in the *ABCA1* gene cause Tangier disease (TGD) (OMIM, 205,400), a rare autosomal recessive disorder characterized by extremely low plasma HDL-C levels (HDL-C < 5 mg/dL) and ApoA-I $\leq$ 10 mg/dL and, increased risk of early-onset CAD [16].

Clinically, TGD is characterized by yellow-orange pharyngeal tonsils, hepatosplenomegaly, corneal opacity, lymphadenopathy, and peripheral neuropathy [35]. The data show that 331 mutations in the *ABC1* gene are reported in the literature [36]. About 1 in 400 individuals in the general population is a heterozygous carrier of a loss-of-function mutation in the *ABCA1* gene (frameshift, nonsense and splicing mutation). In their case, the plasma levels of HDL-C and ApoA-I are variable, being able to be reduced by up to 50% compared with normal levels [35]. Mokuno et al. [37] showed in a Japanese study that *ABCA1* R219K polymorphism (G1051A, rs2230806) K allele is associated with a higher plasma HDL-C levels that may be protective against the risk of CAD in Asian and Caucasian patients [37].

c. *LCAT Gene*

The *LCAT* gene located on chromosome 16q22.1 encodes the enzyme lecithin-cholesterol acyltransferase (LCAT) which is involved in removing cholesterol from the blood and tissues. LCAT catalyzes the esterification of free cholesterol with acyl groups derived from lecithin, an essential step in the maturation of HDL-C. The enzyme LCAT has two major activities: alpha-LCAT activity, which helps attach cholesterol to high density lipoprotein (HDL), and beta-LCAT activity, which facilitates the attachment of cholesterol to other lipoproteins (VLDL and LDL) [38]. Compound homozygous or heterozygous mutations in the *LCAT* gene cause LCAT enzyme deficiency, and two entities are described: Norum disease (OMIM 245,900) and fish-eye disease (FED/Partial LCAT deficiency) (OMIM 136,120) [16].

Norum disease is a rare autosomal recessive condition, characterized by the presence of corneal opacity, hemolytic anemia, proteinuria, renal failure and atherosclerosis. In Norum disease both activities (alpha and beta) of the LCAT enzyme are lost causing very low levels of HDL-C (below the 5th percentile), increased TG and decreased LDL-C [39]. In the FED, only alpha-LCAT activity is lost, beta activity being preserved, allowing the esterification of cholesterol in VLDL and LDL-C, but not in HDL-C [10].

There are few longitudinal follow-up studies of molecular defects associated with LCAT deficiency syndromes. A total of 138 *LCAT* gene mutations were identified, mostly in exons 1 and 4, without a correlation between genotype and phenotype or ethnicity.

It has been observed that there is a significantly higher risk of CAD in the FED compared with Norum disease [38]. This observation is clinically important, suggesting that management must be customized according to the LCAT deficiency phenotype. Thus, in Norum disease the priority is to improve both CVD and progression to end-stage renal disease (ESRD), whereas in FED patients the priority is to reduce cardiovascular risk [38].

5.1.3. Genetic Etiology of Hypertriglyceridemia

Many studies have shown that higher plasma TG levels are a strong independent risk factor for CAD [40]. Among the different types of lipoproteins, chylomicrons (CM) and VLDL particles are the main carriers of TG, whereas LDL-C and HDL-C are mainly involved in cholesterol transport. Plasma TG levels are also influenced by environmental factors (diet, lifestyle, sedentary lifestyle, smoking) [40].

a. LPL Gene

The *LPL* gene (located on chromosome 8p21.3) encodes lipoprotein lipase (LPL), an enzyme that limits the rate at which VLDL convert to LDL-C. Compound homozygous or heterozygous mutations in the *LPL* gene cause Lipoprotein lipase deficiency (LPL deficiency or type I hyperlipoproteinemia) (OMIM, 238,600), a rare autosomal recessive condition [16]. The disease is characterized by an extremely elevated serum triglyceride level, lactescent serum (milky creamy serum), decreased plasma HDL-C and LDL-C levels, eruptive xanthomas, acute abdominal pain, hepatosplenomegaly, and sometimes early-onset atherosclerotic CAD. Heterozygous individuals may have mild hyperlipidemia and reduced postheparin plasma lipolytic activity (PHLA), and early atherosclerosis does not appear to be a feature. It is estimated that approximately 20% of patients with hypertriglyceridemia carry only six common *LPL* gene mutations (Asp9Asn, Asn291Ser, Trp86Arg, Gly188Glu, Pro207Leu, Asp250Asn) associated with type I hyperlipoproteinemia. Testing for these mutations is especially recommended in patients at high risk for premature atherosclerosis. The S447X polymorphism (SX genotype and X allele) has been associated with lower plasma triglyceride levels and higher plasma HDL-C levels compared with those with absent X alleles, and can be considered a protective factor against the development of CAD [41].

b. APOC2 Gene

The *APOC2* gene (located on chromosome 19q13.32) encodes apolipoprotein C-II (ApoC-II) which is a cofactor needed to activate LPL, the enzyme that hydrolyzes plasma triglycerides and transfers fatty acids to tissues. Homozygous mutations in *APOC2* cause Hyperlipoproteinemia, type Ib (OMIM, 608,083), an autosomal recessive disease characterized by extremely elevated serum concentrations of triglycerides (up to 30,000 mg/dL) and chylomicrons (CM), causing recurrent pancreatitis and early atherosclerosis [16,42].

c. ABCG5 and ABCG8 Genes

Sitosterolemia (STSL) is a rare, autosomal recessive disease caused by mutations in the genes *ABCG5* (encoding sterol-1) and *ABCG8* (encoding sterol-2) located on chromosome 2p21. The presence of intestinal hyperabsorption of all sterols derivatives and the reduced ability to excrete sterols into the bile lead to elevated plasma sterol levels (>30 times the normal value), development of tendon xanthomas, accelerated atherosclerosis, and premature CAD. Most patients have homozygous or compound heterozygous mutations of the two genes involved, whereas the prevalence of heterozygous individuals and their phenotypic features are not fully known [6,43]. Mutations in the *ABCG5* gene have been reported frequently in Asian patients, whereas Caucasian patients usually have *ABCG8* mutations. However, Wang et al. [44] reported the presence of *ABCG8* gene mutations in 3 of the 8 patients from unrelated Chinese families, suggesting that *ABCG8* mutations are not present exclusively in Caucasians [44].

5.1.4. Familial Combined Hyperlipidemia and Familial Hypertriglyceridemia
The *APOA1/C3/A4/A5* Gene Cluster and Lipid Metabolism

a. Familial Combined Hyperlipidemia

Familial Combined Hyperlipidemia (FCHL) is the most common form of primary dyslipidemia, affecting 1–2% of the Western population and 14–20% of patients with premature CAD. The manifestations of FCHL are heterogeneous, the disease may manifest itself in the form of mixed hyperlipidemia, isolated hypercholesterolemia, hypertriglyceridemia or in combination with elevated ApoB levels. Although initially considered an autosomal dominant disease with incomplete penetration, linkage analysis and GWAS have suggested that the etiology of FCHL is complex, multifactorial. The characteristic FCHL phenotype is determined by the interaction between genetic factors (several genes, of which 1 or 2 with major effect-oligogenic theory) and environmental factors. Although the etiology of FCHL is not fully elucidated, GWASs have indicated three possible loci involved: 1q21-23, 11p14.1-q12.1, and 16q22-24.1 [4].

Various studies have shown the key role of the *APOA1/C3/A4/A5* haplotype (located on chromosome 11) in modulating lipoprotein metabolism. The conclusion of the study by Liu et al. [45] was that certain variants of the *APOA1/C3/A4/A5* haplotype may be useful markers for predicting the response to fenofibrate therapy, and further confirmation is required in other studies [45]. Eichenbaum-Voline et al. [46] showed in a study that the *APOA5* c.56G>G and *APOC3* c.386G>G alleles are associated with the production of FCHL [46,47].

The prevalence of CAD in patients with FCHL under the age of 60 is approximately 15% [48]. Patients with FCHL have an increased risk of CVD and are frequently associated with other metabolic disorders: type 2 diabetes mellitus (T2DM), non-alcoholic fatty liver disease, steatohepatitis and metabolic syndrome. Hopkins et al. [49] identified metabolic syndrome in 65% of patients with FCHL, compared with 19% of control subjects [49].

b. Familial Hypertriglyceridemia

Familial hypertriglyceridemia (FHTG) (OMIM, 145,750) is a rare hereditary primary dyslipidemia characterized by a moderate increase in serum triglycerides (>400 mg/dL), usually in the absence of significant hypercholesterolemia [16]. FHTG has a prevalence of 5–10% in the general population and is an autosomal dominant monogenic disease that rarely manifests itself in childhood, being usually diagnosed in adulthood. Affected people are associated with obesity and decreased glucose tolerance. The metabolic cause of FHTG is the hepatic secretion of large VLDL particles rich in triglycerides that are slowly catabolized. Although the molecular defect has not yet been identified, some studies have suggested that several loci may be associated with FHTG (e.g.,15q11.2-q13.1, 8q11-q13), but further studies are needed to confirm this association [4]. The *APOA5* SNP rs2075291 (c.553G>T; p.185Gly>Cys) can be considered a susceptibility factor for hypertriglyceridemia and CAD [50].

The *APOA5* G553T allelic variant (which causes cysteine substitution with glycine-185) was identified by Kao et al. [51] in a study that included Chinese patients who had hypertriglyceridemia [51].

Do et al. [52] identified that rare *APOA5* and *LDLR* alleles increase the risk of MI; *APOA5* gene polymorphism was associated with elevated plasma TG levels, whereas carriers of *LDLR* mutations had elevated plasma LDL-C [52]. The prevalence of FHTG in families in which premature CAD occurred was analyzed in two independent studies. Hopkins et al. [50] found FHTG in 20.5% of families with at least one case of CAD; approximately 71% of patients with FHTG had metabolic syndrome, compared with 19% in the control group [50]. Genest et al. [53] identified the presence of hypertriglyceridemia in 1% and hypertriglyceridemia with hypoalphalipoproteinemia in 14.7% of families in whom there was a CAD diagnosed before the age of 60 [53].

5.1.5. Atherosclerosis Susceptibility/Atherogenic Lipoprotein Phenotype

Mutations in the *ATHS* gene (located on chromosome 19p13.3-p13.2) cause Atherosclerosis Susceptibility (ATHS) also called Atherogenic Lipoprotein Phenotype (ALP) (OMIM, 108,725) [16]. ATHS/ALP is an autosomal dominant monogenic disease characterized by the presence of elevated plasma LDL levels, elevated triglyceride-rich lipoproteins levels, and decreased plasma HDL levels, and is associated with an increased risk of CAD and MI. ALP has two phenotypic variants: type A-characterized by the presence of large LDL particles and type B-characterized by the presence of small and dense LDL particles. Current data indicate an association between the presence of the type B phenotype (low, dense LDL) and an increased risk of CAD. Austin et al. [54] concluded that phenotype B may be an independent risk factor for CAD and a 3-fold higher risk of MI [54].

Nishina et al. [55] identified a link between the ALP phenotype and the *LDLR* gene locus (located on chromosome 19p13.3-p13.2) and concluded that the *ATHS* gene that causes ATHS/ALP may be the same as the *LDLR* gene or is located near the *LDLR* locus [55]. The link between the *ATHS* gene and the *LDLR* locus was later confirmed in the study by Rotter et al. [56], which suggested that the specific ALP phenotype is determined, however, by a different gene from the *LDLR* gene [56].

Some studies have provided important evidence for the involvement of the *CETP* gene (located on chromosome 16q13) encoding cholesteryl ester transfer protein-CETP) and the *SOD2* gene (located on chromosome 6q25.3), encoding superoxide dismutase-2-SOD2 in the production of an increased susceptibility to atherogenic dyslipidemia, as well as a possible involvement of the haplotype *APOA1/APOC3/APOA4* (located on chromosome 11p14.1-q12.1) [16,56]. Srisawasdi et al. [57] showed in a study that included 299 Thai patients treated with statins, the polymorphisms of *CETP* rs3764261 (CC genotype) and rs708272 (GG and GA genotypes) may have a higher susceptibility to atherogenic dyslipidemia [57].

Allayee et al. [58] concluded that there are common genetic factors that determine FCH, but also ATS/ALP (type B, small dense LDL particles) associated with early-onset CAD [58].

5.2. Other Monogenic CAD

5.2.1. MEF2A Gene

Mutations in the *MEF2A* gene (located on chromosome 15q26.3) cause coronary artery disease, 1 (ADCAD1) (OMIM, 608,320) [16]. The *MEF2A* gene encodes a transcription factor (myocyte enhancer factor 2A) that acts in the embryonic period. The *MEF2A* gene is thought to contribute to the maintenance of vascular endothelial cell function (being involved in myocyte differentiation and vasculogenesis) and to interact with other factors involved in the pathogenesis of CVD [59].

Wang et al. [60] identified a deletion in exon 11 of the *MEF2A* gene in 10 of the 13 members affected by CAD (9 of whom had a history of MI), belonging to a large family, analyzed by genome-wide linkage analysis. The mutation was not identified in the case of family members unaffected by CAD. Deletion of seven amino acids (D7aa MEF2A) disrupts the activity of the transcription factor MEF2A associated with abnormalities in endothelial cells and vascular smooth muscle cells (VSMc) involved in the processes of atherogenesis. The results obtained led to the identification of a pathogenic mutation of a gene that intervenes in the MEF2A signaling pathway, involved in the etiopathogenesis of familial vascular disease associated with CAD/MI [60].

The involvement of the *MEF2A* gene in the pathogenesis of CAD remains controversial, as in other studies the association with familial/sporadic CAD has not been proven. Cases have been reported in which individuals with D7aa deletion *MEF2A* did not have CAD before the expected age of onset of CAD, whereas members of the same family who had CAD did not have the mutation. In some studies, the *MEF2* gene variants c.704C>A (p.S235Y), c.812C>G (p.P271R), c.836C>T (p.P279L), c.848G>A (p.G283D) mis-senses, c.1315C>T (p.R439X) nonsense, and seven out-of-frame deletions were predicted as disease-causing variants for CAD [59].

The allelic variants that do not alter the activity of the MEF2A transcription factor are not associated with an increased risk of CAD, and the prevalence of pathogenic *MEF2A* mutations in the general population is not yet fully known [6,61]. The phenotypic variability and penetration of the mutant gene may be due to the interaction of *MEF2A* with other modifier genes (epistasis) or environmental factors [59].

Improving or maintaining MEF2A expression in vascular endothelial cells may be a new strategy for developing vascular protection methods and exploring new vascular protective drugs. Liu et al. [62] identified a new mechanism involved in the protective role of resveratrol in promoting the expression of MEF2A in vascular endothelial cells, which in turn would influence the expression of anti-apoptosis and anti-aging genes (eg *SIRT1* gene) and thus inhibit premature apoptosis or senescence of vascular endothelial cells [62].

5.2.2. ST6GALNAC5 Gene

The *ST6GALNAC5* gene located on chromosome 1p31.1 (OMIM, 610,134) encodes sialyltransferase 7e, an enzyme that modifies proteins and ceramides on the cell surface, influencing intercellular interactions and those between cells and the extracellular matrix [16].

InanlooRahatloo et al. [63] analyzed an consanguineous Iranian family, with cases of autosomal dominant premature CAD. GWAS combined with WES allowed the identification of a heterozygous mutation (c.G295A) in the *ST6GALNAC5* gene (which determines p.Val99Met). Targeted sequencing of all family members confirmed the co-segregation between this allelic variant and the CAD phenotype [63]. Analysis of other Iranian families with CAD identified a second heterozygous mutation p.*337Qext*20 identified in two unrelated patients. One of the patients had a brother with CAD and two unaffected siblings. Both mutations have been shown to increase sialyltransferase activity in vitro, possibly in vivo. Increased sialyltransferase activity in blood cells and serum sialic acid levels are associated with atherosclerosis and CAD [64]. Some studies in the United States have provided statistically significant additional evidence for the potential contribution of *ST6GALNAC5* gene mutations to the occurrence of CAD [63]. The evidence provided by these studies supports the idea that sialic acid and sialyltransferase activity are involved in the pathogenesis of atherosclerotic CAD, and that the gain-of-function mutations in the *ST6GALNAC5* gene are an etiological factor for CAD. The pathophysiological mechanism and the prevalence of functional mutations in the *ST6GALNAC5* gene in the general population and in patients with CAD are still unknown [63].

5.2.3. CYP27A1 Gene

Homozygous or compound heterozygous mutations in the *CYP27A1* gene (located on chromosome 2q35) cause cerebrotendinous xanthomatosis (CTX) (OMIM, 213,700), a rare autosomal recessive lipid storage disease [16]. CTX is manifested by progressive neurological dysfunction (cerebellar ataxia with postpubertal onset, systemic damage to the spinal cord and a pseudobulbar phase leading to death), premature atherosclerosis and cataracts [16].

In the study by Inanloo Rahatloo et al. [65], the analysis of CAD patients using WES led to the identification of the *CYP27A1* c.G674A mutation that causes p.Arg225His protein substitution. The mutation of the *CYP27A1* gene affects the function of the enzyme sterol 27-hydroxylase, which is involved in the transport and elimination of cholesterol from cells, and this mechanism can be correlated with CAD phenotype [65]. In another study, the analysis of a group of 100 unrelated CAD patients using WES identified the presence in seven of them of four different *CYP27A1* allelic variants (p.Arg14Gly, p.Arg26Lys, p.Ala27Arg and p.Val86Met) that could cause CAD [65]. Chen at al. [66] identified three new mutations in *CYP27A1* (p.Arg513Cys, c.1477-2A>C and p.Arg188Stop (NM 000784.3) in a study that included four Chinese families with CTX [66]. Lee at al. [67] reported another pathogenic mutation in the *CYP27A1* gene present in two Taiwanese brothers with CTX [67]. Both brothers had a compound heterozygous genotype with a mutation in exon 2 (c.435G>T, cryptic splice site) and a mutation in intron 7 (c.1264A>G, canonical spice site) [67]. In another study that analyzed members of an Iranian family affected by CTX, Rashvand et al. [68] identified a homozygous splicing mutation, NM_000784: exon6: c.1184+1G>A in the *CYP27A1* gene, that was present in most cases [68]. The results of these studies confirm that mutations in the *CYP27A1* gene, which regulate cholesterol homeostasis, can lead to atherosclerosis [66,67].

5.2.4. *LRP6* Gene

Mutations in the *LRP6* gene (located on chromosome 12p13.2) encoding low-density lipoprotein receptor-related protein 6 (LRP6) cause Coronary artery disease, autosomal dominant, 2 (ADCAD2) (OMIM, 610,947) [16]. ADCAD2 is characterized by an increased risk of MI in the presence of increased metabolic risk factors.

Mani et al. [69] analyzed a family with autosomal dominant premature CAD, in which family members had clinical manifestations specific to the metabolic syndrome (hyperlipidemia, hypertension, DM) and osteoporosis [69]. In these patients, they identified a R611C homozygous missense mutation (which substitutes cysteine for arginine) in the *LRP6* gene, which encodes a co-receptor in the Wnt signaling pathway [69]. These could be an important evidence of the influence of Wnt signaling pathway abnormalities on cardiovascular risk factors (CRF). Most heterozygous individuals over the age of 45 had clinical manifestations of metabolic syndrome, suggesting that the impact of *LRP6* mutation on mulftiple CAD risk factors is important, and the ubiquitous expression of *LRP6* gene could explain pleiotropic manifestations in various tissues [69].

Loss-of-function mutations in the *LPR5* and *LPR6* genes cause decreased bone density and osteoporosis.

In addition, recent studies have shown a strong association between osteoporosis and CAD, which may be the pleiotropic effects of mutations in the Wnt signaling pathway. Intronic mutations of *TCFL* gene and other transcription factors involved in the Wnt signaling pathway are associated with type 2 diabetes mellitus (T2DM) and maturity-onset diabetes of the young (MODY diabetes). In the future, investigating the factors that interfere with the Wnt signaling pathway in patients with premature CAD and metabolic syndrome could provide new perspectives into the pathophysiology of the disease and the use of more effective prophylactic measures [69].

Wang et al. [70] analyzed 766 Chinese patients with CAD and concluded that the *LRP6* gene polymorphism (the C allele of the SNP rs11054731 located in intron 2) is associated with increased susceptibility and severity of CAD [70].

6. Polygenic CAD: Genes and Polymorphisms Associated with CAD

Monogenic mutations explain only a small part of the etiology of CAD/MI, being recognized that the etiology of CAD is complex and the variable phenotype results from the interaction between many genes (polygeny) and environmental factors. The large number of genes, possibly involved, and the insufficient knowledge of the pathophysiological mechanisms through which they intervene in the production of the disease have created difficulties in the attempts to elucidate the etiology of CAD over time. The development of molecular technologies in the last two decades has allowed extensive analysis of the whole genome (GWAS) or exome (WES), which provided important information on the role of genetic factors in the etiology of multifactorial diseases (heritability).

Candidate gene-based association studies (CGS) have made little contribution to elucidating the genetic etiology of CAD or other multifactorial diseases. The cause could be the low reproducibility correlated with the small number of cases analyzed, which lead to results with low statistical power for the identification of less associated allelic variants [10].

Genome-wide association studies (GWAS) examine the co-segregation of polymorphic genetic markers (SNPs-single nucleotide polymorphism) distributed throughout the genome in families affected by CAD. A rare allelic variant present in 1% of the population is considered polymorphism. It is estimated that approximately 3,000,000 SNPs (one SNP in every 1000 base pairs) are present throughout the genome (3 billion base pairs) [10].

Early GWASs showed a reduced association of common allelic variants with CAD with odds ratio (OR) ranging from 1.1 to 1.4. The need to identify these allelic variants and to confirm the results through other independent studies has extended international collaborations, which has allowed the analysis of a very large number of samples [10].

The first two GWASs (2007) identified an association of SNPs located in the 9p21 chromosomal region with CAD and MI, data that were later confirmed by other studies that included large cohorts of patients and a broad ethnic, geographical and demographic spectrum [10,71,72]. Many studies have subsequently confirmed the association with CAD and MI of the 9p21.3 chromosomal region, which contains two cyclin-dependent kinase inhibitors, *CDKN2A* (encoding the prototypic INK4 protein, p16INK4a) and *CDKN2B* (encoding p15INK4b), which are linked to both DM as well as the pathogenesis of atherosclerosis by their role in inhibiting TGF-β-induced cell growth [10,73].

Nikpai et al. [74] performed the largest GWAS meta-analysis that included 185,000 CAD cases and controls, in which they analyzed 6.7 million common (minor allele frequency, MAF > 0.05) and 2.7 million low-frequency (0.005 < MAF < 0.05) variants [74]. In addition to the loci already known to be associated with CAD, they identified 10 new loci containing candidate genes involved in the processes occuring in the vascular wall [74]. They observed the presence of allelic heterogeneity, providing evidence that genetic susceptibility to CAD is determined by common allelic variants (SNPs), without providing evidence of the association between rare alleles and CAD [74].

Another GWAS conducted by the CARDIoGRAMplusC4D Consortium which included a total of 63,746 CAD cases and 130,681 controls identified/confirmed another 15 susceptibility loci for CAD. At that time, the total number of loci known to be associated with CAD was 46. In addition, another 104 independent variants ($r^2 < 0.2$) strongly associated with CAD were identified [6,75]. Together, these variants explain 10.6% of CAD heritability. In total, 12 of the 46 genome-wide significant SNPs showed a significant association with lipid metabolism, and 5 were significantly associated with blood pressure, but none showed a significant association with DM [6,75]. A GWAS by Wang et al. [76] in the Chinese Han population indicated that the SNP variant (rs6903956) in the *C6orf105* gene (located on chromosome 6p24.1) is associated with susceptibility to CAD [76].

In the study published by IBC 50K CAD Consortium, other new susceptibility loci for CAD were reported: *COL4A1/COL4A2, ZC3HC1, CYP17A1* [77]. In a recent large-scale GWAS, Koyama et al. [78] identified 43 new loci associated with increased CAD susceptibility in ethnic Japanese people, not previously reported in other studies [78]. Matsunaga et al. [79] identified three new loci associated with CAD located on chromosomes 1q21 (*CTSS*), 10q26 (*WDR11-FGFR2*) and 11q22 (*RDX TDX1*) highlighting the genetic differences of ethnic Japanese people compared with the European population [79].

In a German study that combined the results of the Wellcome Trust Case Control Consortium (WTCCC) study and the German MI [Myocardial Infarction] Family Study, along with the 9p21.3 locus, two loci were strongly associated with CAD (adjusted $p < 0.05$), being located on chromosomes 6q25.1 (rs6922269) and chromosome 2q36.3 (rs2943634). Combining the results of the two studies, four additional loci were identified that are associated with a high probability (over 80%) with CAD ($p < 1.3 \times 10^{-6}$), located on chromosomes 1p13.3 (rs599839), 1q41 (rs17465637), 10q11.21 (rs501120) and 15q22.33 (rs17228212) [73].

In the chromosomal region 1p13.3 is located the *PSRC1* gene, which encodes a proline-rich protein, and in the chromosomal region 1q41 is the locus of the *MIA3* gene (melanoma 3 inhibitory activity gene), also called *RNA* or *TANGO* [73,80]. Polymorphisms (SNPs) associated with the 10q11.21 chromosomal region are located 100 kb downstream of the *CXCL12* (the stromal cell-derived precursor factor 1) gene. The SNP on chromosome 15q22.33 is an intronic SNP in the *SMAD3* gene, which functions as a transcriptional regulator activated by transforming growth factor β (TGF-β) and activin receptor-like kinase 1 (ALK1) [73,81–83].

Although initially 55 loci associated with CAD/MI were identified, subsequently, starting with 2007, numerous studies have led to the identification of over 321 loci of susceptibility to CAD and MI [78,80–84]. The most common allelic polymorphisms identified by recent GWASs in patients with CAD/MI are shown in Table 2.

Table 2. Candidate genes and CAD-associated genetic polymorphisms identified by GWASs [10,71, 75,78,81,83].

Location/Chromosome	Gene (s)	SNPs	Risk Allele	Risk Allele Frequency
1p32.3	PCSK9	rs112065101	T/C	0.848
1p32.3	PPAP2B	rs9970807	C/T	0.915
1p13.3	SORT1	rs7528419	A/G	0.786
1q21	CTSS	rs6587520	T/C	0.480
1q21.3	IL6R	rs6689306	A/G	0.448
1q41	MIA3	rs67180937	G/T	0.663
2p24.1	AK097927	rs16986953	A/G	0.105
2p24.1	APOB	chr2:21378433:D	D/I	0.746
2p21	ABCG5, ABCG8	chr2:44074126:D	I/D	0.745
2p11.2	VAMP5-VAMP8-GCX	rs7568458	A/T	0.449
2q22.3	ZEB2-ACO74093.1	rs17678683	G/T	0.088
2q33.2	WDR12	chr2:203828796:I	I/D	0.108
3q22.3	MRAS	chr3:138099161:I	I/D	0.163
4q31.22-q31.23	EDNRA	rs4593108	C/G	0.795
4q32.1	GUCY1A3	rs72689147	G/T	0.817
4q12	REST-NOA1	rs17087335	T/G	0.210
5q31.1	SLC22A4-SLC22A5	rs273909	G/A	0.117
6p24.1	ADTRP-C6orf105	rs6903956	A/G	0.354
6p24.1	PHACTR1	rs9349379	G/A	0.432
6p21.31	ANKS1A	rs17609940	G/C	0.824
6p21.2	KCNK5	rs56336142	T/C	0.807
6q23.2	TCF21	rs12202017	A/G	0.700
6q25.3	SLC22A3-LPAL2-LPA	rs55730499	T/C	0.056
6q26	PLG	rs4252185	C/T	0.060
7p21.1	HDAC9	rs2107595	A/G	0.200
7q22.3	BCAP29	rs10953541	C/T	0.783
7q34	ZC3HC1 (PARP12)	rs11556924	C/T	0.687
7q36.1	NOS3	rs17087335	T/C	0.060
8p21.3	LPL	rs264	G/A	0.853
8q24.13	TRIB1	rs2954029	A/T	0.551
9p21.3	CDKN2BAS	rs2891168	G/A	0.489
9q34.2	ABO	rs2519093	T/C	0.191
10p11.23	KIAA1462	rs2487928	A/G	0.418
10q11.21	CXCL12	rs1870634	G/T	0.637
10q23.31	LIPA	rs1412444	T/C	0.369
10q24.32	CYP17A1-CNNM2-NT5C2	rs11191416	T/G	0.873

Table 2. Cont.

Location/Chromosome	Gene (s)	SNPs	Risk Allele	Risk Allele Frequency
10q26	WDR11-FGFR2	rs2257129	C/T	0.900
11q22.3	PDGFD	rs2128739	A/C	0.324
11q22	RDX-FDX1	rs10488763	T/A	0.180
11q23.3	ZNF259-APOA5-APOA1	rs964184	G/C	0.185
11p15.4	SWAP70	rs10840293	A/G	0.550
12q21.33	ATP2B1	rs2681472	G/A	0.201
12q24.12	SH2B3	rs3184504	T/C	0.422
12q24.22-q24.23	KSR2	rs1180803	G/T	0.360
13q12.3	FLT1	rs9319428	A/G	0.314
13q34	COL4A1-COL4A2	rs11838776	A/G	0.263
14q32	HHIPL1	rs10139550	G/C	0.423
15q25.1	ADAMTS7	rs4468572	C/T	0.586
15q26.1	FURIN-FES	rs17514846	A/C	0.440
15q22.33	SMAD3	rs56062135	C/T	0.790
15q26.1	MFGE8-ABHD2	rs8042271	G/A	0.900
17p13.3	SMG6	rs216172	C/G	0.350
17p11.2	RAI1-PEMT-RASD1	rs12936587	G/A	0.611
17q21.32	UBE2Z	rs46522	T/C	0.513
17q23.2	BCAS3	rs7212798	C/T	0.150
18q21.32	PMAIP1-MC4R	rs663129	A/G	0.260
19p13.2	LDLR	rs56289821	G/A	0.900
19q13.32	APOE-APOC1	rs4420638	G/A	0.166
19q13.11	ZNF507-LOC400684	rs12976411	T/A	0.090
21q22.11	KCNE2	rs28451064	A/G	0.121
22q11.23	POM121L9P-ADORA2A	rs180803	G/T	0.970

CAD: Coronary artery disease; A-adenine; C-cytosine; G-guanine; T-thymine; D-deletion; I-insertion; SNP-Single nucleotide polymorphism.

The data obtained were extremely important, because the implementation of polygenic risk scores (PRS) in clinical practice largely depends on the accuracy of predicting the magnitude of the effect of risk alleles, which vary depending on the genetic background [80]. Together, these allelic variants explain approximately 15% of CAD/IHD heritability. Most CAD-associated polymorphisms were from genes involved in lipid metabolism, blood pressure regulation, and inflammation, confirming the importance of these factors in the etiology of CAD. In addition, many of the CAD-associated genes are involved in the metabolism of amino acids, polyamines, innate immunity, and degradation of the extracellular matrix (Figure 2) [10,84].

Most of these mutations are located in intergenic regions, at or near the promoters, indicating a possible influence on gene expression by epigenetic regulation, as a possible mechanism of CAD/IHD [85].

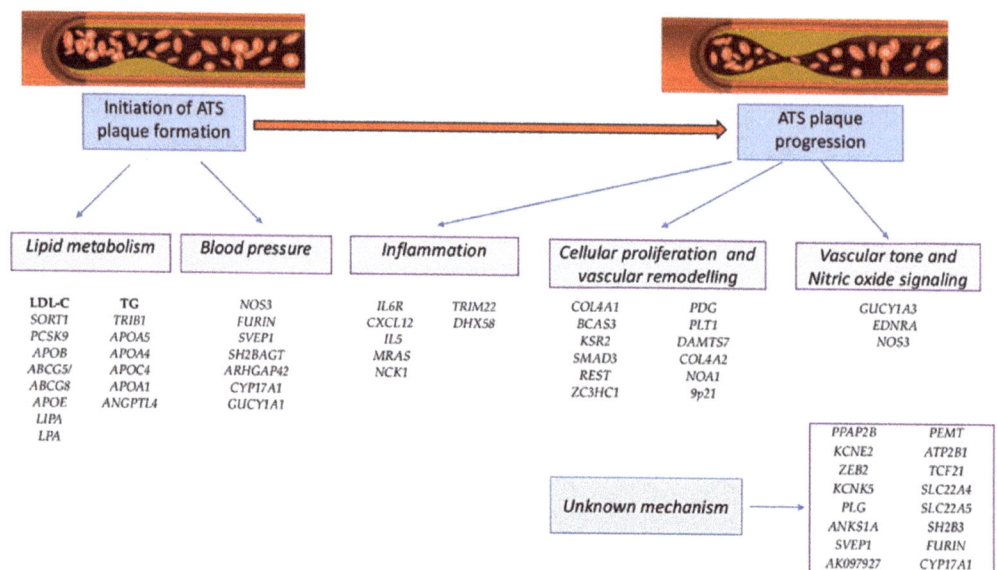

Figure 2. The main genes involved in the pathophysiological mechanism of CAD. CAD: Coronary artery disease; LDL-C: Low-density lipoprotein cholesterol; TG: Triglyceride; ATS plaque: Atherosclerotic plaque.

The consistent results, sometimes achieved through extensive collaborations between different study groups, as well as the availability of data obtained from the scientific community are the main benefits of GWASs. Currently available GWAS databases include IHD-associated genetic variants from the CARDIoGRAMplusC4D consortium, European Genome-phenome Archive and American database of Genotypes and Phenotypes (dbGaP) [10,75]. Identifying the still unknown genetic factors involved in the etiology of complex, multifactorial diseases is one of the major challenges in the case of CAD. Heritability, still unknown, may be due to unidentified variants of the disease associated genes or may be due to factors that do not alter gene structure but wich influence the intensity of gene expression by epigenetic regulation [6].

The major limitations of GWAS are related to the fact that the identified allelic variants could be in a Linkage disequilibrium (LD) with the disease-causing alleles and do not provide any information about the associated pathophysiological mechanism, which must be subsequently identified by specific functional studies. In addition, the definition of the clinical phenotype being studied can vary in different study groups. GWAS sensitivity is limited to high frequency variants (5%). GWASs aim is to identify common allelic variants, which have small, additive effects, being less effective in identifying rare allelic variants with major effects. GWASs (SNPs) have low power to identify structural abnormalities (CNVs caused by deletions, insertions, translocations), as well as a low power to identify both interactions between genes, and the interaction between genetic and environmental factors. To overcome these limits, different strategies have been proposed: the correct definition of the phenotype of the analyzed cases, the increase in the number of patients included in the analyzed groups and the use of groups with extreme phenotypes; development of powerful biostatistical tools to increase the sensitivity of the detection rate, especially of rare allelic variants; fine mapping of SNPs or the use of NGS (next-generation sequencing) for regions of interest to identify rare allelic variants and/or structural variants; taking into account the mechanisms of epigenetic regulation of gene expression [6,10].

6.1. Polymorphism of Genes Involved in Lipid Metabolism: A Novel View

6.1.1. Polymorphisms of *APOE* Gene and CAD

Apolipoprotein E (ApoE) is an LDL receptor (LDLR) ligand and is encoded by the *APOE* gene located on chromosome 19q13.32 that is closely related to the *APOC-I/C-II* gene complex. Through LDLR, ApoE is involved in the elimination of very low density lipoprotein (VLDL) residues and chylomicrons (CM) [84–86]. There are three *APOE* allelic variants (ε2, ε3 and ε4) in the European population, which determine six genotypes (*APOE2/2*, *APOE2/3*, *APOE2/4*, *APOE3/3*, *APOE3/4*, *APOE4/4*), which encode three major ApoE isoforms (ApoE2, ApoE3 and ApoE4) [86,87]. Their presence correlates with a variable affinity for LDLR, resulting in significant differences in plasma total cholesterol (CT) and LDL-C levels. Many studies have shown that *APOE* polymorphism is associated with CAD and increased risk of MI. The frequency of the *APOE*ε4 allele in the European population is about 15% and is associated with early atherosclerosis, increased mortality, risk of ischemic stroke, Alzheimer's disease and MI [86,87]. Heterozygous carriers of the *APOE*ε4 have an 8.3% higher LDL-C levels than individuals *APOE*ε3 homozygotes. Heterozygous carriers of the *APOE*ε2 allele have 14.2% lower plasma LDL-C levels compared with *APOE*ε3 homozygotes [86,87]. Various studies have shown that individual carriers of the *APOE*ε4 allele have a 40% higher risk of death from CAD than people with the *APOE3/3* genotype or *APOE*ε2 carriers [88].

In the study by Gerdes et al. [89], men carrying *APOE*ε4 allele had a 1.8-fold increased risk of death from CAD compared with carriers of other *APOE* alleles [89].

Humphries et al. [90] found that the relative risk of developing CAD is dependent on the interaction between *APOE* genotype and smoking status, suggesting that the interaction between genetic and environmental factors is involved in the variable expressivity of CAD related to *APOE* genotype [90]. These results were not confirmed by the Whitehall II study, which, although confirming the protective effect of the *APOE*ε2 allele, did not reveal a higher risk for CAD in non-smokers carrying the *APOE*ε4 allele, all smokers having a similar risk for CAD, regardless of the *APOE* genotype [91].

6.1.2. Polymorphisms of *APOB* Gene and CAD

The *APOB* gene mutations cause Familial Defective Apolipoprotein B-100 (FDB), an autosomal dominant disease associated with an increased risk of atherosclerosis and CAD [6,21]. Over time, there have been studies that have examined the association between *APOB* polymorphisms and the increased risk of CAD in individuals undiagnosed with FDB. The *APOB* gene has numerous polymorphic loci, three of which (XbaI, EcoRI, SpIns Del) are correlated with elevated plasma total cholesterol (TC), LDL-C, ApoB and triglyceride (TG) levels and an increased risk of developing CAD/MI.

The results obtained by Chiodini et al. [92] demonstrated that *ApoB EcoRI* (although rare) and *SpIns/Del* polymorphisms significantly increase the risk of CAD and MI, but these results need further confirmation by other studies [92].

The *X1*, *R1*, and *ID1* polymorphisms were more common in patients with a history of MI than in the control group, in a study by Hegele et al. [93]; there were no significant differences in plasma LDL-C or ApoB levels between the two groups [93]. A meta-analysis by Chen et al. [94] indicated that *ApoB EcoRI* polymorphism is associated with a moderate risk for CAD, and the E$^-$ allele at this locus could be a susceptibility allele for CAD development [94].

6.1.3. Polymorphisms of *LPL* Gene and Its Modulators Associated with High Risk of CAD

Different types of homozygous or heterozygous compound mutations in the *LPL* gene cause Lipoprotein lipase deficiency (LPLD deficiency), a rare autosomal recessive monogenic disorder. Lipoprotein lipase (LPL) is an enzyme involved in the metabolism of triglycerides-rich lipoproteins and acts on the vascular level. Over time, there have been many studies that have reported an association between *LPL* polymorphisms, and CAD/MI, in some cases the results being contradictory. The *LPL* locus can alternatively be occupied by both common, non-coding and rare allelic variants. Rare loss-of-function mutations in *LPL* gene are associated with an increased risk of CAD, and gain-of-function mutations in *LPL* gene are associated with reduced risk of CAD [80].

Several meta-analyses suggested that, compared with non-carriers, heterozygous individuals with Gly188Glu, Asp9Asn and Asn291Ser substitutions have an atherogenic lipoprotein profile, whereas carriers of Ser447Ter substitution have a protective lipoprotein profile [80].

In a recent meta-analysis, He et al. [95] showed that *LPL* HindIII and S447X polymorphisms but not PvuII could act as protective factors against MI, requiring further confirmation by other case–control studies with a larger number of subjects analyzed [95]. Ma et al. [96] did not identify in their meta-analysis any significant association for *LPL* N291S and PvuII polymorphisms and CAD. Analyzing the results according to ethnicity, they observed a significant correlation between *LPL* S447X polymorphism and CAD susceptibility in Caucasians, an autosomal dominant transmitted variant. The *LPL* D9N polymorphism was associated with an increased risk of CAD, whereas S447X and HindIII polymorphisms showed protective effects. No association was observed between *LPL* N291S and PvuII polymorphisms and risk of CAD [96]. Talmud et al. [97] analyzed 2708 healthy middle-aged European men and found that smokers with *LPL* Asp9Asn polymorphism had a 10.4-fold higher risk of IHD/CAD compared with non-smoker individuals who do not carry that mutation; individuals who smoked but did not carry the allele had a 1.6 times higher risk than non-smokers [97]. No association was identified between the *LPL* Asn291Ser allelic variant and the increased risk of IHD/CAD [97]. Along with the *LPL* gene, the predisposition to CAD is also determined by the genes that regulate its endogenous activity, such as the *APOA5*, *APOC3* and *ANGPTL3* genes [80,98].

6.1.4. Polymorphism of *OLR1* (*LOX1*) Gene and CAD

The *OLR1* (*LOX1*) (oxidized low-density lipoprotein receptor 1) gene is located on chromosome 12p13.2 and encodes a low-density lipoprotein receptor (LDLR) that belongs to the C-type lectin superfamily. The LDLR protein binds, internalizes, and degrades oxidized LDL, and may be involved in the regulation of apoptosis. Gene regulation is mediated by the cAMP signaling pathway. The *OLR1* gene mutations have been associated with atherosclerosis and an increased risk of CAD/MI and Alzheimer's disease in various studies [16].

Earlier studies indicated the association of *OLR1* K167N polymorphism and CAD/MI, as well as a different frequency of the homozygous genotype IVS4–73T/T in individuals with MI and in the control group without MI. These particularities were contradicted by the study of Trabetti et al. [99], which considers that they are correlated with genetic differences between different ethnic groups, as well as with the limited number of patients analyzed [99].

SNPs located in the *OLR1* gene could have clinical significance and could be considered CAD candidate biomarkers, their identification being useful in assessing the genetic risk of CAD. The *OLR1* gene has six non-coding SNPs, which form a haplotype [100]. In a meta-analysis, Salehipour et al. [100] identified a significant association between SNPs rs1050283 (3′UTR*188 C>T) and rs3736235 (IVS4-14 A>G) located in *OLR1* haplotype and the occurrence of CAD [100]. They suggested that the precise determination of CAD association with polymorphisms located in a haplotype requires the analysis of all SNPs located in that specific haplotype [100].

6.1.5. Other Genetic Polymorphisms Involved in Lipid Metabolism Associated with Increased Risk of CAD

a. SORT1 Gene

The *SORT1* gene (sortilin 1), located on chromosome 1p13.3, identified by the first GWASs, encodes sortilin 1, which plays an important role in regulating plasma LDL-C levels by interacting with *APOB* gene in the Golgi apparatus in hepatocytes. Several studies have reported an association between plasma sortilin levels and cardiovascular damage and DM, which led to the idea that circulating sortilin plasma levels should be used as a potential biomarker for cardiovascular disease (CVD) and DM [101]. However, the results obtained in various studies are not conclusive, possibly in correlation with the small number of patients included in the analyzed samples [101]. Møller et al. [101] genotyping and sequencing the entire genome and corroborating the data obtained with plasma sortiline levels in 1173 patients with stable angina pectoris (diagnosed by computer angiography) [101].

Thus, two independent *cis* protein quantitative trait loci (pQTL) on chromosome 1p13.3 were identified, one of which is already known to be associated with CAD. In contrast, there was no association between circulating sortilin levels and coronary artery calcium score (CACS) or disease severity [101]. They concluded that although low sortilin levels are associated with the risk of CAD, its effect size is too small for sortilin to be a useful biomarker for CAD in medium or low-risk chest pain patients [101].

b. *TRIB1 Gene*

The *TRIB1* gene located on chromosome 8q24.13 encodes pseudokinase 1 involved in hepatic lipid metabolism by influencing the expression of lipogenic genes, and is also associated with insulin resistance. However, its mechanisms of action are not fully elucidated. The *TRIB1* locus has been linked to the metabolism of hepatic triglycerides in mice and to plasma triglyceride levels and CAD in humans [16]. GWASs indicated a SNP located at ≈30 kb downstream of *TRIB1* gene, which would have complex regulatory effects on genes or pathways involved in hepatic triglyceride (TG) metabolism. Some studies suggest that *TRIB1* gene suppresses the transcriptional activity of the *FOXO1* gene, thus suppressing the expression of the G6Pase and Phosphoenolpyruvate carboxykinase (PEPCK) enzymes, limiting gluconeogenesis [80,102]. Douvris et al. [103] identified by GWAS the *TRIBAL* locus that interacts with the *TRIB1* locus. The *TRIBAL* locus has a risk SNP that influences the expression of the *TRIB1* gene and is associated with elevated plasma TG levels [103].

6.2. Polymorphism of Genes Involved in Vascular Homeostasis

The formation and growth of atheroma plaque in the coronary wall is a slow and progressive process in which the endothelium is a key player. The number of risk genes which can generate vascular wall dysfunction has increased with deciphering the complex pathophysiological mechanisms of atherosclerosis, including the role of innate immunity and prothrombotic factors. Through synergistic action, they lead to vascular obstruction and cardiomyocyte ischemia [4,6].

6.2.1. Genes Involved in the Function of Vascular Smooth Muscle Cells (VSMc)

Vascular smooth muscle cells (VSMc) can be involved in the formation of atherosclerotic plaque by at least two mechanisms: modulating blood pressure through vascular tone and vascular remodeling, which, together with other factors, lead to either stabilization or progression and rupture of the atherosclerotic plaque [4,6].

a. *Endothelial Cell Nitric Oxide Synthase 3 (NOS3) Gene Polymorphism*

The *NOS3* gene located on chromosome 7q36.1 encodes the nitric oxide endothelial cell synthase (eNOS), an enzymatic protein with 1203 amino acids and 133 kDa, expressed in vascular endothelial cells, cardiomyocytes and platelets. eNOS causes the release of nitric oxide (NO) at the vascular level which causes the relaxation of vascular smooth cells. NO also has the physiological role of preventing the formation of atherosclerotic plaques by inhibiting the proliferation of smooth muscles and the adhesion and aggregation of platelets. Various studies have suggested that changes in vascular NO levels disrupt vascular homeostasis, causing endothelial dysfunction and may play a role in the etiopathogenesis of CAD [104]. Studies in mice have shown that the absence of nitric oxide receptor in vascular smooth muscle cells (VSMc) causes hypertension [4,104].

NOS3 gene polymorphism may influence eNOS enzyme synthesis. *NOS3* expression is regulated by epigenetic mechanisms (DNA methylation) and micro-RNA molecules. The localisation and activity of the eNOS protein is regulated by post-translational mechanisms (phosphorylation or acetylation).

Li at al. [105] analyzed the association between genetic variants of the *NOS3* gene and the risk of CAD in a meta-analysis that included 132 GWASs [105]. Of the thirteen *NOS3* allelic variants analyzed, the polymorphisms rs891512, rs1799983, rs2070744, rs11771443 and rs869109213 had a significant association with CAD and could serve as genetic biomarkers of CAD [105]. Three of these (rs1799983, rs2070744 and rs869109213 polymorphisms) were significantly correlated with the risk of MI and ACS. The rs869109213 polymorphism was common in Caucasians, and rs1799983 and rs2070744 polymorphisms were significant in both Caucasians and the Asians [105].

Gholami et al. [106] analyzed the study of Lin et al. [105] and completed the results obtained by them, concluding that, in the case of the five polymorphisms significantly associated with CAD, major alleles of rs1799983 (G), rs2070744 (T) and rs869109213 (4b) showed protective effect for CAD [105,106].

b. *TCF21 Gene Polymorphysm*

The *TCF21* gene (located on chromosome 6q23.2) encodes a transcription factor (TCF21) expressed in the epicardium during the embryonic period, which plays a role in differentiating epicardial cells. Recently, data on the role of TCF21 in the etiology of atherosclerotic CAD have been published. The loss-of-function mutation of *TCF21* gene during the embryonic period would be associated with premature differentiation of coronary vascular smooth muscle cells (VSMc) into the pericardium, leading to decreased migration of VSMc into the myocardium. The association of *TCF21* polymorphism with CAD has been shown in populations of different ethnicities [80,107].

Wirka et al. [107] showed that *TCF21* deficiency inhibited the VSMc phenotypic switch to fibromyocytes which reduces the number of fibromyocytes in the fibrous cap of atherosclerotic plaques, which thus become unstable [107]. In addition, downstream of the *TCF21* gene there are known susceptibility loci for CAD suggesting that *TCF21* gene could play a major role in the atherosclerotic plaques formation by epigenetic regulation of the expression of other genes [80,108]. A pathogenic mutation in the 3'UTR region of the *TCF21* gene impairs mRNA stability by differentiated binding of a microRNA. Directing the interaction between microRNA and mRNA by oligomers could be an effective therapeutic target for coronary VSMc [80].

c. *ADAMTS7 Gene Polymorphism*

The *ADAMTS7* gene located on chromosome 15q25.1 encodes a zinc-dependent protease expressed in the extracellular matrix. ADAMTS7 is a transmembrane protein that is involved in both the interaction between proteins and in multiple processes in the body, including signaling, adhesion, and cell migration. ADAMTS7 is synthesized in vascular endothelial cells and VSMc and has been shown to degrade several members of the thrombospondin family. Currently, the mechanisms by which ADAMTS7 determines CAD are not fully elucidated. ADAMTS7 protein promotes VSMc migration and neointima formation after injury by degradation of a cartilage oligomeric matrix protein [80]. Mice deficient in Adamts7 develop less atherosclerosis and are resistant to the formation of neointima secondary to vascular damage [80]. Three different GWASs identified the 15.25.1 locus and the *ADAMTS7* gene as being associated with coronary atherosclerosis. The main SNP associated with CAD was rs3825807, which determines the substitution of adenine for guanine, resulting in a serine-proline substitution in the ADAMTS7 prodomene, which would affect the maturation of ADAMTS7 protein. None of the studies reported an association between *ADAMTS7* gene polymorphism and increased mortality in CAD patients [109].

d. HHIPL1 Gene Polymorphism

GWASs have identified a possible new CAD-associated locus on chromosome 14q32, occupied by the *HHIPL1* gene (*hedgehog interacting protein-like 1*) which encodes a homologous sequence of an antagonist of the hedgehog signaling pathway. The function of *HHIPL1* gene and its role in atherosclerosis is not fully understood. The *HHIPL1* gene is involved in the development of coronary vascularization in the embryonic period. HHIPL1 is a proaterogenic protein that enhances hedgehog signaling and regulates VSMc proliferation and migration. In experimental animal models, HHIPL1 deficiency attenuates the development of atherosclerosis by reducing VSMc proliferation and migration. Inhibition of HHIPL1 protein function could provide a new therapeutic strategy for CAD [110].

6.2.2. Genes Involved in Blood Pressure Regulation

a. Angiotensin Converting Enzyme (ACE), Angiotensin II Type I Receptor (AGTR1) and Angiotensinogen (AGT) Genes Polymorphism

The *ACE* gene (located on chromosome 17q23.3) encodes the angiotensin converting enzyme (ACE) that converts angiotensin I to angiotensin II. The effects of angiotensin II are mediated by the angiotensin II type 1 receptor (AGT1R), encoded by the *AGTR1* gene (located on chromosome 3q23). Angiotensinogen (AGT) (encoded by the *AGT* gene located on chromosome 1q42.2) and ACE play an important role in regulating blood pressure, whereas AGTR1 plays a major role in the etiology of many cardiovascular diseases (CVD). Numerous studies have been conducted over time that have analyzed the involvement of the renin-angiotensin system and its components in the development of CAD and MI [80].

The *ACE* I/D polymorphism (rs4646994) is characterized by the presence (I) or absence (D) of a 287 bp Alu repeat sequence in intron 16, resulting in 3 genotypes-DD, II and ID. It is suspected that the presence of the homozygous DD genotype would be associated with the appearance of a severe form of CAD, whereas the homozygous II genotype could have a protective effect on CAD development. In their study, Amara et al. [111] showed that individuals who smoked, homozygous DD and heterozygous I/D had an increased risk of CAD, confirming the results of previous studies [111]. The association of the DD genotype with the increased risk of MI has been supported by some smaller studies, but has not been confirmed by other studies that have included a large number of patients [80].

In a large case–control study, Lindpainter et al. [112] did not identify an association between the presence of the D allele and an increased risk of IHD/CAD or MI [112]. Additionally, in a multicenter case–control study Keavney et al. [113] did not identify an association between the *ACE* DD genotype and an increased risk of MI [113]. On the other hand, Borai et al. [114] identified that the concomitant presence of *ACE* (I/D) and *AGT* (M235T) polymorphisms increases the risk of developing CAD, and each of the *ACE* D and *AGT* T alleles could be considered an independent risk factor for CAD [114].

Many studies have analyzed a possible association between the *AGTR1* gene A1166C polymorphism and CAD, but the results have been controversial. A meta-analysis by Feng et al. [115] showed that the polymorphism of the *AT1R* gene A1166C was associated with the risk of MI, with a significant association between the C allele and susceptibility to MI, whereas the AA genotype played a protective role [115]. The *AGTR1* gene A1166C polymorphism has been associated with an increased risk of hypertension in Asian and Caucasian populations, but not in Africans [116].

b. CYP11B2 Gene Polymorphism

The *CYP11B2* gene (located on chromosome 8q24.3) encodes aldosterone synthetase (ALDOS) and is regulated by angiotensin II. Several recent studies have shown that the *CYP11B2* gene rs1799998 -344C/T polymorphism is correlated with the presence of cardiovascular disease (CVD) [117,118]. A meta-analysis by Wang et al. [118] showed that the allelic variant 344CC is a risk factor for CAD and ischemic stroke in the Chinese population [118]. The presence of the *CYP11B2* -344C allele was associated with an increased risk of MI in smokers and those with dyslipidemia in a Finnish study [119].

6.3. Genes Associated with Vascular Hemostasis: Role of Hemostatic Gene Polymorphisms in CAD

The arterial thrombi formation is a complex and dynamic pathological process that is initiated in a damaged atherosclerotic plaque, which can completely block blood flow, producing MI. The process involves many factors, including collagen plaque components, platelet collagen receptor (glycoprotein Ia/IIa and glycoprotein VI), and blood clotting proteins [4,9].

6.3.1. ITGA2 Gene

The platelet glycoprotein (GP) complex Ia/IIa (GPIa/IIa-integrin alpha-2/integrin beta-2) (especially GPIa) is a major collagen receptor and plays an important role in platelet adhesion and aggregation with the initiation of vascular thrombosis. The phenotypic variability of this complex is closely related to the polymorphism of the *ITGA2* gene (located on chromosome 5q11.2) which encodes GPIa (integrin alfa 2). There are different opinions about the importance of the *ITGA2* gene C807T polymorphism which is thought to be associated with the risk of MI or ischemic stroke. Along with the C807T polymorphism associated with variable expression of the GPIa/IIa receptor, another *ITGA2* A1648G polymorphism was associated with changes in the tertiary structure of GPIa [4]. Kroll et al. [120] analyzed a group of 2163 Caucasian men with CAD (diagnosed by coronary angiography), showing that the *ITGA2* gene A1648G polymorphism plays an important role in the development of CAD [120].

Santoso et al. [121] analyzed a group of 2237 men with CAD (diagnosed by angiography), in which they investigated the association between *GPIa* (C807 and T807 alleles) polymorphisms and CAD/MI. No significant association with CAD/MI was observed in the total sample for any of these variants. However, the T807 allele was strongly associated with non-fatal MI in homozygous or heterozygous patients under the age of 62, with the highest risk in young heterozygous patients under the age of 49 [121].

6.3.2. Glycoprotein IIb/IIIa Platelet Receptor Genes (ITGB2 and ITGB3 Gene Polymorphisms)

Fibrinogen is the major ligand of the platelet receptor GPIIb/IIIa. The polymorphism of the *ITGB2* gene (located on chromosome 21q22.3) encoding glycoprotein IIb (GPIIb-beta-2 integrin) and the *ITGB3* gene (located on chromosome 17q21.32) encoding glycoprotein IIIa (GPIIIa-integrin beta-3) were analyzed, in connection with a possible causal association in patients with CAD/MI [16,122].

The study by Reiner et al. [122] included a group of 68 young women (aged between 18 and 44 years) who have had an MI, in which they analyzed the association with GPIIb polymorphism. The study also included a control group (369 unaffected women under the age of 44) [122]. Women homozygous (Ser843/Ser843) or heterozygous (Ser843/Ile843) for the allelic variant Ser843 of the *ITGB2* gene had a significant risk of MI (1.85 times higher) compared with the control group. The risk was higher among young women who had a positive family history, who smoked, or who had hypercholesterolemia [122]. The *ITGB2* Ser843 allelic variant did not have a significant association with MI in the Japanese male population [123].

The *PlA1/PlA2* (*HPA1-a/HPA-1b*) polymorphisms of the *ITGB3* gene encoding GPIIIa are associated with altered beta-3 subunit conformation and increased fibrinogen binding [124].

In a meta-analysis that included 57 studies eligible for statistical analysis (which included 17,911 patients and 24,584 controls), Floyd et al. [124] showed that individuals carrying the *PlA2* allele (*PlA1/PlA2* heterozygous genotype) had a significantly increased risk of MI ($n = 40,692$; OR 1.077, 95% CI 1.024–1.132; $p = 0.004$). The degree of association with MI increased with decreasing age of subjects (≤ 45 years: $n = 9547$; OR 1.205, 95% CI 1.067–1.360; $p = 0.003$) and with adjustment of data for conventional cardiovascular risk factors (CRF) ($n = 12,001$; OR 1.240, 95% CI 1.117–1.376; $p < 0.001$). The study concluded that in young patients, the relative absence of conventional cardiovascular risk factors (CRF) results in a significant association between the presence of the *PlA2* allele and the risk of MI. The relationship between *PlA1/PlA2* polymorphism and MI still needs further studies [124]. In a Finnish study, young men (<40 years old) with *PlA2/PlA2* homozygous genotype had a 3–4-fold increased risk of IHD and MI [125].

6.3.3. Plasminogen Activator Inhibitor 1 (PAI-1) Gene Polymorphism

The *PAI-1* gene (located on chromosome 7q22.1) encodes the plasminogen activator inhibitor 1 (PAI-1) which plays an important role in regulating thrombosis and intravascular thrombolysis. Many studies have analyzed the association between the 4G/5G polymorphism of *PAI-1* gene promoter and CAD. A common *PAI-1* 4G allele is associated with elevated levels of circulating PAI-1 and allows activator transcription factor binding to the promoter, without binding to transcription inhibitory factors, such as in the case of the 5G allele [126].

In the meta-analysis by Liang et al. [126], which analyzed the results of 53 studies, it is argued that *PAI-1* 4G/5G polymorphism may contribute to individual susceptibility to CAD, but to further evaluate gene-gene and gene-environment interactions on *PAI-1* gene 4G/5G polymorphism and CAD, more studies are needed in selected populations, from different environmental backgrounds or where different risk factors are present [126]. The *PAI-1* 4G/4G polymorphism causes deficient fibrinolytic activity, and may be a useful marker of fibrinolytic activity, increasing the risk of CAD [127].

6.3.4. Thrombospondin (TBHS) Genes Polymorphisms

The thrombospondin family (TSPs) includes 5 multifunctional glycoproteins (subgroup A: TSP-1, TSP-2 and, subgroup B: TSP-3, TSP-4, TSP-5), secreted in the extracellular matrix, with antiangiogenic functions. Zhang et al. [128] performed a meta-analysis that included 13 studies (10,801 cases and 9381 controls) in which they analyzed the association between SNP polymorphism in genes encoding thrombospondin-1 (*THBS1*-located on chromosome 15q14), thrombospondin-2 (*THBS2*-located on chromosome 6q27 and thrombospondin-4 (*THBS4*-located on chromosome 5q14.1) and the risk of CAD. The conclusion of the study was that *THBS1* N700S polymorphism was associated with an increased risk of CAD especially in the European and Asian population, whereas the *THBS4* A387P allelic variant had a significant association with CAD in the American population; no association was observed between *THBS2* 3'UTR polymorphism and CAD risk [128].

6.3.5. Factor V Leiden (F5) Allele Arg506Gln and Prothrombin (F2) Variant G20210A

The role of the Arg506G allele of the *F5* gene (encoding factor V Leiden-F5 Leiden, located on chromosome 1q24.2) and the G20210A allelic variant of the *F2* gene (located on chromosome 11p11.2, encoding prothrombin), in the production of MI, remains controversial. Although the two polymorphisms are associated with an increased risk of venous thrombosis, their role has not been demonstrated in the production of arterial thrombosis. Individuals heterozygous for the *F5* gene Arg506Gln mutation (3–5% of the population) have a seven times higher risk of venous thrombosis, whereas homozygotes have a 100 times higher risk [4].

In the study by Ercan et al. [129], which included 181 patients with angiographically documented CAD and a control group of 107 patients, although the *F5* Arg506G heterozygous mutation and the *F2* G20210A heterozygote mutation were more common in patients with CAD than in the control group, and no statistically significant association was found between their presence and CAD [129]. Most clinical trials have not shown any association between these alleles and the increased risk of CAD/MI, and more studies are needed to reach definitive conclusions [4].

6.4. Metabolic Factors: Hyperhomocysteinemia (MTHFR Gene Polymorphism)

The enzyme methylenetetrahydrofolate reductase (MTHFR) encoded by the *MTHFR* gene (located on chromosome 1q36.22) is involved in the remethylation of homocysteine to methionine [16]. The *MTHFR* gene mutations associated with decreased enzymatic activity, will increase plasma homocysteine levels. Because hyperhomocysteinemia is associated with an increased risk of CAD, it has become necessary to study the genes involved in homocysteine metabolism [16,130].

A meta-analysis by Lewis et al. [130], which included 80 studies (26,000 patients and 31,183 controls), showed that there was no solid evidence to support an association of *MTHFR* C677T (rs1801133) polymorphism with CAD in Europe, North America, or Australia. Geographical variability may be due to higher folic acid intake in North America and Europe or poor data communication. Additionally, there is no clear evidence that folic acid administration decreases plasma homocysteine levels, thus having a protective role in the occurrence of cardiovascular disease (CVD) [130].

Another meta-analysis by Brattström et al. [131] included 23 studies, and the conclusion was that the *MTHFR* C677T mutation is commonly associated with mild hyperhomocysteinemia and does not increase the risk of CVD [131]. Nedelcu et al. [132] analyzed a group of 61 MI patients under the age of 45, with the results showing a strong association between plasma homocysteine levels and the first MI among young patients, pointing out that plasma homocysteine levels could be a possible risk factor for MI [132].

Klerk et al. [133] analyzed 40 studies (including 11,162 IHD/CAD subjects and 12,758 controls), concluding that *MTHFR* TT polymorphism was associated with an increased risk of IHD in cases associated with folate deficiency. The European population with the *MTHFR* TT genotype had a significantly higher risk of IHD (odds ratio 1.14, 1.01–1.28) compared with North Americans in whom no increase in risk for the same genotype was observed (odds ratio 0.87, 0.73–1.05), the differences being partially explained by the different dietary intake of folates in the two analyzed populations [133].

6.5. Genes Associated with Inflammation: IL6 Gene Polymorphism

The *IL6* gene (located on chromosome 7p15.3) encodes interleukin 6 (IL6), a cytokine that regulates the production of C-reactive protein (CRP), an inflammatory marker associated with increased risk of IHD/CAD. The association between *IL6* gene polymorphism and IHD/CAD has been extensively studied. Two common *IL6* gene promoter polymorphisms (-174G>C and -572G>C) were associated in various studies with an increased risk of CAD, in other studies, the results being contradictory [4,80].

In the European HIFMECH study in which patients from two high-risk CAD centers in northern Europe and two low-risk CAD centers in southern Europe were analyzed, the association between *IL6* promoter polymorphisms (-572G>C and -174G>C) with circulating levels of inflammatory markers and the risk of MI. The plasma IL6 and CRP levels were similar in controls in both regions, but were higher in those with CAD. The frequency of the rare -174C allele (-174G>C polymorphism) was higher in the northern European group (0.43 vs. 0.28; $p < 0.0005$), where carriers of the -174C allele had a reduced risk of MI compared with homozygotes -174GG (OR 0.53, 95% CI 0.32, 0.86). This effect was not observed in the southern European population nor in the -572G>C variant (which was not associated with an increase or decrease in the risk of MI). No regional differences of the -572G>C allele frequency were observed. None of the genotypes were associated with a significant effect on plasma IL6 levels, either in patients with CAD or in control groups [134].

6.6. Other Susceptibility Loci for CAD

GWASs have identified other susceptibility loci for CAD in families with premature CAD, located on chromosomes 1, 2, 3, 14, 16 and X [5,80].

A study that included Icelandic families with peripheral arterial occlusive disease (PAOD) provided evidence of the involvement of the locus on chromosome 1p31 (PAOD locus). The PAOD locus has been associated with stroke and MI caused by atherosclerosis. There was no correlation of the PAOD locus with the occurrence of hyperlipidemia, hypertension, or DM [135].

Linkage analysis in families with premature CAD identified two other chromosomal regions: 2q21.1-q22 and Xq23-q26 [136]. Pajukanta et al. [136] identified the locus 2q21.1-q22 (Coronary Heart Disease, Susceptibility To, 2-CHDS2 locus, OMIM 608316) [16] in a study that included Finnish families, in which the proband showed premature CAD, defined by stenosis with more than 50% of at least two coronary arteries. They later identified the second susceptibility locus for CAD located on the Xq23-q26 chromosome (Coronary heart disease, susceptibility to, 3-CHDS3 locus, OMIM 300464) [16,136]. The angiotensin II receptor 2 (*AGTR2*) gene, located in the Xq32 locus, could play a major role in cardiovascular homeostasis [136].

The locus 2q36-q37.3 has been identified by GWAS in families with ACS including MI and unstable angina with onset before the age of 70 years. At this level are located the insulin receptor substrate-1 (*IRS1*) gene, the high-density lipoprotein binding protein (*HDLBP*) gene, and the calpain-10 (*CAPN10*) gene (which determines Non- Insulin Dependent Diabetes Mellitus 1, NIDDM1). Other loci associated with CAD in diabetes mellitus (DM) patients have been located on chromosomes 3q26-q27 and 20q11-q13.82 [5,137]. GWASs in the families of patients with CAD who had coronary artery calcification identified two other loci of interest located on chromosomes 6p21.3 and 10q21.3 [138].

Other loci associated with premature CAD were located on chromosomes 3q13, 14q32, and chromosome 16pter-p13 [5]. Zhu et al. [139] showed that the GA/AA polymorphism of the *ALDH2* gene (located on chromosome 12q24) encoding alcohol dehydrogenase 2 (ADH2) is an independent risk factor for MI [139].

7. Discussion

A complete understanding of the role of genetic factors in the emergence of CAD is one of the goals of modern medicine. Deciphering the complex pathophysiological mechanisms of CAD, identifying all the genetic factors involved, as well as translating the new information obtained through molecular technology in medical practice, are essential for the development of screening methods based on genetic risk scores. This new approach will facilitate the identification of people at high risk for CAD, the implementation of early prophylactic measures and the establishment of new therapeutic targets. Gene therapy strategies are the next step in the treatment and prevention of the disease.

CAD remains a leading cause of death worldwide, despite improved treatment and prophylactic methods. The most common cause of CAD is coronary atherosclerosis, which can have a monogenic or multifactorial etiology. GWASs and WES discovered over 321 CAD risk loci and many risk genes, most of which are linked to the presence of a disorder of lipid metabolism and hypertension [82]. It is estimated that together, all these genetic factors identified by GWASs explain about 40–60% of CAD heritability, suggesting that there are still unidentified genetic factors [6,85,140]. In addition, possible interactions between different genes (epistasis), mechanisms of epigenetic regulation, as well as interactions between genetic and environmental factors, which cannot be identified by GWASs or WES, should be considered.

7.1. Challenges for the Future in the Post-GWAS Era

Identifying all the factors involved is a real challenge for future studies and will certainly contribute to solving this real puzzle represented by the complex genetic architecture of IHD/CAD etiology.

A major challenge in the coming years will be the integration of information from analyses-omics (genomics, epigenomics, transcriptomics, proteomics and metabolomics) and their correlation with phenotypic manifestations (detected by imaging, functional and clinical tests) [10]. Continued progress in this area will depend on the development of new analytical techniques based on large databases. The information obtained will allow a better characterization of specific CAD phenotypes (for each CAD subtype), and the molecular redefinition of the phenotypes will certainly contribute to the development of precision medicine [6,10].

Epidemiological research over the past 50 years has uncovered a multitude of biomarkers often used for CVD risk prediction. However, no conclusions could be drawn to confirm the causal relationship between these biomarkers and CAD, even in the case of strong evidence of their association with the disease.

Mendelian randomization (MR) studies may reveal a causal relationship between a biomarker and CAD, providing evidence of the biomarker's contribution to disease development, specifying whether the observed association is influenced by unrecognized exogenous factors or the disease itself affects the level of the biomarker [10,147,148].

The genetic variant used in this type of study should significantly affect the biomarker investigated, but should not affect other phenotypes that could confound the association between the biomarker and the disease. If this biomarker is a true causal risk factor for CAD, the genotypes of the variant used should be associated with the risk for CAD in the direction predicted by the association of the biomarker with CAD. The analysis of the causal factors of CAD by MR has an extraordinary potential to identify possible therapeutic targets. The opportunities and challenges of MR studies in the case of CAD were discussed, and over time being used several biomarkers involved in lipid metabolism, inflammation, obesity, DM and hypertension [5,10,147,148].

The creation of large, accessible international databases and the sharing of information between different study groups will elucidate the contradictory results of some studies that included small groups of patients. Because early-onset CAD appears to be associated with genetic susceptibility more frequently than CAD in elderly patients, future studies should focus on the study of affected young populations. Clarifying ethnic differences in the risk of CAD and the response to different therapies may indicate genetic differences that will allow the development of targeted and personalized drug therapy [4,5].

As the quantity of data provided by different types of studies increases, it will be necessary to improve the methods of statistical and bioinformatics analysis that will help to decipher the complex etiology of IHD/CAD. Candidate gene-based association studies have identified genetic polymorphisms that are significantly associated with a reduced risk of CAD and MI [4,6]. However, the results obtained for many of these potential genetic loci, which would provide protection against CAD, are contradictory. Their number and distribution in the general population are still unknown and their identification will probably be an important objective of future studies [4].

7.2. Translating the Results of GWASs into Clinical Practice and the Importance of Polygenic Risk Scores (PRS) for Prevention of CAD

Knowledge of the genetic architecture of CAD has clinical applications such as the identification of new therapeutic targets and the improvement of cardiovascular risk estimation, and in pharmacogenomics [4,10]. GWASs have unequivocally shown that complex common diseases have a polygenic etiology and have allowed researchers to identify genetic variants (polymorphisms) associated with these diseases. These allelic variants can be combined into a polygenic risk score (PRS) that includes some of an individual's susceptibility to the disease [149].

Improving CVD risk information could be achieved by using polygenic risk scores (PRS) that could establish from birth the existence of a genetic predisposition to CAD [4,10]. Information on genetic factors provides the only tool to guide the prevention of CAD through targeted interventions, before the emergence of traditional cardiovascular risk factors (CRF) or specific clinical manifestations of the disease. Although initially the results were disappointing, later the discovery of numerous polymorphisms associated with CAD, the analysis of large cohorts and the biostatistical processing of the data obtained (as in the case of UK Biobank), allowed the realization of polygenic risk scores (PRS) (at the level of the whole genome) [80].

A PRS (polygenic risk score) is calculated as the sum of a several weighted genomic variants to estimate their effect, which was determined by GWAS [80] Many small effect size genetic variants contribute to a person's susceptibility to CAD. The PRS prediction quantifies the contributing effects in a score and estimates whether the individual tested has a high and medium risk of CAD [149]. PRS is the aggregate contribution of many common genetic variants (minor alleles with a frequency > 0.01) that have small to moderate individual effects. The PRS are singular, quantitative values for genetic susceptibility to polygenic diseases such as CAD. GWAS demonstrates that several common genetic variants make individuals susceptible to CAD. GWASs allow the systematic and individual comparison of the prevalence of SNPs in individuals with CAD and those without CAD, to generate SNP-level association statistics, these statistics being the central element of PRS [150]. Initially, most PRS for CAD were made for the European population and could not be used for people of other ethnicities. Identifying these ethnic genetic differences was a challenge, along with identifying new genetic risk factors for CAD, in the era of genomic medicine [80].

Subsequently, the predictive power of PRS for CAD has been improved by including evidence of association, linkage disequilibrium, anticipated functional impact, pleiotropy, and cross-ancestral data that allow the use of PRS in populations of different ethnicities (diverse ancestry). In the case of CAD, PRS could be used to identify high-risk individuals who would benefit from early prophylactic measures through intensive lifestyle modification, imaging surveillance and early lipid-lowering therapy (statins). Completed clinical trials have shown that individuals with a high PRS for CAD obtain the maximum benefits from early LDL-C lowering therapy [150].

7.3. Prophylactic Measures in Families at High Risk for CAD

Knowing the genetic risk factors of CAD in certain groups of patients requires customizing prevention and treatment strategies. In their case, adopting a healthy lifestyle with a balanced diet and regular exercise and avoiding traditional CAD risk factors such as excessive lipid consumption and smoking, could reduce the severity of the disease and the onset of acute complications such as MI. The use of risk assessment guidelines as well as the approach of personalized prevention strategies based on family risk is a common practice in the management of patients/families at high risk of CAD [5,14,80].

7.4. Genetic Counseling in Families at High Risk for CAD

Because the disease can have a monogenic etiology (especially in atherosclerotic CAD) or a complex, multifactorial, or polygenic inheritance, the calculation of disease risk and genetic counseling in high-risk CAD families is based on the genetic risk factors present in that family.

Genetic counseling for patients at high risk for CAD should include, in addition to detailed physical examination, family history and pedigree analysis (which may provide important information on family aggregation or for a monogenic inheritance), personal medical history, habits, and medicines used [5,14].

Disease risk assessment and genetic counseling can be difficult because in most cases CAD has a multifactorial etiology and a large number of loci and genes are involved. Moreover, to this is added the variable interaction between different genes (epistasis) as well as the interaction between genetic and environmental factors.

Although we focused on an in-depth analysis of data from the literature on the role of CAD genetic factors, as well as methods of their analysis, we still consider that our study was limited by incomplete data from the literature on CAD etiology (the "missing heritability" of CAD). Deciphering the etiology of CAD/CHD is a fascinating topic, which remains relevant due to the complexity of the possible factors involved and the interaction between them. In addition, future research will most likely identify new CAD candidate biomarkers, which, together with the use of PRS, will improve CAD risk prediction.

8. Conclusions

In the last decade, remarkable progress has been made in elucidating the complex etiology of CAD with the help of increasingly advanced molecular technologies and the processing of data obtained by efficient statistical and bioinformatics methods. Although overall CAD mortality has remained high, the main benefit has been the identification of new therapeutic targets.

In addition, GWASs provided information that offered a new perspective on the complex pathophysiology of CAD, and the newly identified genetic factors, along with those already known, currently represent about 40–50% of CAD heritability.

Future identification of new genetic factors could explain the "missing heritability" of CAD, without ignoring the fact that the interaction between different genes or between genetic and environmental factors could determine the phenotypic variability of CAD. Additionally, the identification of genetic factors that would have a protective role against CAD may be an important objective of future research.

The current use of PRS could improve CAD risk prediction, allowing the identification of people at higher risk for CAD, who could benefit from personalized prevention and treatment.

It is expected that following the sustained efforts of the large international consortiums, new genetic risk factors for CAD will be identified, with translation into clinical practice related to the development of new therapeutic molecules that act on specific targets.

Author Contributions: Conceptualization, L.I.B. and E.V.G.; methodology, L.I.B., E.V.G., L.F., M.C.B., E.Ț. and I.-I.C.; investigation, data curation, E.V.G., L.I.B., L.F., E.Ț. and M.C.B.; writing—original draft preparation, L.I.B. and E.V.G.; writing—review and editing, L.F., M.C.B. and I.-I.C.; visualization, L.F., M.C.B., E.Ț. and I.-I.C.; supervision, L.I.B. and E.V.G. All authors contributed equally to the study. All authors have read and agreed to the published version of the manuscript.

Funding: This research received no external funding.

Institutional Review Board Statement: Not applicable.

Informed Consent Statement: Not applicable.

Data Availability Statement: Not applicable.

Conflicts of Interest: The authors declare no conflict of interest.

Abbreviations

CAD: Coronary artery disease; IHD: Ischemic heart disease; MI: Acute myocardial infarction; ACS: Acute coronary syndrome; SCD: Sudden cardiac death; PA: Angina pectoris (myocardial ischaemia); CVD: Cardiovascular disease; CRF: Cardiovascular risk factors; DM: Diabetes mellitus; T2DM: Type 2 diabetes mellitus; PRS: Polygenic risk scores; TC: Total cholesterol; VSMc: Vascular smooth muscle cells; MAF: Minor allele frequency; HDL-C: High-density lipoprotein cholesterol; LDL-C: Low-density lipoprotein cholesterol; TG: Triglyceride; CGS: Candidate gene-based association studies; GWAS: Genome-wide association studies; LA: Genetic Linkage analysis; WES: Whole exome sequencing.

References

1. European Heart References Network (EHN). European Cardiovascular Disease Statistics. 2017. Available online: https://ehnheart.org/cvd-statistics.html/ (accessed on 21 January 2022).
2. Heart Disease Statistics 2022. Gerardo Sison Editor. Available online: https://www.singlecare.com/blog/news/heart-disease-statistics/ (accessed on 21 January 2022).
3. Muse, E.D.; Chen, S.F.; Torkamani, A. Monogenic and Polygenic Models of Coronary Artery Disease. *Curr. Cardiol. Rep.* **2021**, *23*, 107. [CrossRef] [PubMed]
4. Nordlie, M.A.; Wold, L.E.; Kloner, R.A. Genetic contributors toward increased risk for ischemic heart disease. *J. Mol. Cell. Cardiol.* **2005**, *39*, 667–679. [CrossRef] [PubMed]
5. Scheuner, M.T. Genetic evaluation for coronary artery disease. *Genet. Med.* **2003**, *5*, 69–85. [CrossRef] [PubMed]
6. Dai, X.; Wiernek, S.; Evans, J.P.; Runge, M.S. Genetics of coronary artery disease and myocardial infarction. *World J. Cardiol.* **2016**, *8*, 1–23. [CrossRef]

7. Mach, F.; Baigent, C.; Catapano, A.L.; Koskinas, K.C.; Casula, M.; Badimon, L.; Chapman, M.J.; De Backer, G.G.; Delgado, V.; Ference, B.A.; et al. ESC Scientific Document Group. 2019 ESC/EAS Guidelines for the Management of Dyslipidaemias: Lipid Modification to Reduce Cardiovascular Risk. *Eur. Heart J.* **2020**, *41*, 111–188; Erratum in *Eur. Heart J.* **2020**, *41*, 4255. [CrossRef]
8. Visseren, F.L.J.; Mach, F.; Smulders, Y.M.; Carballo, D.; Koskinas, K.C.; Bäck, M.; Benetos, A.; Biffi, A.; Boavida, J.M.; Capodanno, D.; et al. ESC Scientific Document Group. 2021 ESC Guidelines on cardiovascular disease prevention in clinical practice: Developed by the Task Force for cardiovascular disease prevention in clinical practice with representatives of the European Society of Cardiology and 12 medical societies with the special contribution of the European Association of Preventive Cardiology (EAPC). *Rev. Esp. Cardiol.* **2022**, *75*, 429. [CrossRef]
9. Fedele, F.; Pucci, M.; Severino, P. Genetic Polymorphisms and Ischemic Heart Disease. In *Genetic Polymorphisms*; Parine, N.R., Ed.; IntechOpen: London, UK, 2017; pp. 205–219. [CrossRef]
10. Elosua, R.; Sayols-Baixeras, S. The Genetics of Ischemic Heart Disease: From Current Knowledge to Clinical Implications. *Rev. Esp. Cardiol.* **2017**, *70*, 754–762. (In English) [CrossRef]
11. Whelton, P.K.; Carey, R.M.; Aronow, W.S.; Casey, D.E., Jr.; Collins, K.J.; Dennison Himmelfarb, C.; DePalma, S.M.; Gidding, S.; Jamerson, K.A.; Jones, D.W.; et al. 2017 ACC/AHA/AAPA/ABC/ACPM/AGS/APhA/ASH/ASPC/NMA/PCNA Guideline for the Prevention, Detection, Evaluation, and Management of High Blood Pressure in Adults: Executive Summary: A Report of the American College of Cardiology/American Heart Association Task Force on Clinical Practice Guidelines. *Hypertension* **2018**, *71*, 1269–1324; Erratum in *Hypertension* **2018**, *71*, e136–e139; Erratum in *Hypertension* **2018**, *72*, e33. [CrossRef]
12. Yusuf, S.; Hawken, S.; Ounpuu, S.; Dans, T.; Avezum, A.; Lanas, F.; McQueen, M.; Budaj, A.; Pais, P.; Varigos, J.; et al. Effect of potentially modifiable risk factors associated with myocardial infarction in 52 countries (the INTERHEART study): Case-control study. *Lancet* **2004**, *364*, 937–952. [CrossRef]
13. Pechlivanis, S.; Lehmann, N.; Hoffmann, P.; Nöthen, M.M.; Jöckel, K.H.; Erbel, R.; Moebus, S. Risk prediction for coronary heart disease by a genetic risk score—Results from the Heinz Nixdorf Recall study. *BMC Med. Genet.* **2020**, *21*, 178. [CrossRef]
14. Knuuti, J.; Wijns, W.; Saraste, A.; Capodanno, D.; Barbato, E.; Funck-Brentano, C.; Prescott, E.; Storey, R.F.; Deaton, C.; Cuisset, T.; et al. ESC Scientific Document Group. 2019 ESC Guidelines for the diagnosis and management of chronic coronary syndromes. *Eur. Heart J.* **2020**, *41*, 407–477; Erratum in *Eur. Heart J.* **2020**, *41*, 4242. [CrossRef] [PubMed]
15. Brown, J.C.; Gerhardt, T.E.; Kwon, E. Risk Factors for Coronary Artery Disease. In *StatPearls*; StatPearls Publishing: Treasure Island, FL, USA, 2021. Available online: https://www.ncbi.nlm.nih.gov/books/NBK554410/ (accessed on 22 January 2022).
16. OMIM—Online Mendelian Inheritance in Man. Available online: https://www.omim.org (accessed on 14 February 2022).
17. Gabcova-Balaziova, D.; Stanikova, D.; Vohnout, B.; Huckova, M.; Stanik, J.; Klimes, I.; Raslova, K.; Gasperikova, D. Molecular-genetic aspects of familial hypercholesterolemia. *Endocr. Regul.* **2015**, *49*, 164–181. [CrossRef] [PubMed]
18. Abifadel, M.S.; Rabès, J.H.; Boileau, C.R. Genetic Testing in Familial Hypercholesterolemia: Strengthening the Tools, Reinforcing Efforts, and Diagnosis. *JACC Basic Transl. Sci.* **2021**, *6*, 831–833. [CrossRef] [PubMed]
19. Soria, L.F.; Ludwig, E.H.; Clarke, H.R.; Vega, G.L.; Grundy, S.M.; McCarthy, B.J. Association between a specific apolipoprotein B mutation and familial defective apolipoprotein B-100. *Proc. Natl. Acad. Sci. USA* **1989**, *86*, 587–591. [CrossRef] [PubMed]
20. Andersen, L.H.; Miserez, A.R.; Ahmad, Z.; Andersen, R.L. Familial defective apolipoprotein B-100: A review. *J. Clin. Lipidol.* **2016**, *10*, 1297–1302. [CrossRef] [PubMed]
21. Pullinger, C.R.; Hennessy, L.K.; Chatterton, J.E.; Liu, W.; Love, J.A.; Mendel, C.M.; Frost, P.H.; Malloy, M.J.; Schumaker, V.N.; Kane, J.P. Familial ligand-defective apolipoprotein B. Identification of a new mutation that decreases LDL receptor binding affinity. *J. Clin. Investig.* **1995**, *95*, 1225–1234. [CrossRef]
22. Thomas, E.R.; Atanur, S.S.; Norsworthy, P.J.; Encheva, V.; Snijders, A.P.; Game, L.; Vandrovcova, J.; Siddiq, A.; Seed, M.; Soutar, A.K.; et al. Identification and biochemical analysis of a novel APOB mutation that causes autosomal dominant hypercholesterolemia. *Mol. Genet. Genom. Med.* **2013**, *1*, 155–161. [CrossRef]
23. Schmidt, R.J.; Beyer, T.P.; Bensch, W.R.; Qian, Y.-W.; Lin, A.; Kowala, M.; Alborn, W.E.; Konrad, R.J.; Cao, G. Secreted proprotein convertase subtilisin/kexin type 9 reduces both hepatic and extrahepatic low-density lipoprotein receptors in vivo. *Biochem. Biophys. Res. Commun.* **2008**, *370*, 634–640. [CrossRef]
24. Abifadel, M.; Rabès, J.P.; Devillers, M.; Munnich, A.; Erlich, D.; Junien, C.; Varret, M.; Boileau, C. Mutations and polymorphisms in the proprotein convertase subtilisin kexin 9 (PCSK9) gene in cholesterol metabolism and disease. *Hum. Mutat.* **2009**, *30*, 520–529. [CrossRef]
25. Kathiresan, S.; Voight, B.F.; Purcell, S.; Musunuru, K.; Ardissino, D.; Mannucci, P.M.; Anand, S.; Engert, J.C.; Samani, N.J.; Schunkert, H.; et al. Genome-wide association of early-onset myocardial infarction with single nucleotide polymorphisms and copy number variants. *Nat. Genet.* **2009**, *1*, 334–341. [CrossRef]
26. Cohen, J.C.; Boerwinkle, E.; Mosley, T.H.; Hobbs, H.H. Sequence variations in PCSK9, low LDL, and protection against coronary heart disease. *N. Engl. J. Med.* **2006**, *354*, 1264–1272. [CrossRef] [PubMed]
27. Chuan, J.; Qian, Z.; Zhang, Y.; Tong, R.; Peng, M. The association of the PCSK9 rs562556 polymorphism with serum lipids level: A meta-analysis. *Lipids Health Dis.* **2019**, *18*, 105. [CrossRef] [PubMed]
28. D'Erasmo, L.; Di Costanzo, A.; Arca, M. Autosomal recessive hypercholesterolemia: Update for 2020. *Curr. Opin. Lipidol.* **2020**, *31*, 56–61. [CrossRef] [PubMed]

29. Arca, M.; Zuliani, G.; Wilund, K.; Campagna, F.; Fellin, R.; Bertolini, S.; Calandra, S.; Ricci, G.; Glorioso, N.; Maioli, M.; et al. Autosomal recessive hypercholesterolaemia in Sardinia, Italy, and mutations in ARH: A clinical and molecular genetic analysis. *Lancet* **2002**, *359*, 841–847. [CrossRef]
30. Novo, S. Low HDL-cholesterol concentrations cause atherosclerotic disease to develop. ESC European Society of Cardiology. *E-J. ESC Counc. Cardiol. Pract.* **2009**, *7*, 32. Available online: https://www.escardio.org/Journals/E-Journal-of-Cardiology-Practice/Volume-7/Low-HDL-cholesterol-concentrations-cause-atherosclerotic-disease-to-develop (accessed on 26 January 2022).
31. Rader, D.J.; deGoma, E.M. Approach to the patient with extremely low HDL-cholesterol. *J. Clin. Endocrinol. Metab.* **2012**, *97*, 3399–3407. [CrossRef]
32. Yamakawa-Kobayashi, K.; Yanagi, H.; Fukayama, H.; Hirano, C.; Shimakura, Y.; Yamamoto, N.; Arinami, T.; Tsuchiya, S.; Hamaguchi, H. Frequent occurrence of hypoalphalipoproteinemia due to mutant apolipoprotein A-I gene in the population: A population-based survey. *Hum. Molec. Genet.* **1999**, *8*, 331–336. [CrossRef]
33. Haase, C.L.; Frikke-Schmidt, R.; Nordestgaard, B.G.; Tybjærg-Hansen, A. Population-based resequencing of APOA1 in 10,330 individuals: Spectrum of genetic variation, phenotype, and comparison with extreme phenotype approach. *PLoS Genet.* **2012**, *8*, e1003063. [CrossRef]
34. Bielicki, J.K.; Oda, M.N. Apolipoprotein A-I(Milano) and apolipoprotein A-I(Paris) exhibit an antioxidant activity distinct from that of wild-type apolipoprotein A-I. *Biochemistry* **2002**, *41*, 2089–2096. [CrossRef]
35. Koseki, M.; Yamashita, S.; Ogura, M.; Ishigaki, Y.; Ono, K.; Tsukamoto, K.; Hori, M.; Matsuki, K.; Yokoyama, S.; Harada-Shiba, M. Current Diagnosis and Management of Tangier Disease. *J. Atheroscler. Thromb.* **2021**, *28*, 802–810. [CrossRef]
36. The Human Gene Mutation Database at the Institute of Medical Genetics in Cardiff. Available online: http://www.hgmd.cf.ac.uk/ac/gene.php?gene=ABCA1/ (accessed on 26 January 2022).
37. Mokuno, J.; Hisida, A.; Morita, E.; Sasakabe, T.; Hattori, Y.; Suma, S.; Okada, R.; Kawai, S.; Naito, M.; Wakai, K. ATP-binding cassette transporter A1 (ABCA1) R219K (G1051A, rs2230806) polymorphism and serum high-density lipoprotein cholesterol levels in a large Japanese population: Cross-sectional data from the Daiko Study. *Endocr. J.* **2015**, *62*, 543–549. [CrossRef] [PubMed]
38. Mehta, R.; Elías-López, D.; Martagón, A.J.; Pérez-Méndez, O.A.; Sánchez, M.L.O.; Segura, Y.; Tusié, M.; Aguilar-Salinas, C.A. LCAT deficiency: A systematic review with the clinical and genetic description of Mexican kindred. *Lipids Health Dis.* **2021**, *20*, 70. [CrossRef] [PubMed]
39. McIntyre, N. Familial LCAT deficiency and fish-eye disease. *J. Inherit. Metab. Dis.* **1988**, *11*, 45–56. [CrossRef] [PubMed]
40. Reiner, Ž. Hypertriglyceridaemia and risk of coronary artery disease. *Nat. Rev. Cardiol.* **2017**, *14*, 401–411. [CrossRef] [PubMed]
41. Gehrisch, S. Common mutations of the lipoprotein lipase gene and their clinical significance. *Curr. Atheroscler. Rep.* **1999**, *1*, 70–78. [CrossRef] [PubMed]
42. Cox, D.W.; Breckenridge, W.C.; Little, J.A. Inheritance of apolipoprotein C-II deficiency with hypertriglyceridemia and pancreatitis. *N. Engl. J. Med.* **1978**, *299*, 1421–1424. [CrossRef]
43. Yoo, E.G. Sitosterolemia: A review and update of pathophysiology, clinical spectrum, diagnosis, and management. *Ann. Pediatr. Endocrinol. Metab.* **2016**, *21*, 7–14. [CrossRef]
44. Wang, Z.; Caom, L.; Sum, Y.; Wang, G.; Wang, R.; Yu, Z.; Bai, X.; Ruan, C. Specific macrothrombocytopenia/hemolytic anemia associated with sitosterolemia. *Am. J. Hematol.* **2014**, *89*, 320–324. [CrossRef]
45. Liu, Y.; Ordovas, J.M.; Gao, G.; Province, M.; Straka, R.J.; Tsai, M.Y.; Lai, C.Q.; Zhang, K.; Borecki, I.; Hixson, J.E.; et al. Pharmacogenetic association of the APOA1/C3/A4/A5 gene cluster and lipid responses to fenofibrate: The genetics of lipid-lowering drugs and diet network study. *Pharm. Genom.* **2009**, *19*, 161–169. [CrossRef]
46. Eichenbaum-Voline, S.; Olivier, M.; Jones, E.L.; Naoumova, R.P.; Jones, B.; Gau, B.; Patel, H.N.; Seed, M.; Betteridge, D.J.; Galton, D.J.; et al. Linkage and association between distinct variants of the APOA1/C3/A4/A5 gene cluster and familial combined hyperlipidemia. *Arter. Thromb. Vasc. Biol.* **2004**, *24*, 167–174. [CrossRef]
47. Timpson, N.J.; Walter, K.; Min, J.L.; Tachmazidou, I.; Malerba, G.; Shin, S.Y.; Chen, L.; Futema, M.; Southam, L.; Iotchkova, V.; et al. UK1OK Consortium Members. A rare variant in APOC3 is associated with plasma triglyceride and VLDL levels in Europeans. *Nat. Commun.* **2014**, *5*, 4871. [CrossRef] [PubMed]
48. Taghizadeh, E.; Esfehani, R.J.; Sahebkar, A.; Parizadeh, S.M.; Rostami, D.; Mirinezhad, M.; Poursheikhani, A.; Mobarhan, M.G.; Pasdar, A. Familial combined hyperlipidemia: An overview of the underlying molecular mechanisms and therapeutic strategies. *IUBMB Life* **2019**, *71*, 1221–1229. [CrossRef] [PubMed]
49. Hopkins, P.N.; Heiss, G.; Ellison, R.C.; Province, M.A.; Pankow, J.S.; Eckfeldt, J.H.; Hunt, S.C. Coronary artery disease risk in familial combined hyperlipidemia and familial hypertriglyceridemia: A case-control comparison from the National Heart, Lung, and Blood Institute Family Heart Study. *Circulation* **2003**, *108*, 519–523. [CrossRef] [PubMed]
50. Bogari, N.M.; Aljohani, A.; Amin, A.A.; Al-Allaf, F.A.; Dannoun, A.; Taher, M.M.; Elsayed, A.; Rednah, D.I.; Elkhatee, O.; Porqueddu, M.; et al. A genetic variant c.553G>T (rs2075291) in the apolipoprotein A5 gene is associated with altered triglycerides levels in coronary artery disease (CAD) patients with lipid lowering drug. *BMC Cardiovasc. Disord.* **2019**, *19*, 2. [CrossRef]
51. Kao, J.T.; Wen, H.C.; Chien, K.L.; Hsu, H.C.; Lin, S.W. A novel genetic variant in the apolipoprotein A5 gene is associated with hypertriglyceridemia. *Hum. Mol. Genet.* **2003**, *12*, 2533–2539. [CrossRef]
52. Do, R.; Project, N.E.S.; Stitziel, N.; Won, H.-H.; Jørgensen, A.B.; Duga, S.; Merlini, P.A.; Kiezun, A.; Farrall, M.; NHLBI Exome Sequencing Project; et al. Exome sequencing identifies rare LDLR and APOA5 alleles conferring risk for myocardial infarction. *Nature* **2015**, *518*, 102–106. [CrossRef]

53. Genest, J.J., Jr.; Martin-Munley, S.S.; McNamara, J.R.; Ordovas, J.M.; Jenner, J.; Myers, R.H.; Silberman, S.R.; Wilson, P.W.; Salem, D.N.; Schaefer, E.J. Familial lipoprotein disorders in patients with premature coronary artery disease. *Circulation* **1992**, *85*, 2025–2033. [CrossRef]
54. Austin, M.A.; Breslow, J.L.; Hennekens, C.H.; Buring, J.E.; Willett, W.C.; Krauss, R.M. Low-Density Lipoprotein Subclass Patterns and Risk of Myocardial Infarction. *JAMA* **1988**, *260*, 1917–1921. [CrossRef]
55. Nishina, P.M.; Johnson, J.P.; Naggert, J.K.; Krauss, R.M. Linkage of atherogenic lipoprotein phenotype to the low density lipoprotein receptor locus on the short arm of chromosome 19. *Proc. Natl. Acad. Sci. USA* **1992**, *89*, 708–712. [CrossRef]
56. Rotter, J.I.; Bu, X.; Cantor, R.M.; Warden, C.H.; Brown, J.; Gray, R.J.; Blanche, P.J.; Krauss, R.M.; Lusis, A.J. Multilocus genetic determinants of LDL particle size in coronary artery disease families. *Am. J. Hum. Genet.* **1996**, *58*, 585–594.
57. Srisawasdi, P.; Rodcharoen, P.; Vanavanan, S.; Chittamma, A.; Sukasem, C.; Na Nakorn, C.; Dejthevaporn, C.; Kroll, M.H. Association of CETP Gene Variants with Atherogenic Dyslipidemia Among Thai Patients Treated with Statin. *Pharmgenom. Pers. Med.* **2021**, *14*, 1–13. [CrossRef] [PubMed]
58. Allayee, H.; Aouizerat, B.E.; Cantor, R.M.; Dallinga-Thie, G.M.; Krauss, R.M.; Lanning, C.D.; Rotter, J.I.; Lusis, A.J.; de Bruin, T.W. Families with familial combined hyperlipidemia and families enriched for coronary artery disease share genetic determinants for the atherogenic lipoprotein phenotype. *Am. J. Hum. Genet.* **1998**, *63*, 577–585. [CrossRef] [PubMed]
59. Omidi, S.; Ghasemi, S.; Kalayinia, S. Is There Any Association Between the MEF2A Gene Changes and Coronary Artery Disease? *Acta Med. Iran.* **2020**, *58*, 366–375. [CrossRef]
60. Wang, L.; Fan, C.; Topol, S.E.; Topol, E.J.; Wang, Q. Mutation of MEF2A in an inherited disorder with features of coronary artery disease. *Science* **2003**, *302*, 1578–1581. [CrossRef] [PubMed]
61. Huang, X.C.; Wang, W. Association of MEF2A gene 3'UTR mutations with coronary artery disease. *Genet. Mol. Res.* **2015**, *14*, 11073–11078. [CrossRef]
62. Liu, B.; Pang, L.; Ji, Y.; Fang, L.; Tian, C.W.; Chen, J.; Chen, C.; Zhong, Y.; Ou, W.C.; Xiong, Y.; et al. MEF2A Is the Trigger of Resveratrol Exerting Protection on Vascular Endothelial Cell. *Front. Cardiovasc. Med.* **2022**, *8*, 775392. [CrossRef]
63. InanlooRahatloo, K.; Parsa, A.F.; Huse, K.; Rasooli, P.; Davaran, S.; Platzer, M.; Kramer, M.; Fan, J.B.; Turk, C.; Amini, S.; et al. Mutation in ST6GALNAC5 identified in family with coronary artery disease. *Sci. Rep.* **2014**, *4*, 3595. [CrossRef]
64. Cheeseman, J.; Kuhnle, G.; Stafford, G.; Gardner, R.A.; Spencer, D.I.; Osborn, H.M. Sialic acid as a potential biomarker for cardiovascular disease, diabetes and cancer. *Biomark. Med.* **2021**, *15*, 911–928. [CrossRef]
65. Inanloorahatloo, K.; Zand Parsa, A.F.; Huse, K.; Rasooli, P.; Davaran, S.; Platzer, M.; Fan, J.B.; Amini, S.; Steemers, F.; Elahi, E. Mutation in CYP27A1 identified in family with coronary artery disease. *Eur. J. Med. Genet.* **2013**, *56*, 655–660. [CrossRef]
66. Chen, C.; Zhang, Y.; Wu, H.; Sun, Y.W.; Cai, Y.H.; Wu, J.J.; Wang, J.; Gong, L.Y.; Ding, Z.T. Clinical and molecular genetic features of cerebrotendinous xanthomatosis patients in Chinese families. *Metab. Brain Dis.* **2017**, *32*, 1609–1618. [CrossRef]
67. Lee, C.W.; Lee, J.J.; Lee, Y.F.; Wang, P.W.; Pan, T.L.; Chang, W.N.; Tsai, M.H. Clinical and molecular genetic features of cerebrotendinous xanthomatosis in Taiwan: Report of a novel CYP27A1 mutation and literature review. *J. Clin. Lipidol.* **2019**, *13*, 954–959.e1. [CrossRef] [PubMed]
68. Rashvand, Z.; Kahrizi, K.; Najmabadi, H.; Najafipour, R.; Omrani, M.D. Clinical and Genetic Characteristics of Splicing Variant in CYP27A1 in an Iranian Family with Cerebrotendinous xanthomatosis. *Iran. Biomed. J.* **2021**, *25*, 132–139. [CrossRef] [PubMed]
69. Mani, A.; Radhakrishnan, J.; Wang, H.; Mani, A.; Mani, M.A.; Nelson-Williams, C.; Carew, K.S.; Mane, S.; Najmabadi, H.; Wu, D.; et al. LRP6 mutation in a family with early coronary disease and metabolic risk factors. *Science* **2007**, *315*, 1278–1282. [CrossRef] [PubMed]
70. Wang, H.; Liu, Q.J.; Chen, M.Z.; Li, L.; Zhang, K.; Cheng, G.H.; Ma, L.; Gong, Y.Q. Association of common polymorphisms in the LRP6 gene with sporadic coronary artery disease in a Chinese population. *Chin. Med. J.* **2012**, *125*, 444–449.
71. McPherson, R.; Pertsemlidis, A.; Kavaslar, N.; Stewart, A.; Roberts, R.; Cox, D.R.; Hinds, D.A.; Pennacchio, L.A.; Tybjaerg-Hansen, A.; Folsom, A.R.; et al. A common allele on chromosome 9 associated with coronary heart disease. *Science* **2007**, *316*, 1488–1491. [CrossRef]
72. Helgadottir, A.; Thorleifsson, G.; Manolescu, A.; Gretarsdottir, S.; Blondal, T.; Jonasdottir, A.; Jonasdottir, A.; Sigurdsson, A.; Baker, A.; Palsson, A.; et al. A common variant on chromosome 9p21 affects the risk of myocardial infarction. *Science* **2007**, *316*, 1491–1493. [CrossRef]
73. Samani, N.J.; Erdmann, J.; Hall, A.S.; Hengsterberg, C.; Mangino, M.; Mayer, B.; Dixon, R.J.; Meitinger, T.; Braund, P.; Wichmann, H.E.; et al. WTCCC and the Cardiogenics Consortium Genomewide association analysis of coronary artery disease. *N. Engl. J. Med.* **2007**, *357*, 443–453. [CrossRef]
74. Nikpay, M.; Goel, A.; Won, H.H.; Hall, L.M.; Willenborg, C.; Kanoni, S.; Saleheen, D.; Kyriakou, T.; Nelson, C.P.; Hopewell, J.C.; et al. A comprehensive 1,000 Genomes-based genome-wide association meta-analysis of coronary artery disease. *Nat. Genet.* **2015**, *47*, 1121–1130. [CrossRef]
75. Deloukas, P.; Kanoni, S.; Willenborg, C.; Farrall, M.; Assimes, T.L.; Thompson, J.R.; Ingelsson, E.; Saleheen, D.; Erdmann, J.; Goldstein, B.A.; et al. Large-scale association analysis identifies new risk loci for coronary artery disease. *Nat. Genet.* **2013**, *45*, 25–33. [CrossRef]
76. Wang, F.; Xu, C.Q.; He, Q.; Cai, J.P.; Li, X.C.; Wang, D.; Xiong, X.; Liao, Y.H.; Zeng, Q.T.; Yang, Y.Z.; et al. Genome-wide association identifies a susceptibility locus for coronary artery disease in the Chinese Han population. *Nat. Genet.* **2011**, *43*, 345–349. [CrossRef]

77. IBC 50K CAD Consortium. Large-scale gene-centric analysis identifies novel variants for coronary artery disease. *PLoS Genet.* **2011**, *7*, e1002260; Erratum in *PLoS Genet.* **2012**, *8*, 2–12. [CrossRef]
78. Koyama, S.; Ito, K.; Terao, C.; Akiyama, M.; Horikoshi, M.; Momozawa, Y.; Matsunaga, H.; Ieki, H.; Ozaki, K.; Onouchi, Y.; et al. Population-specific and trans-ancestry genome-wide analyses identify distinct and shared genetic risk loci for coronary artery disease. Population-specific and trans-ancestry genome-wide analyses identify distinct and shared genetic risk loci for coronary artery disease. *Nat. Genet.* **2020**, *52*, 1169–1177. [CrossRef] [PubMed]
79. Matsunaga, H.; Ito, K.; Akiyama, M.; Takahashi, A.; Koyama, S.; Nomura, S.; Ieki, H.; Ozaki, K.; Onouchi, Y.; Sakaue, S.; et al. Transethnic Meta-Analysis of Genome-Wide Association Studies Identifies Three New Loci and Characterizes Population-Specific Differences for Coronary Artery Disease. *Circ. Genom. Precis. Med.* **2020**, *13*, e002670. [CrossRef] [PubMed]
80. Kessler, T.; Schunkert, H. Coronary Artery Disease Genetics Enlightened by Genome-Wide Association Studies. *JACC Basic Transl. Sci.* **2021**, *6*, 610–623. [CrossRef]
81. Shadrina, A.S.; Shashkova, T.I.; Torgasheva, A.A.; Sharapov, S.Z.; Klarić, L.; Pakhomov, E.D.; Alexeev, D.G.; Wilson, J.F.; Tsepilov, Y.A.; Joshi, P.K.; et al. Prioritization of causal genes for coronary artery disease based on cumulative evidence from experimental and in silico studies. *Sci. Rep.* **2020**, *10*, 10486. [CrossRef]
82. Chen, Z.; Schunkert, H. Genetics of coronary artery disease in the post-GWAS era. *J. Intern. Med.* **2021**, *290*, 980–992. [CrossRef]
83. LeBlanc, M.; Zuber, V.; Andreassen, B.K.; Witoelar, A.; Zeng, L.; Bettella, F.; Wang, Y.; McEvoy, L.K.; Thompson, W.K.; Schork, A.J.; et al. Identifying Novel Gene Variants in Coronary Artery Disease and Shared Genes with Several Cardiovascular Risk Factors. *Circ. Res.* **2016**, *118*, 83–94. [CrossRef]
84. Ghosh, S.; Vivar, J.; Nelson, C.P.; Willenborg, C.; Segrè, A.V.; Mäkinen, V.P.; Nikpay, M.; Erdmann, J.; Blankenberg, S.; O'Donnell, C.; et al. Systems Genetics Analysis of Genome-Wide Association Study Reveals Novel Associations Between Key Biological Processes and Coronary Artery Disease. Arteriosclerosis, thrombosis, and vascular biolog. *Arter. Thromb. Vasc. Biol.* **2015**, *35*, 1712–1722. [CrossRef]
85. Won, H.H.; Natarajan, P.; Dobbyn, A.; Jordan, D.M.; Roussos, P.; Lage, K.; Raychaudhuri, S.; Stahl, E.; Do, R. Disproportionate Contributions of Select Genomic Compartments and Cell Types to Genetic Risk for Coronary Artery Disease. *PLoS Genet.* **2015**, *11*, e1005622. [CrossRef]
86. Blum, C.B. Type III Hyperlipoproteinemia: Still Worth Considering? *Prog. Cardiovasc. Dis.* **2016**, *59*, 119–124. [CrossRef]
87. Atis, O.; Sahin, S.; Ceyhan, K.; Ozyurt, H.; Akbas, A.; Benli, I. The Distribution of Apolipoprotein E Gene Polymorphism and Apolipoprotein E Levels among Coronary Artery Patients Compared to Controls. *Eurasian J. Med.* **2016**, *48*, 90–94. [CrossRef] [PubMed]
88. Eichne, J.E.; Dunn, S.T.; Perveen, G.; Thompson, D.M.; Stewart, K.E.; Stroehla, B.C. Apolipoprotein E polymorphism and cardiovascular disease: A HuGE review. *Am. J. Epidemiol.* **2002**, *155*, 487–495. [CrossRef] [PubMed]
89. Gerdes, L.U.; Jeune, B.; Ranberg, K.A.; Nybo, H.; Vaupel, J.W. Estimation of apolipoprotein E genotype-specific relative mortality risks from the distribution of genotypes in centenarians and middle-aged men: Apolipoprotein E gene is a "frailty gene", not a "longevity gene". *Genet. Epidemiol.* **2000**, *19*, 202–210. [CrossRef]
90. Humphries, S.E.; Talmud, P.J.; Hawe, E.; Bolla, M.; Day, I.N.; Miller, G.J. Apolipoprotein E4 and coronary heart disease in middle-aged men who smoke: A prospective study. *Lancet* **2001**, *358*, 115–119. [CrossRef]
91. Talmud, P.J.; Lewis, S.J.; Hawe, E.; Martin, S.; Acharya, J.; Marmot, M.G.; Humphries, S.E.; Brunner, E.J. No APOEepsilon4 effect on coronary heart disease risk in a cohort with low smoking prevalence: The Whitehall II study. *Atherosclerosis* **2004**, *177*, 105–112. [CrossRef]
92. Chiodini, B.D.; Barlera, S.; Franzosi, M.G.; Beceiro, V.L.; Introna, M.; Tognoni, G. APO B gene polymorphisms and coronary artery disease: A meta-analysis. *Atherosclerosis* **2003**, *167*, 355–366. [CrossRef]
93. Hegele, R.A.; Huang, L.S.; Herbert, P.N.; Blum, C.B.; Buring, J.E.; Hennekens, C.H.; Breslow, J.L. Apolipoprotein B-gene DNA polymorphisms associated with myocardial infarction. *N. Engl. J. Med.* **1986**, *315*, 1509–1515. [CrossRef]
94. Chen, Y.; Zeng, J.; Tan, Y.; Feng, M.; Qin, J.; Lin, M.; Zhao, X.; Zhao, X.; Liang, Y.; Zhang, N.; et al. Association between apolipoprotein B EcoRI polymorphisms and coronary heart disease: A meta-analysis. *Wien. Klin. Wochenschr.* **2016**, *128*, 890–897. [CrossRef]
95. He, K.; Zhu, Z.; Chen, Y. Lipoprotein Lipase Gene Polymorphisms Are Associated with Myocardial Infarction Risk: A Meta-Analysis. *Genet. Test. Mol. Biomark.* **2021**, *25*, 434–444. [CrossRef]
96. Ma, W.Q.; Wang, Y.; Han, X.Q.; Zhu, Y.; Liu, N.F. Associations between LPL gene polymorphisms and coronary artery disease: Evidence based on an updated and cumulative meta-analysis. *Biosci. Rep.* **2018**, *38*, BSR20171642. [CrossRef]
97. Talmud, P.J.; Bujac, S.R.; Hall, S.; Miller, G.J.; Humphries, S.E. Substitution of asparagine for aspartic acid at residue 9 (D9N) of lipoprotein lipase markedly augments risk of ischaemic heart disease in male smokers. *Atherosclerosis* **2000**, *149*, 75–81. [CrossRef]
98. Chen, Y.Q.; Pottanat, T.G.; Zhen, E.Y.; Siegel, R.W.; Ehsani, M.; Qian, Y.W.; Konrad, R.J. ApoA5 lowers triglyceride levels via suppression of ANGPTL3/8-mediated LPL inhibition. *J. Lipid Res.* **2021**, *62*, 100068. [CrossRef] [PubMed]
99. Trabetti, E.; Biscuola, M.; Cavallari, U.; Malerba, G.; Girelli, D.; Olivieri, O.; Martinelli, N.; Corrocher, R.; Pignatti, P.F. On the association of the oxidised LDL receptor 1 (OLR1) gene in patients with acute myocardial infarction or coronary artery disease. *Eur. J. Hum. Genet.* **2006**, *14*, 127–130. [CrossRef] [PubMed]

100. Salehipour, P.; Rezagholizadeh, F.; Mahdiannasser, M.; Kazerani, R.; Modarressi, M.H. Association of OLR1 gene polymorphisms with the risk of coronary artery disease: A systematic review and meta-analysis. *Heart Lung* **2021**, *50*, 334–343. [CrossRef] [PubMed]
101. Møller, P.L.; Rohde, P.D.; Winther, S.; Breining, P.; Nissen, L.; Nykjaer, A.; Bøttcher, M.; Nyegaard, M.; Kjolby, M. Sortilin as a Biomarker for Cardiovascular Disease Revisited. *Front. Cardiovasc. Med.* **2021**, *8*, 652584. [CrossRef] [PubMed]
102. Tsuzuki, K.; Itoh, Y.; Inoue, Y.; Hayashi, H. TRB1 negatively regulates gluconeogenesis by suppressing the transcriptional activity of FOXO1. *FEBS Lett.* **2019**, *593*, 369–380. [CrossRef]
103. Douvris, A.; Soubeyrand, S.; Naing, T.; Martinuk, A.; Nikpay, M.; Williams, A.; Buick, J.; Yauk, C.; McPherson, R. Functional analysis of the TRIB1 associated locus linked to plasma triglycerides and coronary artery disease. *J. Am. Heart Assoc.* **2014**, *3*, e000884; Erratum in *J. Am. Heart Assoc.* **2016**, *5*, e002056. [CrossRef]
104. Aimo, A.; Botto, N.; Vittorini, S.; Emdin, M. Polymorphisms in the eNOS gene and the risk of coronary artery disease: Making the case for genome-wide association studies. *Eur. J. Prev. Cardiol.* **2019**, *26*, 157–159. [CrossRef]
105. Li, X.; Lin, Y.; Zhang, R. Associations between endothelial nitric oxide synthase gene polymorphisms and the risk of coronary artery disease: A systematic review and meta-analysis of 132 case-control studies. *Eur. J. Prev. Cardiol.* **2019**, *26*, 160–170. [CrossRef]
106. Gholami, M.; Amoli, M.M.; Sharifi, F.; Khoshnevisan, K. Comments on and assessments of 'Associations between endothelial nitric oxide synthase gene polymorphisms and the risk of coronary artery disease: A systematic review and meta-analysis of 132 case-control studies. *Eur. J. Prev. Cardiol.* **2020**, *27*, 660–663. [CrossRef]
107. Wirka, R.C.; Wagh, D.; Paik, D.T.; Pjanic, M.; Nguyen, T.; Miller, C.L.; Kundu, R.; Nagao, M.; Coller, J.; Koyano, T.K.; et al. Atheroprotective roles of smooth muscle cell phenotypic modulation and the TCF21 disease gene as revealed by single-cell analysis. *Nat. Med.* **2019**, *25*, 1280–1289. [CrossRef] [PubMed]
108. Zhao, Q.; Wirka, R.; Nguyen, T.; Nagao, M.; Cheng, P.; Miller, C.L.; Kim, J.B.; Pjanic, M.; Quertermous, T. TCF21 and AP-1 interact through epigenetic modifications to regulate coronary artery disease gene expression. *Genome Med.* **2019**, *11*, 23. [CrossRef] [PubMed]
109. Pereira, A.; Palma Dos Reis, R.; Rodrigues, R.; Sousa, A.C.; Gomes, S.; Borges, S.; Ornelas, I.; Freitas, A.I.; Guerra, G.; Henriques, E.; et al. Association of ADAMTS7 gene polymorphism with cardiovascular survival in coronary artery disease. *Physiol. Genom.* **2016**, *48*, 810–815. [CrossRef] [PubMed]
110. Aravani, D.; Morris, G.E.; Jones, P.D.; Tattersall, H.K.; Karamanavi, E.; Kaiser, M.A.; Kostogrys, R.B.; Ghaderi Najafabadi, M.; Andrews, S.L.; Nath, M.; et al. HHIPL1, a Gene at the 14q32 Coronary Artery Disease Locus, Positively Regulates Hedgehog Signaling and Promotes Atherosclerosis. *Circulation* **2019**, *140*, 500–513. [CrossRef]
111. Amara, A.; Mrad, M.; Sayeh, A.; Lahideb, D.; Layouni, S.; Haggui, A.; Fekih-Mrissa, N.; Haouala, H.; Nsiri, B. The Effect of ACE I/D Polymorphisms Alone and with Concomitant Risk Factors on Coronary Artery Disease. *Clin. Appl. Thromb. Hemost.* **2018**, *24*, 157–163. [CrossRef]
112. Lindpaintner, K.; Lee, M.; Larson, M.G.; Rao, V.S.; Pfeffer, M.A.; Ordovas, J.M.; Schaefer, E.J.; Wilson, A.F.; Wilson, P.W.; Vasan, R.S.; et al. Absence of association or genetic linkage between the angiotensin-converting-enzyme gene and left ventricular mass. *N. Engl. J. Med.* **1996**, *334*, 1023–1028. [CrossRef]
113. Keavney, B.; McKenzie, C.; Parish, S.; Palmer, A.; Clark, S.; Youngman, L.; Delépine, M.; Lathrop, M.; Peto, R.; Collins, R. Large-scale test of hypothesised associations between the angiotensin-converting-enzyme insertion/deletion polymorphism and myocardial infarction in about 5000 cases and 6000 controls. International Studies of Infarct Survival (ISIS) Collaborators. *Lancet* **2000**, *355*, 434–442. [CrossRef]
114. Borai, I.H.; Hassan, N.S.; Shaker, O.G.; Ashour, E.E.; Badrawy, M.E.I.; Olfat, M.; Fawzi, L.; Mageed, L. Synergistic effect of ACE and AGT genes in coronary artery disease. *J. Basic Appl. Sci.* **2018**, *7*, 111–117. [CrossRef]
115. Feng, X.; Zheng, B.S.; Shi, J.J.; Qian, J.; He, W.; Zhou, H.F. A systematic review and meta-analysis of the association between angiotensin II type 1 receptor A1166C gene polymorphism and myocardial infarction susceptibility. *J. Renin-Angiotensin-Aldosterone Syst.* **2014**, *15*, 307–315. [CrossRef]
116. Liu, D.X.; Zhang, Y.Q.; Hu, B.; Zhang, J.; Zhao, Q. Association of AT1R polymorphism with hypertension risk: An update meta-analysis based on 28,952 subjects. *J. Renin-Angiotensin-Aldosterone Syst.* **2015**, *16*, 898–909. [CrossRef]
117. Sun, J.; Zhao, M.; Miao, S.; Xi, B. Polymorphisms of three genes (ACE, AGT and CYP11B2) in the renin-angiotensinaldosterone system are not associated with blood pressure salt sensitivity: A systematic meta-analysis. *Blood Press.* **2016**, *25*, 117–122. [CrossRef] [PubMed]
118. Wang, L.; Zhang, Z.; Liu, D.; Yuan, K.; Zhu, G.; Qi, X. Association of -344C/T polymorphism in the aldosterone synthase (CYP11B2) gene with cardiac and cerebrovascular events in Chinese patients with hypertension. *J. Int. Med. Res.* **2020**, *48*, 300060520949409. [CrossRef] [PubMed]
119. Hautanen, A.; Toivanen, P.; Mänttäri, M.; Tenkanen, L.; Kupari, M.; Manninen, V.; Kayes, K.M.; Rosenfeld, S.; White, P.C. Joint effects of an aldosterone synthase (CYP11B2) gene polymorphism and classic risk factors on risk of myocardial infarction. *Circulation* **1999**, *100*, 2213–2218. [CrossRef] [PubMed]
120. Kroll, H.; Gardemann, A.; Fechter, A.; Haberbosch, W.; Santoso, S. The impact of the glycoprotein Ia collagen receptor subunit A1648G gene polymorphism on coronary artery disease and acute myocardial infarction. *Thromb. Haemost.* **2000**, *83*, 392–396.

121. Santoso, S.; Kunicki, T.J.; Kroll, H.; Haberbosch, W.; Gardemann, A. Association of the platelet glycoprotein Ia C807T gene polymorphism with nonfatal myocardial infarction in younger patients. *Blood* **1999**, *93*, 2449–2453. [CrossRef]
122. Reiner, A.P.; Schwartz, S.M.; Kumar, P.N.; Rosendaal, F.R.; Pearce, R.M.; Aramaki, K.M.; Psaty, B.M.; Siscovick, D.S. Platelet glycoprotein IIb polymorphism, traditional risk factors and non-fatal myocardial infarction in young women. *Br. J. Haematol.* **2001**, *112*, 632–636. [CrossRef]
123. Hato, T.; Minamoto, Y.; Fukuyama, T.; Fujit, S. Polymorphisms of HPA-1 through 6 on platelet membrane glycoprotein receptors are not a genetic risk factor for myocardial infarction in the Japanese population. *Am. J. Cardiol.* **1997**, *80*, 1222–1224. [CrossRef]
124. Floyd, C.N.; Mustafa, A.; Ferro, A. The PlA1/A2 polymorphism of glycoprotein IIIa as a risk factor for myocardial infarction: A meta-analysis. *PLoS ONE* **2014**, *9*, e101518. [CrossRef]
125. Bojesen, S.E.; Juul, K.; Schnohr, P.; Tybjaerg-Hansen, A.; Nordestgaard, B.G. Copenhagen City Heart Study. Platelet glycoprotein IIb/IIIa Pl(A2)/Pl(A2) homozygosity associated with risk of ischemic cardiovascular disease and myocardial infarction in young men: The Copenhagen City Heart Study. *J. Am. Coll. Cardiol.* **2003**, *42*, 661–667. [CrossRef]
126. Liang, Z.; Jiang, W.; Ouyang, M.; Yang, K. PAI-1 4G/5G polymorphism and coronary artery disease risk: A meta-analysis. *Int. J. Clin. Exp. Med.* **2015**, *8*, 2097–2107.
127. Khaki-Khatibi, F.; Karimian, A. Association of PAI-1 serum levels and polymorphism of gene of Plasminogen Activator Inhibitor-1 in patient of Non-diabetic and Non-smoker with Coronary Artery Disease. *Med. J. Tabriz Univ. Med. Sci.* **2018**, *40*, 43–48.
128. Zhang, X.J.; Wei, C.Y.; Li, W.B.; Zhang, L.L.; Zhou, Y.; Wang, Z.H.; Tang, M.X.; Zhang, W.; Zhang, Y.; Zhong, M. Association between single nucleotide polymorphisms in thrombospondins genes and coronary artery disease: A meta-analysis. *Thromb. Res.* **2015**, *136*, 45–51. [CrossRef] [PubMed]
129. Ercan, B.; Tamer, L.; Sucu, N.; Pekdemir, H.; Camsari, A.; Atik, U. Factor VLeiden and prothrombin G20210A gene polymorphisms in patients with coronary artery disease. *Yonsei Med. J.* **2008**, *49*, 237–243. [CrossRef] [PubMed]
130. Lewis, S.J.; Ebrahim, S.; Smith, G.D. Meta-analysis of MTHFR 677->T polymorphism and coronary heart disease: Does totality of evidence support causal role for homocysteine and preventive potential of folate? *BMJ* **2005**, *331*, 1053. [CrossRef]
131. Brattström, L.; Wilcken, D.E.; Ohrvik, J.; Brudin, L. Common methylenetetrahydrofolate reductase gene mutation leads to hyperhomocysteinemia but not to vascular disease: The result of a meta-analysis. *Circulation* **1998**, *98*, 2520–2526. [CrossRef]
132. Nedelcu, C.; Ionescu, M.; Pantea-Stoian, A.; Niță, D.; Petcu, L.; Mazilu, L.; Suceveanu, A.I.; Tuță, L.A.; Parepa, I.R. Correlation between plasma homocysteine and first myocardial infarction in young patients: Case-control study in Constanta County, Romania. *Exp. Ther. Med.* **2021**, *21*, 101. [CrossRef]
133. Klerk, M.; Verhoef, P.; Clarke, R.; Blom, H.J.; Kok, F.J.; Schouten, E.G. MTHFR Studies Collaboration Group. MTHFR 677C->T polymorphism and risk of coronary heart disease: A meta-analysis. *JAMA* **2002**, *288*, 2023–2031. [CrossRef]
134. Kelberman, D.; Hawe, E.; Luong, L.A.; Mohamed-Ali, V.; Lundman, P.; Tornvall, P.; Aillaud, M.F.; Juhan-Vague, I.; Yudkin, J.S.; Margaglione, M.; et al. HIFMECH study group. Effect of Interleukin-6 promoter polymorphisms in survivors of myocardial infarction and matched controls in the North and South of Europe. The HIFMECH Study. *Thromb. Haemost.* **2004**, *92*, 1122–1128. [CrossRef]
135. Gudmundsson, G.; Matthiasson, S.E.; Arason, H.; Johannsson, H.; Runarsson, F.; Bjarnason, H.; Helgadottir, K.; Thorisdottir, S.; Ingadottir, G.; Lindpaintner, K.; et al. Localization of a gene for peripheral arterial occlusive disease to chromosome 1p31. *Am. J. Hum. Genet.* **2002**, *70*, 586–592. [CrossRef]
136. Pajukanta, P.; Cargill, M.; Viitanen, L.; Nuotio, I.; Kareinen, A.; Perola, M.; Terwilliger, J.D.; Kempas, E.; Daly, M.; Lilja, H.; et al. Two loci on chromosomes 2 and X for premature coronary heart disease identified in early- and late-settlement populations of Finland. *Am. J. Hum. Genet.* **2000**, *67*, 1481–1493. [CrossRef]
137. Harrap, S.B.; Zammit, K.S.; Wong, Z.Y.; Williams, F.M.; Bahlo, M.; Tonkin, A.M.; Anderson, S.T. Genome-wide linkage analysis of the acute coronary syndrome suggests a locus on chromosome 2. *Arter. Thromb. Vasc. Biol.* **2002**, *22*, 874–878. [CrossRef] [PubMed]
138. Lange, L.A.; Lange, E.M.; Bielak, L.F.; Langefeld, D.; Kardia, S.L.; Royston, P.; Turner, S.T.; Sheedy, P.F., 2nd; Boerwinkle, E.; Peyser, P.A. Autosomal genome-wide scan for coronary artery calcification loci in sibships at high risk for hypertension. *Arter. Thromb. Vasc. Biol.* **2002**, *22*, 418–423. [CrossRef] [PubMed]
139. Zhu, L.P.; Yin, W.L.; Peng, L.; Zhou, X.H.; Zhou, P.; Xuan, S.X.; Luo, Y.; Chen, C.; Cheng, B.; Lin, J.D.; et al. Association of Aldehyde Dehydrogenase 2 Gene Polymorphism with Myocardial Infarction. *J. Inflamm. Res.* **2021**, *14*, 3039–3047. [CrossRef] [PubMed]
140. Stevens, H.Y.; Melchior, B.; Bell, K.S.; Yun, S.; Yeh, J.C.; Frangos, J.A. PECAM-1 is a critical mediator of atherosclerosis. *Dis. Model. Mech.* **2008**, *1*, 175–181. [CrossRef]
141. Thomas, C.B.; Cohen, B.H. The familial occurrence of hypertension and coronary artery disease, with observations concerning obesity and diabetes. *Ann. Intern. Med.* **1955**, *42*, 90–127. [CrossRef]
142. Brown, D.; Giles, W.H.; Burke, W.; Greenlund, K.J.; Croft, J.B. Familial aggregation of early-onset myocardial infarction. *Community Genet.* **2002**, *5*, 232–238. [CrossRef]
143. Schildkraut, J.M.; Myers, R.H.; Cupples, L.A.; Kiely, D.K.; Kannel, W.B. Coronary risk associated with age and sex of parental heart disease in the Framingham Study. *Am. J. Cardiol.* **1989**, *64*, 555–559. [CrossRef]
144. Chacko, M.; Sarma, P.S.; Harikrishnan, S.; Zachariah, G.; Jeemon, P. Family history of cardiovascular disease and risk of premature coronary heart disease: A matched case-control study. *Wellcome Open Res.* **2020**, *5*, 70. [CrossRef]

145. Zdravkovic, S.; Wienke, A.; Pedersen, N.L.; Marenberg, M.E.; Yashin, A.I.; De Faire, U. Heritability of death from coronary heart disease: A 36-year follow-up of 20966 Swedish twins. *J. Intern. Med.* **2002**, *252*, 247–254. [CrossRef]
146. Wienke, A.; Holm, N.V.; Skytthe, A.; Yashin, A.I. The heritability of mortality due to heart diseases: A correlated frailty model applied to Danish twins. *Twin Res.* **2001**, *4*, 266–274. [CrossRef]
147. Jansen, H.; Samani, N.J.; Schunkert, H. Mendelian randomization studies in coronary artery disease. *Eur. Heart J.* **2014**, *35*, 1917–1924. [CrossRef] [PubMed]
148. Kjeldsen, E.W.; Thomassen, J.Q.; Frikke-Schmidt, R. HDL cholesterol concentrations and risk of atherosclerotic cardiovascular disease—Insights from randomized clinical trials and human genetics. *Biochim. Biophys. Acta Mol. Cell Biol. Lipids* **2022**, *1867*, 159063. [CrossRef] [PubMed]
149. Lewis, C.M.; Vassos, E. Polygenic risk scores: From research tools to clinical instruments. *Genome Med.* **2020**, *12*, 44. [CrossRef] [PubMed]
150. Klarin, D.; Natarajanm, P. Clinical utility of polygenic risk scores for coronary artery disease. *Nat. Rev. Cardiol.* **2021**, *19*, 291–301. [CrossRef]

MDPI
St. Alban-Anlage 66
4052 Basel
Switzerland
Tel. +41 61 683 77 34
Fax +41 61 302 89 18
www.mdpi.com

Life Editorial Office
E-mail: life@mdpi.com
www.mdpi.com/journal/life

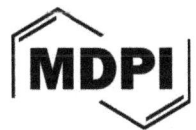

www.ingramcontent.com/pod-product-compliance
Lightning Source LLC
LaVergne TN
LVHW070431100526
838202LV00014B/1573